Management for the Health Information Professional

Janette R. Kelly, MBA, RHIA
Pamela S. Greenstone, M.Ed., RHIA

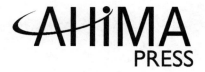

AHiMA
PRESS

ISBN: 978-1-58426-507-8
AHIMA Product No.: AB124014

AHIMA Staff:
Caitlin Wilson, Assistant Editor
Megan Grennan, Senior Production Development Editor
Jason O. Malley, Vice President, Business and Innovation
Pamela Woolf, Director of Publications

For more information, including updates, about AHIMA Press publications, visit
http://www.ahima.org/publications/updates.aspx

American Health Information Management Association
233 North Michigan Avenue, 21st Floor
Chicago, Illinois 60601-5809
http://ahima.org

Brief Table of Contents

Detailed Table of Contents

About the Authors

Janette R. Kelly, MBA, RHIA is an associate professor in the Health Information Management program at the University of Cincinnati. Ms. Kelly earned her master's degree from Xavier University and bachelor's degree from The Ohio State University. She has more than 25 years of HIM management and consulting experience in a variety of healthcare settings including teaching hospitals, community hospitals, skilled nursing facilities, physician offices, and vendors. She is active within her state and local HIM associations and is a past president of the Ohio Health Information Management Association and the Greater Cincinnati Health Information Management Association.

Pamela S. Greenstone, MEd, RHIA is an assistant professor and program director of the Health Information Management program at the University of Cincinnati. Ms. Greenstone earned her master's degree from the University of Cincinnati and bachelor's degree from Ferris State University. She has more than 25 years of HIM management experience in a variety of healthcare settings including freestanding rehabilitation facilities, long-term acute hospitals, skilled nursing facilities, and a pediatric acute-care hospital. She is active within her state and local HIM associations and is a past president of the Ohio Health Information Management Association.

Preface

This textbook is intended to provide practical instruction in management principles from a health information management (HIM) perspective with both theory and practice examples given. It is written for HIM professionals at the undergraduate level and is specifically intended for bachelor's level students in a four-year program. The career goal for most RHIA-eligible students is a management position in the healthcare field. HIM managers are found in all healthcare settings: acute-care, outpatient, long-term care, rehabilitation, and even as vendors. The principles introduced here will provide a foundation and path for sound management practice and decision making. At the same time, there is recognition of the importance that the human resources (HR) department plays in today's healthcare management environment. Organizations differ on the extent to which managers are requested or required to seek the consult of HR, and a new HIM manager must be aware of the situations that will require input from the HR department. This textbook identifies those situations and offers guidance as to when a new HIM manager should include HR in their decision-making process.

Each chapter includes learning objectives and key terms, Check Your Understanding questions to test comprehension of chapter material, references applicable to chapter content, and a case study that covers comprehensive chapter content.

In addition to a case study for each chapter, appendix E provides three additional case studies to provide comprehensive scenarios integrating content from all chapters. Each case study includes learning objectives, a real-world scenario, assumptions, and deliverables. The case studies are written from a manager's perspective and require critical thinking and, in some cases, additional research to support answers. The case studies may be used in their entirety as presented, or faculty may modify or enhance the case studies to fit their needs.

Ancillaries include the instructor manual to accompany the textbook, PowerPoint presentations, a test bank, discussion questions to be utilized within the classroom or online discussion boards, crosswalks to RHIA domains, and answer keys as appropriate. The student workbook includes end-of-chapter review questions, answers to review and Check Your Understanding questions, and crosswalks to RHIA domains.

Chapter 1, "Traditional Theories of Management and Leadership," addresses the historical perspective as a precipitating factor to the understanding of management practices. Major management and leadership theories are identified and their concepts are discussed. Scientific, administrative, humanistic, operational, and contemporary management theorists and their research are presented as a foundation for the HIM manager. Leadership theories such as behavioral, contingency, transformational, values-based, and servant-based are discussed in relation to leadership practices within healthcare organizations.

Chapter 2, "Management Functions of HIM," introduces the management functions of planning, organizing, leading, and controlling in relation to an HIM manager's job responsibilities. The chapter serves as a guide to the management functions discussed in later chapters by referencing topics and the chapters in which they are covered. Also detailed are the levels of management most seen in healthcare organizations. The chapter concludes with a discussion of the ethical aspects of HIM in healthcare organizations.

Chapter 3, "Leadership Concepts in HIM," addresses the trends that HIM professionals must keep abreast of in management practice. It is not enough to understand changes to coding guidelines or privacy matters; an HIM manager must be aware of concepts in the business world and their potential impact on healthcare in general and HIM specifically. Leadership concepts discussed in this chapter are diversity in the workplace, the increasing use of teams in healthcare, and the importance of motivation and morale in the work place. Motivation theories are presented to lay the groundwork for a discussion on motivation.

Chapter 4, "Change Management in HIM," addresses strategic planning in healthcare organizations and how developing new strategic initiatives is necessary to meet the changing needs of today's healthcare environment. Change management theories and notable change management techniques are also discussed as the ability to successfully manage change is a skill necessary for all HIM professionals. HIM managers also need to understand the critical conversations and conflict management skills required to overcome the resistance evident in a changing environment. Negotiation techniques and the collaborative skills necessary to manage change in a healthcare organization are also covered.

Chapter 5, "Legal Aspects of Healthcare Management," discusses major laws impacting the United States workforce. Understanding the laws that affect the workplace is the responsibility of each HIM manager. This chapter provides a description of workforce legislation and the implications that the laws have on interviewing, counseling, and progressive discipline practices in the workplace. Knowledge of employment law allows a manager to act with confidence and assurance, but should never be a substitute for advice and recommendations from human resources professionals or legal counsel.

Chapter 6, "Job Descriptions and Roles in HIM," outlines the basic components of job analysis and job design such as techniques for assessing job needs, reviewing job analysis methods, and designing jobs that will attract highly-skilled individuals. Job roles and responsibilities are changing at a rapid pace within HIM. HIM professionals are assuming jobs in nontraditional workplaces that require job descriptions reflective of the skills necessary in these new workplaces. The chapter includes a review of the components of job descriptions and job specifications. There is also a discussion of job crafting and job redesign as methods of improving HIM employee job satisfaction and retaining motivated HIM processionals.

Chapter 7, "Recruitment, Selection, and Retention in HIM," examines the recruiting tools available to managers, details the selection process of new employees, and discusses the impact of turnover and retention on the HIM workforce. Recruitment, selection, and retention are basic functions of any HIM manager's responsibilities. As the electronic health record becomes the standard in healthcare organizations, HIM positions continue to change and develop. The need for file clerks disappears, but the need for scanning clerks increases. Voice recognition technology means that transcriptionists do less typing and more editing. Coding personnel develop new skills as they work with physicians and other healthcare providers to improve clinical documentation in the record. Population statistics indicate that the younger workforce is declining, so there will be increased competition among organizations to hire younger workers. An organization must hire and retain qualified individuals as part of any strategic plan.

Chapter 8, "Performance Management in HIM," discusses the role that the human resource department plays in the performance management process and outlines the components of performance management within healthcare organizations. HIM managers are involved in the performance appraisal process both as recipients and providers of evaluations, so this chapter includes the performance appraisal life cycle and performance management tools. The development of performance standards is discussed in detail as is the rating of employee performance. The assessment of performance in terms of short- and long-term performance variability is delineated along with the contributing factors to performance variability. The chapter discusses the completion of performance appraisal documents and the HIM manager's role in this process. Different appraisal methods that can be adopted, and the advantages and disadvantages of each are also addressed.

Chapter 9, "Training and Development in HIM," provides the fundamentals of staff training and development. As the recent transition from ICD-9-CM to ICD-10-CM/PCS has illustrated, the opportunities for training and developing are plentiful and HIM managers need to assume the teaching role. This chapter covers orientation and training as well as staff development related to continuing education and career development. Training and development may be coordinated organization-wide through an education department, but in an HIM department or work section area the HIM manager is responsible for these activities. HIM managers have the technical expertise, education, and practical experience to carry out necessary training, but they must also possess the skills to perform needs assessments, understand learning styles, and choose appropriate methods of instruction. This chapter discusses all of the necessary components of a training and development program.

Chapter 10, "Organizational Structure of HIM," provides guidance in assessing a healthcare organization's landscape in relation to internal and external influences and how these influences impact the HIM department's organizational model. HIM students and practitioners need to keep pace with changes that are significantly impacting the HIM field. HIM managers need to be cognizant of the environmental factors that are impacting the profession and know how to adapt to these changes. HIM managers also need to be aware of the committee structures that exist within healthcare organizations, and how these committees impact the management of HIM departments. This chapter will also discuss the external influences related to government initiatives that impact the management of health information. A review of competitors for HIM roles and how HIM professionals must stay current and relevant in today's competitive healthcare market is provided. The chapter concludes with a summarization of the textbook.

Acknowledgements

Jan Kelly, MBA, RHIA

I would like to thank my husband Tom, and daughters Emily and Caroline, for their patience and understanding during the writing of this textbook. I am sure they are sick of hearing, "Sorry, I have to work on the book." I would like to thank my mother, Lois Richard, for introducing me to the profession of health information management during my freshman year in college. Mothers always know best. I would like to thank the many administrators, bosses, peers, and employees who have helped to shape my management style and philosophy over the years. Finally, a special thanks to Pam Greenstone. I could and would have never done this without her!

Pam Greenstone, MEd, RHIA

I would like to thank my husband Mike for his patience and encouragement throughout the many weekends and evening hours that I spent writing this textbook. I am also thankful for all the management experiences that I encountered within my HIM career that allowed me to embark on this writing endeavor. It was wonderful having Jan Kelly as a collaborative partner and I would not have done this journey without her.

We both would like to thank editor Megan Grennan and technical reviewer Braden Michael B. Tabisula, MBA, RHIA, for their invaluable input to the writing process for this textbook. Their knowledge, suggestions, and ideas added greatly to the content of the textbook.

1

Traditional Theories of Management and Leadership

Learning Objectives

- Identify the traditional theories of management
- Describe the impact of traditional theories of management on health information functions
- Compare and contrast traditional theories of management within healthcare organizations
- Describe the traditional theories of leadership
- List the key functions and skills of traditional leadership theories
- Compare and contrast traditional theories of leadership within healthcare organizations

Key Terms

Acceptance view of authority
Administrative management
Authoritarian leader
Authoritarian management
Authority
Autocratic leadership style
Backcasting
Behavioral theories of leadership
Charismatic authority

Collaborative performance appraisals
Consultative leadership
Contemporary management
Contingency approach
Democratic leader
DMAIC approach
Gantt chart
Great man theory
Humanistic management
Job enlargement

Laissez-faire leader
Leadership
Leadership continuum
Lean
Legitimate authority
Management
Management by objectives (MBO)
Management theory
Managerial grid
Maslow's hierarchy of human needs
Normative decision model

Operations management
Participative leadership
Participatory management
Path-goal theory
Rational-legal authority
Scientific management
Servant leadership
Situational leadership theory
Six Sigma
The Iowa Studies

The Michigan studies	Theory Y	Transformational	Weber's theory of
The Ohio State leadership	Traditional authority	leadership	bureaucratic
study	Trait theory of leadership	Value	management
Theory X	Transactional leadership	Values-based leadership	Zone of indifference

Management is an essential component of the health information management (HIM) profession; understanding management from a historical perspective is the precipitating factor behind the creation of this first chapter. Research of management and leadership theories provides a strong foundation for health information management and leadership within today's healthcare environment. Management is the judicious use of means to accomplish an end (Merriam-Webster 2015). It is also the "organization and coordination of the activities of a business in order to achieve defined objectives" (Business Dictionary 2015). Management is also the group of those who manage or direct an organization. Within the context of healthcare, the American Health Information Management Association (AHIMA) provides a definition of **management** as the process of planning, organizing and leading organizational activities. This is the standardized definition for understanding the study of management within this chapter and is the fundamental definition throughout this text.

The following are a few other terms that must be defined in order to study the history of management theories and leadership styles:

- **Manager:** An individual who is in charge of a business or department
- **Leader:** An individual who has commanding authority or influence
- **Follower:** An individual who is in the service of another
- **Employee:** An individual who works for another person or for an organization for wages or a salary
- **Subordinate:** An individual in a position of less power or authority than someone else (Merriam-Webster 2015)

Management theory is a collection of ideas which set forth general rules on how to manage a business or organization. Management theory addresses how managers and supervisors relate to their organizations in the knowledge of its goals, the implementation of effective means to achieve the set goals, and how to motivate employees to perform to the highest standard (Business Dictionary 2015). Historical management theories are concepts that made a significant impression on the management practices utilized within healthcare organizations. Discernment of the historical management theories and the correct context in which these theories evolved is an important learning component for HIM professionals. In this first chapter, the individuals associated with early management and leadership theories are identified along with the concepts most closely related to their research. The first section of this chapter outlines the scientific, administrative, humanistic, contemporary, and operations management theorists who impacted the study of management and addresses the management concepts most closely related to each of theorists. Figure 1.1 depicts a timeline of management theories and the notable individuals associated with each theory.

The second section of this chapter addresses behavioral, contingency, transformational, values-based, and servant leadership theories that impact the development of leadership practices within organizations.

The final section of this chapter provides a case study that can be utilized by HIM professionals to apply, compare, and contrast the management and leadership theories outlined here.

Scientific Management

Early in the 20th century, scientific management was one of the first-identified forms of management because it is a discipline that can be studied and tested within organizations. Scientific management evolved with the advent of the United States' industrial revolution and is considered one of the classic approaches to understanding the role of management within organizations. **Scientific management** is studying work processes and how they impact workers' productivity (Schachter 2010). Scientific management theory is primarily concerned with improving the efficiency of individual employees in the work environment by assessing the distribution of work, studying time and

Figure 1.1.   The evolution of management theory

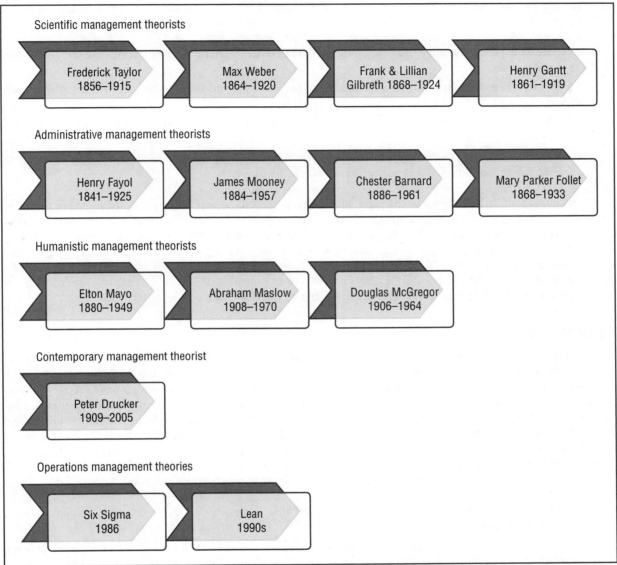

Scientific management theorists

Frederick Taylor
1856–1915

Max Weber
1864–1920

Frank & Lillian
Gilbreth 1868–1924

Henry Gantt
1861–1919

Administrative management theorists

Henry Fayol
1841–1925

James Mooney
1884–1957

Chester Barnard
1886–1961

Mary Parker Follet
1868–1933

Humanistic management theorists

Elton Mayo
1880–1949

Abraham Maslow
1908–1970

Douglas McGregor
1906–1964

Contemporary management theorist

Peter Drucker
1909–2005

Operations management theories

Six Sigma
1986

Lean
1990s

© AHIMA

motion of job tasks as well as measuring work actually performed. (Business Dictionary 2015). The key players in the development of scientific management theories—Frederick Taylor, Max Weber, Frank and Lillian Gilbreth, and Henry Gantt—are discussed along with their notable scientific management contributions.

Frederick Taylor

Management theorist Frederick Taylor introduced time and motion studies for assessing the efficiency of performed work. Taylor felt managers needed more knowledge about work processes in order to motivate employees to perform well. Taylor published *The Principles of Scientific Management* in 1911, in which he established the Taylor "management style" that believed managers could improve employees' work efficiencies by streamlining work motions and hiring employees who were amenable to performing job tasks in this type of environment. Taylor's principles were founded on his research of employees in the workplace and how work performed impacted employees' productivity. Taylor's time and motion studies provided a foundation for managers to understand the time and efforts required to complete a task (Schachter 2010). Taylor has been labeled the father of scientific management and the four scientific principles outlined as follows are often associated within management circles as *Taylorisms* (Parker and Ritson 2005). The four guiding management principles identified in Taylor's work are to:

- Evaluate work performed utilizing the scientific method in order to determine the most efficient way for workers to complete tasks
- Match employees to their jobs based on capability and motivate and train employees to work at maximum efficiency
- Monitor employee performance and provide instructions and supervision to ensure they use the most efficient ways of working
- Allocate the work between managers and subordinates so managers spend their time on planning and training, allowing subordinates to perform tasks efficiently (Eyre 2015)

The principles identified by Taylor in the early 20th century can still be applied in a modified fashion to today's workforce. Today, many HIM tasks require employees to complete their tasks in an efficient manner, utilizing productivity measures outlined by healthcare organizations. For example, chart completion analysts in HIM are required to review all inpatient discharges to ensure that documentation is both present and complete. Analysts must adhere to productivity measures established by the HIM department; for example, documentation review must take place within three days of discharge and six charts per hour must be analyzed. Productivity statistics are collected on a weekly basis and the HIM manager benchmarks each analyst's performance on a regular basis.

Max Weber

Max Weber, another scientific management theorist, introduced the bureaucracy theory around 1904, although much of his work was not published until after his death in 1920. Weber's theory revolved around concepts of legitimate authority in an organization. **Authority** is the right to make decisions and take actions necessary to carry out assigned tasks. **Legitimate authority** identifies individuals who have the right to demonstrate power over other individuals within a bureaucratic organization (Houghton 2010). **Weber's theory of bureaucratic management** outlined a hierarchical or pyramidal structure to help achieve the most rational and efficient operation at the lowest cost along with providing authority to those who had management positions within the hierarchy. Weber's theory viewed bureaucracy in an organization positively as he attempted to explain management practices within this environment. Weber noted there are two essential components to a bureaucratic organization:

- Organizations are structured into hierarchies arranged at an organizational level of authority as demonstrated in an organizational chart.
- The organization and its workgroup are governed by clearly defined decision-making rules that are outlined in policies and procedures that are managed by levels of authority within an organization (Houghton, 2010).

Through his research, Max Weber identified three types of legitimate authority within organizations: traditional, rational-legal, and charismatic authority. **Traditional authority** is when authority is inherently understood within an organization or group. Examples of traditional authority are a corporate business owner, tribal chief, or royal monarch like the Queen of England; each is clearly seen as a leader in authoritative command of a group. Traditional authority "rests on the established belief of sanctity of traditions and legitimacy of those exercising authority under them" (Houghton 2010). **Rational-legal authority** is displayed as boundaries outlined within organizations, which rely on the rules and laws imposed by those in authoritative management positions. Examples of rational-legal authority are the President of the United States and the Chief Executive Officer of a healthcare organization. **Charismatic authority** embodies a leader who has the capacity to influence subordinates. Weber saw charismatic authority as valuable and effective during times of instability.

These three types of authority impact management within organizations in both positive and negative ways. Traditional and rational-legal authority bring stability and order to organizations but allow for very little flexibility within organizational management. Within traditional and rational-legal management situations, managers oversee employees utilizing laws and rules that have been established and handed down from generation to generation.

Charismatic authority, on the other hand, is perceived as bringing disorder to organizations as sometimes charisma is exhibited by those who are not in traditional management roles and do not necessarily follow the traditional lines of authority. Charismatic authority is necessary for allowing change to occur within organizations because it allows those who are willing to change to be role models for those who are not changing (Houghton 2010). Weber's concepts of authority helped organizations understand the impact of management hierarchy from within and his thoughts on charismatic authority may do well in managerial applicability for today's changing healthcare environment. With the advent of healthcare information technology, a medical student or resident may readily embrace and utilize the technology when documenting patient encounters. The individual may exhibit some charismatic authority just by being an advocate for the technology but the medical student or resident most likey does not have any traditional-rational authority within the organization. This charismatic authority will assist the healthcare organization through the change initiative because these individuals will lead the change by example rather than in a traditional authoritative manner.

Frank and Lillian Gilbreth

Frank and Lillian Gilbreth were innovators who followed closely in Taylor's footsteps by continuing scientific management research. However, their perspective on studying work and workers differed from Taylor's. In 1907, Frank Gilbreth performed time and motion studies on workers within the manufacturing industry to assess efficiency of workers' performance. Gilbreth used stopwatch time studies to evaluate how workers performed tasks and how body mechanics impacted the time required to complete tasks. Later in his research, the stopwatch was replaced with recorded motion picture film and called "micromotion study" (Baumgart and Neuhaser 2009). The micromotion study allowed the Gilbreths to film workers completing tasks, review these tasks by playing back the film clips, and then analyze workers' performance for efficiencies that could be obtained by modifying different components of the tasks. Frank Gilbreth introduced new scientific management concepts into the workplace such as "re-organization and improvement of the routing of work, introduction of planning departments, and cost accounting" (Baumgart and Neuhauser 2009). Together in 1916, Frank and Lillian published a paper titled "Fatigue Study," relaying that the aim of the motion study was to accurately determine fatigue resulting from job tasks, to design the tasks so that unnecessary movements are removed, and to design efficient work stations to decrease worker fatigue (Price 1989).

The Gilbreths introduced standardization into healthcare by placing motion picture cameras within hospital operating rooms where motion studies were performed on filmed operations. Operational tasks performed by physicians were analyzed in order to decrease fatigue within the operating room and to gain efficiencies within operation procedures. The findings of these studies were published in two papers by the Gilbreths, "Scientific Management in the Hospital" in 1914, and "Hospital Efficiency from the Standpoint of the Efficiency Effort" in 1915. The findings documented in these papers recommended standardization of hospital design, medical equipment, and patient records to enhance efficiencies of work for healthcare workers as well as decreasing work fatigue (Baumgart and Neuhauser 2009).

Henry Gantt

Another disciple of Taylor's who worked closely with him in the 20th century was Henry Gantt whose legacy is the innovation of the Gantt chart. The **Gantt chart** is a bar chart that allows project managers to plan and control projects at a glance. The Gantt chart defines the steps of a project and the completion dates of each step (Thompson 2015). Figure 1.2 (on the following page) is an example of a Gantt chart. Gantt made three other contributions to the development of scientific management through his research:

- *The task and bonus system.* Gantt found that if workers were given a specific stated reward if they could perform the tasks within the time allotted, and then a further bonus if they could significantly better that time, overall productivity increased immensely within organizations.

- *The perspective of the worker.* Gantt took into account the role the supervisor played in getting subordinates to perform. He encouraged the supervisor to be a "helper and teacher of subordinates" because if all workers met or exceeded the required work standards, the supervisor in turn received a bonus.

- *The social responsibility of business.* "Gantt believed increasingly that management had obligations to the community at large and that the profitable organization had a duty toward the welfare of society" (Witzel 2006).

Figure 1.2.   Example of a Gantt chart

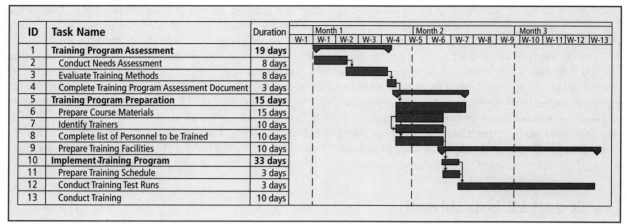

Source: Seidl 2013.

Gantt differed from Taylor's theory in that he believed work was empowering to workers and managers rather than adversarial. Gantt also identified the technique of **backcasting** which is the process of deciding on a goal and then working backwards to determine from the current state what steps need to be taken to achieve the goal. The Gantt chart is a visual display of the backcasting process (Business Dictionary 2015).

Administrative Management

Administrative management is another management theory developed in the early 20th century. It overlaps with the scientific management theory in trying to understand how work is performed but it incorporates assessing the organization as a whole in relation to the work being performed. Administrative management theory attempts to identify the design of an organization and is associated with the following principles:

- Requires a formalized administrative structure where there are clear lines of authority marked as a hierarchical structure.
- Defines a clear division of labor among workers.
- Reflects delegation of power and authority to upper management (Wren et al. 2002).

The following individuals impacted research on administrative management and provide another layer in the evolution of management theories for organizations.

Henry Fayol

Henry Fayol was the first administrative management theorist and is often thought of as the father of modern management. Fayol identified five key managerial functions: forecasting and planning, organization, commanding, coordinating, and controlling the work of the organization (Parker and Ritson 2005). Fayol noted that within the organization, workers performed the technical components and managers performed administrative functions. The differences that Fayol notes between technical and administrative skills for managers are the foundational concepts of administrative management (Wren et al. 2002). Henry Fayol is credited for developing the 14 principles of management for structure and organization that were designed to fit all organizations (Parker and Ritson 2005). Table 1.1 depicts Fayol's 14 principles of management.

Fayol appreciated that an employee's motivation to participate in the workplace included additional factors than just the need for payment of services. Like Taylor, Fayol assumed that management concepts could be applied universally and that the practice of management should only be exhibited by upper level executives within an

Table 1.1. Fayol's 14 principles of management

Principal	Relevance to Healthcare Organizations
Division of labor or work	Understanding how tasks are distributed within a department and who is responsible for the completion of what tasks.
Authority	The right to make decisions and take actions necessary to carry out assigned tasks.
Discipline	Self-control employees display within the context of the work environment which results in an orderly pattern of work behavior.
Unity of command	A principle that assumes each employee reports to only one specific management position.
Unity of direction	The actions of employees are related and are pointing toward the same path or outcome.
Subordination of the individual to the common good	Each individual employee is subject to the well-being of the entire organization.
Remuneration	Employees are rewarded for performing work which includes monetary or non-monetary rewards.
Centralization	The power and authority of an organization is concentrated within a core management group.
Scalar chain	Uninterrupted lines of management are evident within the organization and these lines reflect directly-linked reporting mechanisms for employees.
Order	Relates to the structure and the authoritative direction throughout the organization. Everything has its place and there is a semblance of uniformity.
Equity	Relates to the fairness and impartiality toward all employees within an organization.
Stability	The ability of an organization to remain constant and provide the perception of balance and security to employees.
Initiative	A trait exhibited by employees who perform a task without being directed to do so by management.
Esprit de corps	Employees' feelings of loyalty, enthusiasm, and devotion to a group among others who are members of an organization.

Source: BusinessDictionary.com 2015 and Merriam-Webster 2015.

organization (Parker and Ritson 2005). Fayol's traditional principles of management functions still hold true for certain components of a manager's tasks, but 21st century management must incorporate other management and leadership skills described within this chapter.

James D. Mooney

James D. Mooney was employed by the General Motors Car Company and is most noted for his unpublished paper, "The Science of Industrial Organization." Mooney's paper suggests six principles of organization:

- Division of duties: A natural division of labor occurs because some individuals are better at certain tasks than other tasks.
- Coordination of effort: Because of the natural division of labor, coordination must occur to achieve the objective of work efforts.
- Leadership: Authority resides in formal positions of responsibility such as management roles thus leadership within these roles provides guidance for the coordination of efforts.
- Delegation of duties: The responsibility of completing work efforts requires delegation of duties by management roles to employees within an organization.

- The functional definition of duties: Because of the coordination and delegation of work required in day-to-day operations, a vertical division of labor is necessary outlining authority and responsibility within the organization.
- Line-and-staff principle: Makes a distinction between the line managers who make work decisions and the staff managers who provide advice about how work is to be performed (Wren 2013).

Mooney theorized that these six concepts impacted the management functions within an organization and different management styles were needed to manage diverse organizations. Mooney incorporated the line–staff principles of management of operations because staff managers had the authority for creation of ideas and line managers had the authority to carry out the ideas based on their hierarchical positions within the organization. Mooney utilized an organizational chart to depict the hierarchical management structure within GM's overseas operations (Wren 2013). An organizational chart is described in chapter 10 along with graphic ways to reflect hierarchical management structures within an organization.

Chester Barnard

Chester Barnard developed his management theories while working for AT&T (formerly the American Telephone and Telegraph Company). Throughout the mid-1900s, Bernard provided a management foundation that not only addressed organizational structure but also considered the managerial skills required to obtain cooperation from subordinates within the organization (Malcom and Hartley 2010). Barnard assessed that organizations contained a social entity and not just an organizational chart. He noted that goals within an organization could be achieved by:

- Cooperative attitudes between units
- Cross-training of personnel
- Interdepartmental instruction
- Organizational efficiency and effectiveness
- Creating authentic and realistic goals for the organization
- Developing trust throughout all levels of the organization between employees and management
- Personal responsibility
- Leadership flexibility and balance

Barnard not only published his administrative management theories, he also strived to practice the theories while working at AT&T for 40 years. He was successful as a manager and teacher within the workplace and his ability to persuade others to perform within their jobs allowed him to move up within the company (Malcom and Hartley 2010).

Two management concepts associated with Barnard are the acceptance view of authority and the zone of indifference. The **acceptance view of authority** is evident in organizations when an employee considers a request by the manager to be in the best interest of the group, is understandable, and meets the employee's personal interests. In addition, the request from the manager must not be outside of the employee's mental and physical abilities for compliance (Malcom and Hartley 2010). The **zone of indifference** proves a manager's concept of power; this is the range in which a manager's orders will be perceived as legitimate and the employee will act on or perform the request without a great deal of thought. Managers strive to expand the zone of indifference by being knowledgeable about their workgroup, making requests that fall within the an acceptable range of employee expectation and maximizing requests from employees for which cooperation is most expected (Malcom and Hartley 2010). Both of these theories are dependent on the communication skills of the manager and his or her ability to facilitate cooperation within the workgroup.

Mary Parker Follett

Mary Parker Follett was the first theorist within the administrative management group to be concerned with the psychosocial approach to industry and organizational management rather than a more scientific approach to management. Her early 20th century writings and research centered on the philosophical and psychological foundations of workers and the interdisciplinary approach workers contribute to an organization. The management terms most associated with Follett's work are *togetherness* and *group thinking*. Follett's theory revolved around productive management practices where the manager exercised power *with* others rather than *over* others. She favored a management style where managers worked with subordinates to get work done rather than managers dictating the work to be accomplished by subordinates (Parker and Ritson 2005).

Humanistic Management

Humanistic management was a shift from the scientific management theories in that individual human needs and human values were considered within the management of an organization. For a management style to be considered humanistic, three key dimensions must be considered: (1) human dignity is the key element of consideration, (2) ethical complexities are evaluated, and (3) all stakeholders must be involved in the decision-making process (Humanistic Management Center 2014). The following individuals impacted the study of humanistic management.

Elton Mayo

In 1927, Elton Mayo began his research in human relations management at the Hawthorne plant of Western Electric in Cicero, Illinois. Mayo's thoughts differed from Taylor's scientific management theory in that he assumed that employees were not only interested in receiving remuneration for services, but also that employees wanted to be considered unique individuals with goals and aspirations that match those of the organization (Bruce 2006). The "Hawthorne studies" examined productivity and work conditions for a group of female workers at the Hawthorne plant for almost a year. The study parameters evaluated were the impact of change to hours, wages, rest periods, lighting conditions, organization and degree of supervision, and what specific conditions impacted the group's work performance and productivity (Encyclopedia Britannica 2014). There are four general conclusions that resulted from the Hawthorne studies in regards to management of individuals within an organization and these concepts are related to what has been labeled as the "Hawthorne Effect":

- The aptitudes of individuals (as measured by industrial psychologists) are imperfect predictors of job performance.
- Informal organization affects productivity.
- Workgroup norms affect productivity.
- The workplace is a social system (Encyclopedia Britannica 2014).

Based on the Hawthorne investigations, Mayo suggested that collaboration rather than competition was important to workers. Mayo's Hawthorne findings labeled him as the founder of the human relations movement in management (Bruce 2006).

Abraham Maslow

Abraham Harold Maslow, psychologist and researcher, provides a theory to the management body of knowledge that addresses employees' motivation in terms of human relations. Maslow's research in terms of human relations management addressed a behavioral scientific approach to employee motivation and motivational theory (Ozguner and Ozguner 2014). The theory, **Maslow's hierarchy of human needs**, strived to understand the needs of people at work and what motivated employees to perform within an organization. In this theory, an employee's needs are arranged in hierarchy from low-level psychological needs such as staying alive and being safe to the highest level of needs for self-actualization such as self-fulfillment and achievement (Stum 2001). It is important to include Maslow's impact to the development of management theories within this chapter but his contributions in terms of employee motivation and how this relates to the hierarchy of needs is discussed in more depth within chapter 3.

Douglas McGregor

Douglas McGregor was a management theorist concerned with the observation of managers' behaviors in real work situations. His original writing on "The Human Side of Enterprise," published in 1960, addressed the X and Y theories of management (Burke 2011). McGregor simplistically noted that management concepts can be divided into two categories: Theory X and Theory Y. **Theory X** is a management style that is based on a set of assumptions that managers have toward employees and it leans toward a more authoritarian type of management style. Theory X managers assume that most employees do not like to work and that they must have direct oversight in order to perform their jobs. **Authoritarian management** is a management style in which the "leader dictates policies and procedures, decides what goals are to be achieved, and directs and controls all activities without any meaningful participation by the subordinates" (Business Dictionary 2015). **Theory Y** is the opposite of Theory X in that managers assume that employees enjoy to work and that they are self-motivated in completing their job tasks. Theory Y managers lean toward a more participatory management style. **Participatory management** is a style in which management allows employees to take an active role in decision-making processes that relates directly to their jobs (McQuerrey 2015). Both of these theories provide insight into group dynamics within an organization and provide rationale for behaviors exhibited by managers and subordinates (Burke 2011). Figure 1.3 outlines Theory X and Theory Y manager beliefs regarding employees. McGregor's Theory Y concepts and management ideas provide a view into the impact of different management styles on organizational development (Head 2011).

Additionally, two distinct management concepts addressed by McGregor include job enlargement and collaborative performance appraisals between managers and employees. **Job enlargement** is the concept that adding a variety of job tasks to an individual's job will decrease job monotony and thereby allow more job flexibility. McGregor's research reflected that employees may perform better in an environment where jobs offer a variety of tasks and where evaluations for performance of the tasks are completed by a variety of individuals. **Collaborative performance appraisals** engage employees within the process of evaluating work performed. Collaborative performance appraisals require managers to solicit input from employees about actual work performance. McGregor built his research on the basic premises of Maslow's hierarchy of needs, reflecting that individuals will perform in association with how their needs are being met within the organization and that with job enlargement and collaborative performance appraisals these individuals will perform above and beyond the minimum requirements (Head 2011).

Operations Management

The next wave of management study focused on **operations management**, which is "management that deals with the design and management of products, processes, services, and supply chains. It considers the acquisition, development, and utilization of resources that firms need to deliver the goods and services clients want" (Barrow

Figure 1.3. McGregor's X and Y management theory

McGregor's Humanistic Management Theory	
Theory X managers believe employees are:	**Theory Y managers believe employees are:**
• Lazy	• Motivated
• Resist change	• Open to change
• Do not like responsibility	• Can handle responsibility
• Need play incentives or threats	• Prefer rewards over threats
• Disloyal	• Loyal

2013). Operations management evaluates tools that are needed to manage processes of interrelated activities. Operations managers need to focus on forecasting, planning, scheduling, managing inventories, assuring quality, and motivating employees so as to guide the organization in decision making (Barrow 2013).

Two operations management theories that assist management with improving processes within an organization are Six Sigma and lean. These theories are utilized by organizations (and recently by healthcare organizations) for improving the quality and streamlining operations.

Six Sigma

Created in 1986 by the Motorola Company, **Six Sigma** is a set of techniques and tools utilized to improve the capability of organizational business processes. Six Sigma was created to identify defects as a result of manufacturing processes and improve the variability of product outcomes upon implementation of process improvement initiatives. Both quantitative and qualitative techniques are utilized to improve quality through process improvement. Examples of techniques that are utilized to map out current processes that will be evaluated during a Six Sigma project are *control charts* and *process mapping*. The Six Sigma problem-solving framework is called the **DMAIC approach**. DMAIC is an acronym that stands for: define the opportunity for improvement, measure current performance, analyze the opportunity, improve the opportunity, and control performance after improvements are made. The DMAIC approach is led by a Six Sigma trainer for processes being studied for performance improvement. Organizations may elect either to contract Six Sigma consultants or to have key individuals attend Six Sigma training to become certified trainers (Liberatore 2013).

In healthcare, Six Sigma is most frequently associated with focusing on application of the DMAIC problem-solving framework and process changes as a result of utilizing the framework; outcome and metrics are a result of the process changes, and cost and revenue improves as a result of utilizing the Six Sigma method (Liberatore 2013). A study in 2011 comprehensively assessed Six Sigma within the healthcare industry and the results indicated the following:

- A significant number of healthcare organizations are utilizing Six Sigma and the DMAIC approach for quality improvement initiatives.
- Outcomes from utilizing the Six Sigma approach need to be embraced by healthcare staff and change management techniques need to be incorporated into the process (Liberatore 2013).

Lean

Lean is a management strategy that utilizes less to do more and is a process improvement strategy that can be utilized in any type of organization. Lean thinking is derived from the Japanese auto industry and process improvement initiatives that took place within the Toyota Production System in the 1990s. The basic concept behind lean management is to create more value for customers while utilizing fewer resources. Lean thinking requires management to strategically assess all work processes and eliminate as much waste of in terms of human effort, space, capital, and time while still delivering a quality product (Lean Enterprise Institute 2015). Lean thinking requires that managers change their practices and behaviors by committing to the tools and thought processes required to develop a "lean" organization. A lean management strategy necessitates that all levels of leadership be involved in the process in order for the strategy to be effective (Institute for Healthcare Improvement 2005).

Lean management differs from traditional management practices. It is a high-maintenance approach that requires leaders to review actual work, assess best practices, and provide accountability for streamlining work as necessary. Value-added jobs within an organization are established when workers and managers spend 100 percent of their time on standardized processes that are directly related to assigned job tasks. Healthcare organizations are embracing lean strategies more frequently to reduce costs, reduce duplicity of work, and enhance patient safety initiatives (Institute for Healthcare Improvement 2005). Healthcare organizations implementing lean management practices evaluate the management structure required to most effectively provide services to patient populations and eliminate redundancy in job roles and tasks as necessitated to become more efficient or "lean" in providing these services.

Contemporary Management

Contemporary management uses current practices to plan, organize, and control individuals within an organization. Given their complexity, today's healthcare organizations rely on managers who can assess an organization's culture and utilize the best of the best managerial skills to lead within the organization. One of the most notable theorists associated with contemporary management research is Peter Drucker.

Peter Drucker was an author, teacher, writer, and management consultant and was nicknamed the "father of modern management" (Business Dictionary 2015). Drucker spent many years studying a variety of topics associated with management. Drucker's philosophy of management noted that a business is not only an economic organization but a human social organization as well. He believed that it was up to management to maintain a positive work environment in order for employees to stay motivated to perform (Kurzynski 2009).

Drucker originally introduced **management by objectives (MBO)** within an early writing entitled "The Practice of Management" in 1954 (Fernandez 2009). Management by objectives is a management style in which the objectives of an organization are agreed upon by management and employees so that everyone is working toward common goals (Business Dictionary 2015). Management by objectives is a very structured approach whereby objectives are written from the top down within an organization and each manager has a set of prescribed performance objectives. The manager works with his or her employees to create performance objectives that roll up under the manager's objectives.

Drucker was concerned with the concepts of business management and structure and he focused primarily on two key elements of an organization: the employee as a whole (referred to as a knowledge worker) and the organization as a whole. Drucker believed that management is concerned with individuals who are working interdependently toward common goals and values. Management should provide the right structure, training, and development so employees can succeed at their jobs. In MBO, managers must challenge themselves and their team to achieve goals by utilizing self-control and self-discipline. Managers must have a vision and lead responsibly. The knowledge worker within an MBO organization is concerned with self-directed productivity and the quality of work performed (Kurzynski 2009).

Drucker was also an advocate for understanding and valuing diversity within the workplace. He examined how managerial and diversity issues affected countries, industries, organizations, and individuals. From these studies, Drucker provided extensive prescriptions for understanding the changing demographics of the United States workforce to assist organizations in leveraging diversity within organizations (Oyler and Pryor 2009). Many of Drucker's management concepts have been incorporated into the management of healthcare organizations at some point in time. Many departments within healthcare organizations utilize MBO to achieve strategic goals throughout the year. Diversity is an important management concept when hiring staff within healthcare organizations and Drucker's research provides excellent guidance for improving the workforce diversity within an organization.

Check Your **Understanding**

1. What management theorist is coined the "father of modern management"?
2. Describe two characteristics that differentiate administrative management theories from scientific management theories.
3. Define one term closely related to Max Weber's bureaucracy theory.
4. Identify the first scientific manager(s) that assessed work fatigue within healthcare.
5. Name the graphic tool that was developed by Henry Gantt and how this tool is utilized today.

Leadership

The second part of this chapter addresses the evolution of leadership theories and the individuals or theories that have served to provide a basis for leadership practices. Although leadership is delineated as one of the attributes of management, it has been studied by scholars as a significant singular contribution to the overall workings of an organization. **Leadership** is the activity of guiding a group of people to a definite result. Many theorists feel that leadership is not a skill that can be taught to individuals but, rather, is an innate quality that appears within individuals. In most organizations, management is the formal structure of the organization and people in management have the authority to ensure tasks are accomplished by employees' efforts. Leadership can be an inherent component of management but also can be exhibited both formally and informally within a healthcare organization. No matter what level of leadership, leaders need cooperation with the assistance of others within the organization in order to obtain extraordinary results.

Classic approaches to leadership focus on the traits and behaviors of the leader. The theories of leadership outlined are:

- Trait theories of leadership
- Behavioral theories of leadership
- Contingency theories of leadership
- Transformational theory of leadership
- Values-based leadership
- Servant leadership

Figure 1.4 reflects an evolution of leadership theories. This diagram suggests that each leadership theory builds on the next and no distinct leadership style fits all management situations within an organization.

Trait Theory of Leadership

Trait theory of leadership attempts to define the general qualities or traits that need to be present within an individual to be a leader. The **great man theory** is the most documented trait theory and notes that certain traits within individuals can be identified as predictors for effective leadership and that by studying great historical leaders, individual traits can clearly be identified as keys for success in leadership. Although traits do seem to play a role in effective leadership, the great man theory has proven to be too simplistic of an explanation for effective leadership in today's society (Ronald 2014).

Figure 1.4.   Evolution of management theories

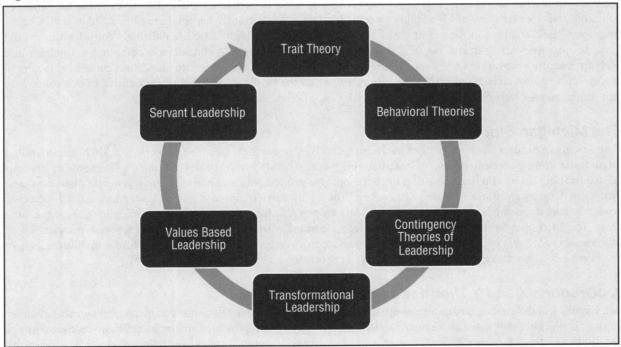

© AHIMA

Behavioral Theories of Leadership

Behavioral theories of leadership focus on the study of specific behaviors of leaders. In the previous section of this text, leadership theories were discussed in terms of leadership traits rather than behavior. In this section, the following studies and leadership theorists that have developed behavioral leadership theories are discussed: The Iowa Studies, The Ohio State Leadership Studies, The Michigan Studies, Theory X and Y, the continuum of leader behavior, and the managerial grid (Ronald 2014).

The Iowa Studies

The Iowa Studies were conducted in 1939 at the Child Welfare Research Station within Iowa State University by Kurt Lewin, Ronald Lippitt, and Ralph K. White (notable researchers from the Iowa University) (Lewin et al. 1939). The Iowa Studies were one of the first behavioral research studies focusing on leadership roles rather than the traits exhibited by leaders. These experimental research studies identified three leadership styles that are representative of the relations between leaders and the individuals being led: authoritarian, democratic, and laissez-faire. The **authoritarian leader** dictates activities to the workgroup but he or she does not participate in the completion of the activities. The authoritarian is very critical of the team's results. The **democratic leader** assists and encourages the workgroup, allows the workgroup to select activities to be completed as a group, and praises the group at completion of the work. The **laissez-faire leader** does not participate in the selection of the group activities and does not provide praise or criticism to the workgroup. The laissez-faire leader provides the resources for the group's activities but does not interfere with how the group performs. The three representative styles of leadership denoted by The Iowa Studies are still evident in today's business environment (Ronald 2014).

The Ohio State Leadership Studies

In the 1950s and 1960s, **The Ohio State Leadership Studies** were conducted by the researchers who were a part of the personnel research board at The Ohio State University (Shartle 1979). This research delineated a two-dimensional theory of leadership behavior and assessed the dimensions of leadership concern over the task objectives (job tasks to be completed by followers) and the concern for relationship objectives (the relationship between leader and follower). A leader behavior description questionnaire was deployed by researchers from The Ohio State University to leaders within actual workplaces. This questionnaire was used to determine the two dimensions of leadership exhibited by leaders within actual workplaces. Figure 1.5 depicts a leader's low or high ability for initiating structure for employee job tasks and a leader's low or high ability to consider employee relations when initiating low or high structure for employees' task completion. For example, a leader exhibiting both high structure and high consideration would provide employees a strong task organization at the same time taking into consideration employees' thoughts and feelings regarding the tasks. The two main limitations of this research were that situational and contextual factors of leadership were not considered within the research and that the two leadership behaviors defined in this study were not proven to positively correlate with effective leadership (Ronald 2014).

The Michigan Studies

The Michigan Studies were undertaken in the early 1950s by researchers from the University of Michigan interested in understanding leadership behaviors in actual workplaces. The Michigan Studies built on the Ohio Studies in terms of determining leadership behaviors that impact employee productivity and enhance employee job satisfaction. The Michigan Studies are more of a one-dimensional theory in that employee-centered leadership and job-centered leadership are opposing leadership styles and leaders are not able to focus on production and employees at the same time. The Michigan Studies do not take into effect situational variances that may impact leadership styles. These studies also noted that effective leaders utilized a participatory style of leadership where the leader involved a team of workers in decision making and problem solving in regards to work decisions (Ronald 2014).

McGregor's X and Y Theories as Behavioral Theories

McGregor's X and Y theories are more closely related to the study of human relationship management (addressed earlier in this chapter) but they can also be linked to leadership. McGregor's opinion of an employee's basic motivation to be led can be identified by either Theory X where employees are only motivated to perform through rewards or sanctions, or Theory Y where employees are motivated to perform through self-control and self-direction (Ronald 2014).

Figure 1.5. The Ohio State Leadership Studies matrix

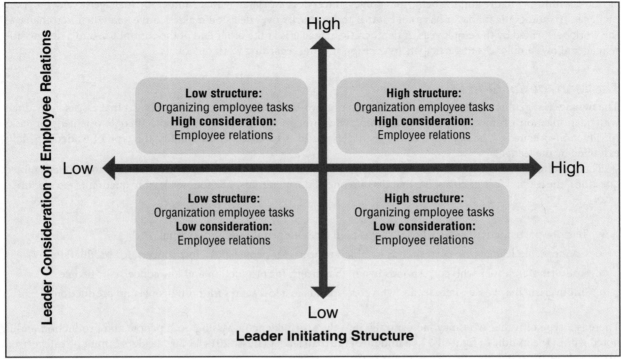

© AHIMA

The Leadership Continuum

The **leadership continuum** is another behavioral theory of leadership that made a significant impact on leadership research within the United States. In 1958, a leadership theory was developed by Robert Tannenbaum and Warren Schmidt based on the earlier Iowa Studies (Ronald 2014). The leadership continuum assumed that leadership behavior can be explained in seven steps of behavioral styles ranging from authority (boss-centered leadership) to delegation (team-centered leadership). This theory noted that leadership styles depend on the characteristics of leaders and followers within a situational context (Ronald 2014). Figure 1.6 depicts the one dimensional continuum

Figure 1.6. Continuum of leadership behavior

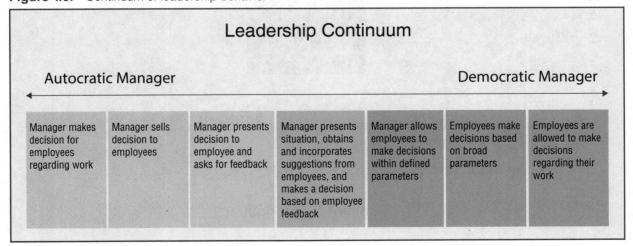

© AHIMA

of leadership behavior. The leadership behaviors associated within this continuum are divided into seven categories as noted within the figure and the behaviors range from styles associated with an autocratic manager to a democratic manager. An autocratic manager has total control and authority over decision making and essentially micromanages the work performed by the employees. A democratic manager is at the other end of the continuum and a democratic manager allows employees to participate in decision making regarding work outcomes.

The Managerial Grid

The **managerial grid** is a behavioral theory that offers a two-dimensional behavioral approach that assists individuals with identification of an appropriate leadership style through the concern for people (people-oriented) or tasks (production-oriented). The objective of the managerial grid is to analyze and identify the type of leadership skills exhibited by the leader.

There are four distinct quadrants within the grid (figure 1.7). Based on the leader's answer to pre-determined questions, the leader is assigned a score that fits into one of the quadrants. The four leadership quadrants are identified as a:

- Team or participative leader whose score is high for both people and production.
- Country club leader who corresponds to a high concern for people and a low concern for production.
- Authoritarian leader who corresponds to a high concern for production and low concern for people.
- Impoverished or laissez-faire leader who corresponds to a low scores for both people and production.

There is a type of leader who may fall centrally into the scoring, encompassing both people and production and is noted within the middle of figure 1.7 as a middle of the road leader (Busse 2014). Many leaders cannot be categorized to one side or the other but are a blend of the two approaches.

Figure 1.7. The managerial grid

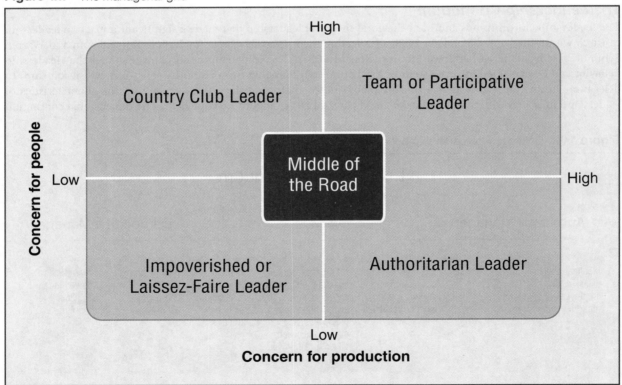

Contingency Approach to Leadership

"Contingency theories hold that leadership effectiveness is related to the interplay of a leader's traits or behaviors and situational factors" (Seyranian 2009). The **contingency approach** to effective leadership is dependent on matching the leader's style to the workplace situation. The following contingency approaches are discussed: Fiedler's contingency model, the path-goal theory, the normative decision model, and the situational theory.

Frederick Fiedler's Contingency Model

Frederick Fiedler studied group performance by utilizing the contingency theory of leadership effectiveness, which he coined in the early 1960s. The theory is dependent on the leader's task or relationship motivational style and situational control. Fiedler identified two styles of leadership: task-motivated, in which a leader is more focused on the worker's tasks, and relationship-motivated, in which a leader is more focused on the relationships associated with workers. Fiedler utilized the "least preferred co-worker scale" to identify the relationship between a leader's orientation or style and the group performance under differing situational conditions. The findings from Fiedler's work proposed that task or relationship motivations are contingent on whether the leader can control and predict a group's outcome, referred to as "situational favorability" (Seyranian 2009). Fiedler's theory has been tested by a number of researchers over the years and his theory has held up well in terms of predicting group outcomes based on the assessment of leadership styles.

The Path-Goal Theory

The **path-goal theory** was originally developed by Martin Evans in 1970 and the theory was further expanded upon by Robert House in 1971. It suggests that a leader should develop a path for followers to achieve group goals. The leadership effectiveness in this model depends on the leader's behaviors, the follower's expectations, and the organizational situation. There are four different leadership styles identified in the path-goal theory:

- Directive leaders provide specific instructions to followers
- Supportive leaders provide emotional support to followers
- Participative leaders allow followers to participate in decision-making processes associated with their work
- Achievement-oriented leaders set goals for their followers and assist followers in achieving their goals

The effectiveness of the leader is dependent on the characteristics of the followers within the workgroup and how closely the follower's characteristics match those of the leader (Seyranian 2009). Figure 1.8 (on the following page) depicts the employee situations or employee expectations versus the appropriate leadership style within the path-goal theory.

The path-goal theory has not been analytically tested by researchers and many leadership theorists feel that developing a path based on a group's expectations is highly complex and there are too many individual variables to actually make any predictions on group outcomes (Ronald 2014).

Normative Decision Model

In 1973, Victor Vroom and Phillip Yetton developed the **normative decision model**, which focuses on situational factors rather than leadership behaviors and it guides managers through the decision-making processes depending on the type of problem encountered. The model attempts to provide leadership style prescriptions to optimize a leader's decision making based on five different methods (Seyranian 2009). The five different methods vary in the degree to which the decision strategy permits subordinates to participate in the decision-making process. The five methods are described as follows:

- An **autocratic leadership style** is characterized by leader control over all decisions with no or very little input from the workgroup. This style is beneficial when decisions need to be made quickly by the leader. Vroom and Yetton prescribe two levels of autocratic leadership—Authority I and Authority II. Authority I level permits no subordinate involvement in the decision-making process. Authority II permits subordinates to respond to specific requests for information from the leader or decision maker (Jago and Vroom 1980).

Figure 1.8.   Employee job attributes within the path-goal theory

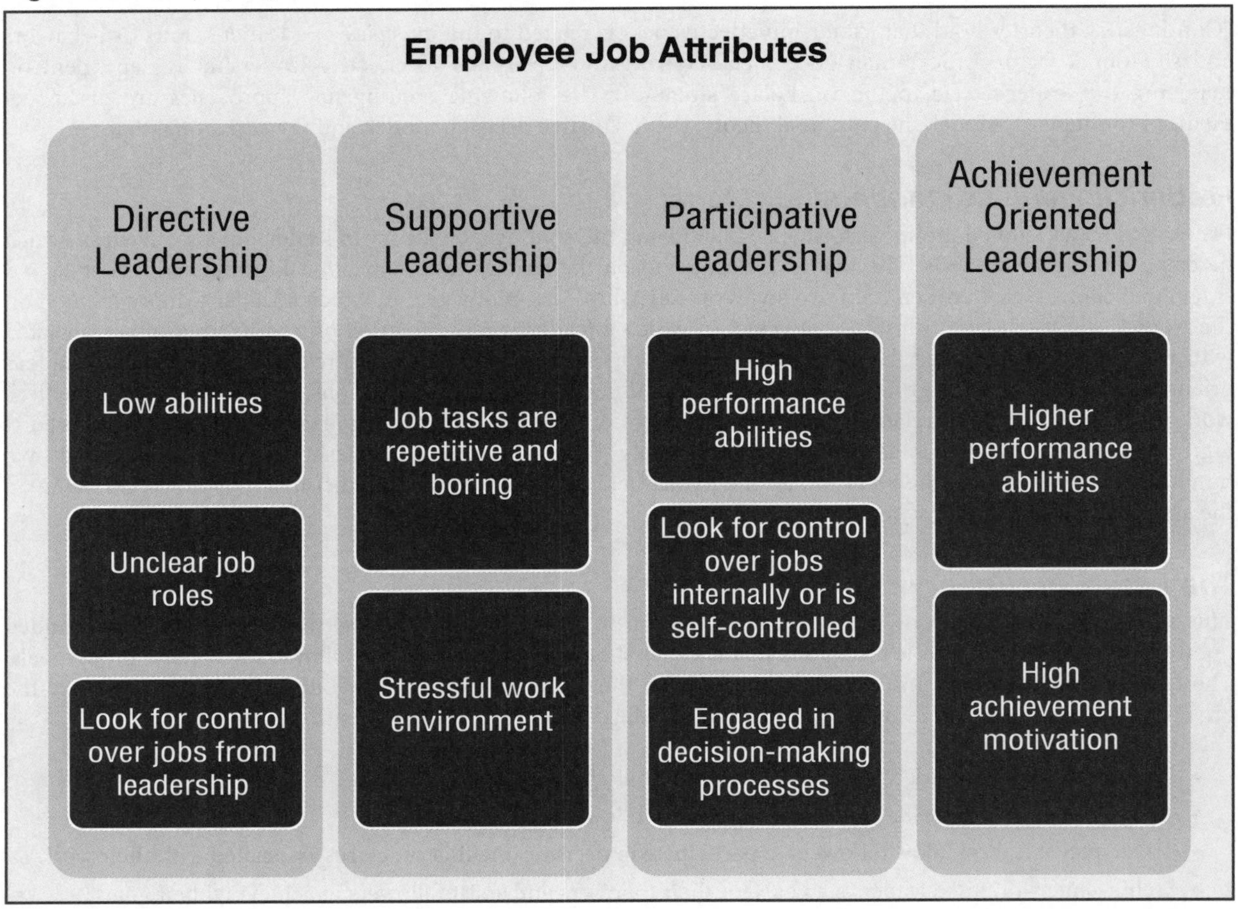

Employee Job Attributes

Directive Leadership	Supportive Leadership	Participative Leadership	Achievement Oriented Leadership
Low abilities	Job tasks are repetitive and boring	High performance abilities	Higher performance abilities
Unclear job roles		Look for control over jobs internally or is self-controlled	
Look for control over jobs from leadership	Stressful work environment	Engaged in decision-making processes	High achievement motivation

© AHIMA

- **Consultative leadership** is task-oriented and focuses on getting input from those who perform the tasks; the ultimate decisions for the group are still made by the leader but this leadership style takes into account the feedback provided by individual workers (Gill 2013). Vroom and Yetton prescribe two levels of consultative leadership within the normative decision model—Consultative I and Consultative II. Consultative I demonstrates one-on-one consultation from the leader with individual subordinates prior to the decision being made. Consultative II describes the process when group consultation is performed prior to the final decision (Jago and Vroom 1980).

- **Participative leadership** is a style in which the leader allows the workers to provide input and make decisions about their work (Seyranian 2009).

Within the normative decision model, leaders utilize a complex decision tree, answering eight different questions about the management situation in order to select a leadership style that most closely fits the situation. The precept behind the normative decision model is that the leader's style relies heavily on the situation and it is beneficial to utilize a systematic method for assessing the situation before deploying a leadership style (Ronald 2014).

Situational Leadership Theory

Paul Hershey and Ken Blanchard developed the **situational leadership theory** in 1969, which proposed that leadership effectiveness depends on the leader's ability to change his or her behavior to meet the demands of the situation. This theory also takes into account the maturity of the followers in terms of their job ability and psychological willingness to work. The behavior of the leader fluctuates depending on the level of maturity exhibited by the follower and the leader adjusts his or her leadership style based on this maturity. For example, if a follower has a low task ability or maturity, the leader would have to utilize a more directive type of leadership style providing more instructions on how to complete the task. A follower with a higher level of task maturity would be able to complete the work with very little direction from the leader (Ronald 2014).

Transformational and Transactional Theories of Leadership

In the 1970s, James MacGregor Burns performed descriptive research on political leaders and their leadership styles. Burns noted that two different styles of leadership were inherent: transformational and transactional. **Transformational leadership** is the act of changing or transforming from one current state to another state. It focuses on leaders' attempts to motivate followers to achieve at a higher level or to perform at a level beyond expectations. Leaders and followers in a transformational model bring one another to higher levels of motivation and morality. The leader creates an environment of trust and therefore followers feel "safe" within their work environment (Kendrick 2011).

There are four important components of transformational leadership that must be considered in order for a change or transformation to take place within an organization.

- The first component is idealized influence in which the leaders are role models for followers. Charisma is a personal quality of leadership arousing popular loyalty or enthusiasm and charisma is often a characteristic seen within those leaders who provide idealized influence over followers (Merriam-Webster 2015).

- The second component is the leader provides inspirational motivation by encouraging followers to achieve at higher levels based on high expectations. The leader creates a shared organizational vision that motivates followers to perform at a higher level.

- The third component is that a transformational leader provides intellectual stimulation by allowing followers to participate in problem-solving and decision-making activities within the organization.

- The fourth factor is individualized consideration that allows followers to develop new skills and enables them to act through collaboration with others to improve performance. This last factor of transformational leadership connects with Maslow's management theory (Avolio and Bass 1995).

Research has shown that transformational leadership styles have a positive effect on followers' work performance and job satisfaction. Transformational leadership behaviors can be developed through training. A research study indicated that psychological and behavioral changes will be exhibited by a leader who participates in transformational leadership training. This is an important finding in that transformational leadership training should include development interventions that address both aspects of psychological and behavioral leadership functions (Mason et al. 2014).

Burns also addressed **transactional leadership**, which is performed through structure and process. There is a hierarchy within the organization where leaders clarify goals and objectives for followers and followers receive some kind of reward in exchange for performing work satisfactorily. The types of rewards elicited within this leadership model are items such as a promotion, pay raise, or personal recognition. The model of transactional leadership is very similar to McGregor's X and Y theories of management (Lowe et al. 1996).

Bernard Bass (1925–2007) was a distinguished professor of management and leadership studies who performed research, conducted workshops, and lectured on leadership throughout the country. Bass was inspired by Burns to study transformational leadership and the abilities of transformational leaders. He characterized transactional leaders as those who avoid risk and attempt to work within the system by maintaining status quo. Bass then characterized transformational leaders as those who seek new or innovative ways to perform work, are willing to take risks, and do not like the status quo. Bass notes that effective leaders are both transactional and transformational rather than polar opposites as identified by Burns. The *multifactor leadership questionnaire* is a tool utilized to measure the components of transactional and transformation leadership and Bass and his colleagues utilized this tool within their research to further assess different leadership styles more accurately. Many scholars have utilized and continue to utilize the tool as a basis for assessing leadership styles (Lowe et al. 1996).

Values-Based Leadership

Values-based leadership is a style of leadership built on a foundation of personal values, principles, or ethics. Values are a key component of effective leadership. A **value** is a principle or ideal intrinsically valuable or desirable (human rather than material) (Merriam-Webster 2015). Values-based leadership makes certain that leaders effectively communicate values of integrity and responsibility to employees within the organization (Snell 2010). In order for values-based leadership to take hold within an organization, leaders should be motivated and committed to the values of the organization. This is particularly true in healthcare where all leaders should embrace the values included within the mission and vision of the organization (Graber and Kilpatrick 2008). Leaders must work on the following elements in order to represent a values-based leadership style:

- Self-reflection: A leader should reflect on his or her personal and professional values and incorporate these values into his or her leadership style.
- Organizational balance: A leader should embrace the values represented by the organization and reflect these values within his or her sphere of influence.
- Values of a team of followers: A leader should take note of the values of the individuals within his or her team and incorporate these values within his or her leadership style.
- Commit to values-based leadership: As a leader, he or she must commit to this leadership style (Kraemer 2011).

Values-based leadership takes commitment from all management and leadership roles within an organization. This type of leadership style is inherent to all stakeholders when it is practiced on a regular basis within organizations. Values-based leadership requires leaders to stand by the organization's values and not compromise personal values if conflict occurs among leaders when values collide (Frost 2014). Figure 1.9 reflects the overlay of values that a health information manager needs to assess in order to become an effective values-based leader.

Figure 1.9. Values-based leadership model

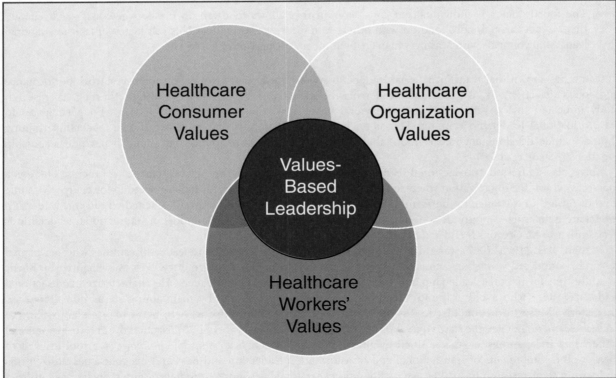

Servant Leadership

Robert Greenleaf was employed at AT&T for 28 years and provided many management contributions to the organization. Throughout Greenleaf's work life at AT&T, he realized that organizations that thrive have able leadership that provides support to employees and serves both the employees and the organization (Spears 1996). In 1970, Greenleaf defined **servant leadership** as a philosophy and set of practices that enriches the lives of individuals, builds better organizations, and ultimately creates a more just and caring world (Spears 1996). Servant leaders, unlike traditional leaders, share the power of leadership with those they serve. Servant-leadership emphasizes increased service to others, a holistic approach to work, promoting a sense of community, and the sharing of power in decision making (Spears 1996). There are 10 characteristics associated with successful servant leaders:

- Listening
- Empathy
- Awareness
- Stewardship
- Commitment to people
- Persuasion
- Foresight
- Healing
- Conceptualization
- Community building (Gill 2013)

The philosophy of servant leadership fits well with a healthcare environment as caregivers must put the needs of whom they serve first. Although this is a leadership style that theoretically fits within healthcare, it is a difficult style to embrace and most healthcare leaders utilize other leadership skills and characteristics when developing within a healthcare organization.

Check Your **Understanding**

1. Describe the great man theory of leadership.
2. Compare and contrast values-based leadership versus servant leadership.
3. Identify the three major studies that impacted the development of behavioral leadership theories.
4. Delineate the characteristics of a transformational leader versus a transactional leader.

Case Study

Objectives

- Assess a variety of management theories to identify solutions for improving the management of operations within an HIM department
- Assess a variety of leadership theories to identify solutions for improving the management of operations within an HIM department
- Create a manager or leader improvement plan, given a template

Instructions

Review the following case study and answer the questions for the scenario by creating a manager or leader improvement plan. Use the template in figure 1.10 to complete this manager or leader plan.

Scenario

Jamie was recently hired as the director of HIM operations within a 500-bed teaching facility. Jamie is a recent graduate of an online HIM bachelor's program and she successfully obtained her registered health information administrator (RHIA) certification within the last month. The director of HIM operations is responsible for the following functions within the HIM department as well as managing the 25 employees that perform these functions:

- Release of information (ROI)
- Management of outsourced transcription
- Patient education for the use and access to patient portals

The management issues present within the operations workgroup that Jamie will be managing are:

- High employee turnover rate
- Lack of standardized training programs for new employees
- Distrust of previous management by employees
- Turnaround times for ROI requests exceed the required benchmarks

Figure 1.10. Manager or leader plan template

<table>
<tr><td colspan="4" align="center">**Manager or Leader Plan Template**</td></tr>
<tr><td colspan="4">**Manager:** [Last name, First name]</td></tr>
<tr><td colspan="4">**Management or Leader Goal:** [Identify two management or leadership theories that Jamie will utilize to manage the operations workgroup over the next year and explain how Jamie will utilize these theories to motivate her team toward the improvement goals]</td></tr>
<tr><td>**Operations workgroup area**</td><td>**Improvement goals**</td><td>**Management or leadership theory** [Provide support by identifying an appropriate management or leadership theory]</td><td>**Projected date of completion**</td></tr>
<tr><td>Release of information</td><td>1.</td><td></td><td></td></tr>
<tr><td></td><td>2.</td><td></td><td></td></tr>
<tr><td></td><td>3.</td><td></td><td></td></tr>
<tr><td>Outsourced transcription</td><td>1.</td><td></td><td></td></tr>
<tr><td></td><td>2.</td><td></td><td></td></tr>
<tr><td></td><td>3.</td><td></td><td></td></tr>
<tr><td>Patient portals</td><td>1.</td><td></td><td></td></tr>
<tr><td></td><td>2.</td><td></td><td></td></tr>
<tr><td></td><td>3.</td><td></td><td></td></tr>
</table>

- Job descriptions for the employees are outdated
- Customer service skills are not optimal as evidenced by the number of complaints received by the senior director of HIM

Assumptions

- The director of HIM operations reports to the senior director of HIM. The senior director of HIM has a very hands-off management style and allows her management team to function independently.
- Jamie has four years of HIM work experience as an inpatient and outpatient coder for this same healthcare organization.
- The manager or leader plan will include goals that incorporate a variety of management and leadership theories.
- Benchmarking data will be collected upon Jamie's hire and improvement must be shown within the goals for each area of the operations workgroup (including transcription, ROI, and patient portals) after one year. If improvements are not noted, Jamie's role as director will be reassessed (note that creation of benchmarks is not an objective of this manager or leader plan).

Deliverables

Create a one-year manager or leader plan for Jamie to utilize as she improves the deficiencies as noted within her workgroup. The plan should include three improvement goals for each area that reports to her and should incorporate improvements for the items that are noted as deficiencies for the operations workgroup. The improvement goals should include support from a variety of management and leadership theories outlined within the chapter. The goals should also include realistic time frames for completion.

Components of the plan should include the following:

1. One example of how a scientific management theory can be utilized to improve the management of ROI turnaround times within this scenario.

2. One example of how a humanistic management theory can be utilized to improve the employee relations within this scenario.

3. Identification of a leadership theory that Jamie should embrace in order to effectively lead her team.

Review Questions

1. _____ is identified as the "father of scientific management."

   a. Henry Fayol
   b. Henry Gantt
   c. Frederick Taylor
   d. Max Weber

2. This management theory is identified by a formalized hierarchical structure with a clear division between workers and management.

   a. Scientific management
   b. Operations management
   c. Humanistic management
   d. Administrative management

3. This management theory includes three key dimensions: human dignity is an important element, ethical complexities are evaluated, and all stakeholders (managers and employees) are involved in the decision-making process.

   a. Humanistic management
   b. Operations management
   c. Administrative management
   d. Scientific management

4. The Hawthorne effect was categorized by _____ after his observations regarding management in the Western Electric Plan, Cicero, IL.

   a. Frederick Taylor
   b. Elton Mayo
   c. Henry Gantt
   d. Abraham Maslow

5. _____ performed human relations management research that was geared toward a behavioral scientific approach in regards to employee motivation.

   a. Abraham Maslow
   b. Frank Gilbreth
   c. Mary Parker Follett
   d. Elton Mayo

6. _____ is a method that provides organizations tools to improve the capability of their business processes and some examples of these techniques are control charts, failure mode, effects analysis, and process mapping.

   a. Lean
   b. Six Sigma
   c. Management by objectives (MBO)
   d. Servant leadership

7. This is a leadership theory that is associated with matching the leader's style to the situation.

   a. Contingency theory
   b. Behavioral theory
   c. Trait theory
   d. Transactional leadership

8. The _____ theory proposed that leadership effectiveness depends on the leader's ability to change his or her behavior to meet the demands of the situation. This theory also takes into account the maturity of the followers in terms of their job ability and psychological willingness to work.

   a. Contingency leadership
   b. Trait leadership
   c. Situational leadership
   d. Behavioral leadership

9. A _____ is defined as a principle or ideal intrinsically valuable or desirable (human rather than material) and is embraced within _____ leadership.

   a. Trait, great man theory
   b. Value, values-based
   c. Service, servant
   d. Behavior, behavioral

10. Transformational leaders are those who:

    a. Avoid risk
    b. Attempt to work within the system by maintaining status quo
    c. Focus on the act of changing from one current state to another
    d. Never want to change

References

Avolio, B. and B. Bass. 1995. Individual consideration viewed at multiple levels of analysis: A multi-level framework for examining the diffusion of transformational leadership. *The Leadership Quarterly.* 16(2):199–218.

Barrow, C. 2013. Operations Management. *The 30 Day MBA=: Your Fast Track Guide to Business Success,* 3rd ed. Philadelphia: Kogan Page Publishers.

Baumgart, A. and D. Neuhauser. 2009. Frank and Lillian Gilbreth: Scientific management in the operation room. *Quality and Safety in Health Care* 18(5):413–415.

Bruce, K. 2006. Henry Dennison, Elton Mayo, and human relations historiography. *Management and Organizational History* 1(2):177–199.

Burke, W. 2011. On the legacy of Theory Y. *Journal of Management History,* 17(2): 193–201.

Business Dictionary. 2015. http://www.businessdictionary.com.

Eyre, E. 2015. Frederick Taylor and Scientific Management—Understanding Taylorism and Early Management Theory. http://www.mindtools.com/pages/article/newTMM_Taylor.htm.

Fernandez, S. 2009. Peter Drucker's leap to faith: Examination the origin of his purpose-driven life and its impact on his views of management. *Journal of Management History* 15(4): 404–441.

Frost, J. 2014. Values based leadership. *Industrial and Commercial Training* 46(3):124–129.

Gill, E. 2013. Servant Leadership: Quotes and Definition of Model. Concordia Online Education. http://www.concordiaonline.net/what-is-servant-leadership/.

Graber, D and A.O. Kilpatrick. 2008. Establishing values-based leadership and value systems in healthcare organizations. *Journal of Health and Human Services Administration* 31(2):179–197.

Encyclopedia Britannica. 2014. http://www.britannica.com/EBchecked/topic/257609/Hawthorne-research.

Head, T.C. 2011. Douglas McGregor's legacy: Lessons learned, lessons lost. *Journal of Management History* 17(2):202–216.

Houghton, J. 2010. Does Max Weber's notion of authority still hold in the twenty-first century? *Journal of Management History* 16(4):449–454.

Humanistic Management Center. 2014. The Three Stepped Approach to Humanistic Management. http://humanisticmanagement.org/cgi-bin/adframe/about_humanistic_management/the_three_stepped_approach_to_humanistic_management/index.html.

Institute for Healthcare Improvement. 2005. Going Lean in Health Care. IHI Innovation Series white paper. Cambridge, MA: Institute for Healthcare Improvement. http://www.ihi.org/resources/Pages/IHIWhitePapers/GoingLeaninHealthCare.aspx.

Jago, A.G. and V.H. Vroom. 1980. An evaluation of two alternatives to the Vroom/Yetton normative model. *Academy of Management Journal* 23(2):347.

Kendrick, J. 2011. Transformational leadership changing individuals and social systems. *Professional Safety* 56(11):14.

Kraemer, H. 2011. Values-based leadership. *Leadership Excellence* 28(7):17.

Kurzynski, M. 2009. Peter Drucker: Modern day Aristotle for the business community. *Journal of Management History* 15(4):357–374.

Lean Enterprise Institute. 2015. What is Lean? http://www.lean.org/WhatsLean/.

Lewin, K., R. Lippitt, and R.K. White. 1939. Patterns of aggressive behavior in experimentally created "social climates." *Journal of Social Psychology* 10(2): 271-99. Print.

Liberatore, M.J. 2013. Six Sigma in healthcare delivery. *International Journal of Health Care Quality Assurance* 26(7): 601–626.

Lowe, K.B., K. Galen Kroeck, and N. Sivasubramaniam. 1996. Effectiveness correlates of transformational and transactional leadership: A meta-analytic. *The Leadership Quarterly* 7(3):385–425.

Malcom, S.B. and N.T. Hartley. 2010. Chester Barnard's moral persuasion, authenticity, and trust: Foundations for leadership. *Journal of Management History* 16(4):454–467.

Mason, C., M. Griffin, and S. Parker. 2014. Transformational leadership development: Connecting psychological and behavioral change. *Leadership and Organizational Development Journal* 35(3):174–194.

McQuerrey, L. 2015. Participatory management styles. *Houston Chronicle.* http://smallbusiness.chron.com/participatory-management-styles-50412.html.

Merriam-Webster. 2015. http://www.merriam-webster.com.

Oyler, J.D. and M.G. Pryor. 2009. Workplace diversity in the United States: The perspective of Peter Drucker. *Journal of Management History* 15(4):420–451.

Ozguner, Z. and M. Ozguner. 2014. A managerial point of view on the relationship between Maslow's hierarchy of needs and Herzberg's dual factor theory. *International Journal of Business and Social Science* 5(7):207–215.

Parker, L.D. and P. Ritson. 2005. Fads, stereotypes and management gurus: Fayol and Follett today. *Management Decision* 43(10):1335–1357.

Price, B. 1989. Frank and Lillian Gilbreth and the manufacture and marketing of motion study, 1908–1924. *Business and Economic History* 2(18):1–12.

Ronald, B. 2014. Comprehensive leadership review: Literature, theories and research. *Advances in Management* 7(5):52–66.

Schachter, H. L. 2010. The role played by Frederick Taylor in the rise of the academic management fields. *Journal of Management History* 16(4):437–448.

Seidl, Patricia B. 2013. Chapter 27 in *Health Information Management: Concepts, Principles, and Practice*, 4th ed. K.M. LaTour, S. Eichenwald Maki, and P.K. Oachs, editors. Chicago: AHIMA.

Seyranian, V. 2009. Contingency Theories of Leadership. *Encyclopedia of Group Processes and Intergroup Relations.* Edited by J.M. Levine and M.A. Hogg. Thousand Oaks, CA: Sage.

Shartle, C. 1979. Early years of The Ohio State University leadership studies. *Journal of Management* 5(2):127–134.

Snell, R. 2010 (Oct). Values-based leadership. *Internal Auditor* 67(5):72.

Spears, L. 1996. Reflections on Robert K. Greenleaf and servant-leadership. *Leadership and Organization Development Journal* 17(7):33–35.

Stum, D. 2001. Maslow Revisited: Building the Employee Commitment Pyramid. *Strategy & Leadership* 29(4): 4–9.

Thompson, S. 2015. Challenges of Humanistic Management. *Houston Chronicle.* Demand Media 2015. http://smallbusiness.chron.com/challenges-humanistic-management-64545.html.

"Weber, Max"Capstone Encyclopedia of Business. 2003. United Kingdom: CapstonePress.

Witzel, M., ed. 2006. *Encyclopedia of the History of American Management.* London: Continuum.

Wren, D.A. 2013. James D. Mooney and General Motors' Multinational Operations, 1922–1940. *Business History Review* 87(3):515–543.

Wren, D., A.G. Bedeian, and J.D. Breeze. 2002. The foundations of Henri Fayol's administrative theory. *Management Decision* 40(9):906–918.

Chapter

2

The Management Functions of Health Information Management

Learning Objectives

- Explain the management functions of planning, organizing, leading, and controlling in relation to a health information management (HIM) manager's job responsibilities
- Discuss policy and procedure development to HIM functions as a management tool
- Explain HIM fiscal responsibilities in relation to budgeting
- Identify the levels of management most exhibited in healthcare organizations
- Discuss ethical concerns in regards to HIM management

Key Terms

Authority	Environmental scan	Operational plans	Scorecard
Budget	Ethics	Organizational chart	Social power
C-suite	Expert power	Organizing	Staffing
Coercive power	Informational power	Planning	Strategic plans
Controlling	Key indicators	Procedure	SWOT analysis
Dashboard	Leading	Referent power	Tactical plans
Delegation	Legitimate power	Reward power	Upward communication
Downward communication			

Health information managers spend their days in the practice of management. Chapters in this textbook discuss the various features of management activities, but this chapter presents these activities together for a discussion of the functions of management. Also covered are the levels of management most seen in healthcare organizations. The chapter concludes with a discussion of the ethical aspects of health information management (HIM) in healthcare organizations.

Functions of Management

The functions of management as identified by Henry Fayol were presented in chapter 1. And while Fayol was considered to be the "father of modern management," over time other researchers tried and tested his theories. There are now variations on what the functions are called, but most sources refer to the four functions of management as planning, organizing, leading, and controlling. These are functions all managers perform, regardless of their business or industry. Each function has a set of independent skills and competencies, but when they are all brought together they form the structure for a manager's core roles and responsibilities. Throughout this text, the skills and competencies successful managers must possess are reviewed. In this chapter, the actions and processes included in each management function are looked at in detail. It is important for new managers to have a firm understanding of how the four functions of management combine to define the manager's role in order to move into a managerial position.

Planning

Planning is an examination of the future and preparation of action plans to attain goals. Of the four traditional management functions, planning must be done first; it is the foundation on which the other functions operate. To effectively manage a department a manager must know what the plan for the future is. Planning is done at all levels within healthcare organizations. The organization's board of trustees, with the help of senior administration, is responsible for putting together a **strategic plan** for the entire organization. This process starts with the organization's mission and vision statements and communication of these to all employees. The organization's overall mission, vision, and goals set the long-term direction of the organization (see chapter 4). Strategic plans are generally in place for three to five years, with annual evaluations. Once the organizational goals are in place, departments create their own strategic plan to match them. While based on the strategic plans, **tactical plans** are short term with a focus of one to three years and are created at the division and departmental level. **Operational plans** are carried out within the departments, cover daily operations, and are in place for one year or less. The departments and other functional areas of the facility create their plans based on the organizational plans. These plans are further broken down by supervisors as they plan and set goals for their functional areas. Finally, individual employees work on their own performance goals using the organizational and departmental plans as their basis for action.

Regardless of whether the planning is done at a strategic, tactical, or operational level, there are activities and tools that contribute to the success of any plan. Planning tools such as policies, procedures, budgets, and environmental scans are then used to carry out the plan successfully.

Environmental Scanning

A planning activity essential in any organization is an environmental scan. An **environmental scan** is a systematic and continuous effort to search for important cues about how the world is changing outside and inside the organization. An environmental scan is an activity that is done at any level; it should be done early in the planning process to gather data that will impact the creation of a plan. With knowledge obtained through a scan, goals and objectives can be developed that focus on how the organization will meet the challenges of the proposed changes. Environmental scanning should be performed at both organizational and departmental levels. One way to perform environmental scanning is a SWOT analysis. A **SWOT analysis** looks at the internal strengths and weaknesses of an organization (or department), and the external opportunities and threats. Internally, the elements over which you have control are examined; and externally, the elements examined are those over which the organization has little, if any, control. External elements pertain to the industry rather than the organization, and may also include market analysis and trends. A SWOT analysis is not a task list of things to do, but rather a description of the factors that will impact a plan or project. A SWOT analysis should be done with input from all those affected by the plan. The transition from ICD-9 to ICD-10 is an example that helps illustrate the SWOT concept (see figure 2.1).

Planning Tools

Once the environmental scan is complete, results are used to develop goals and objectives to lead the work of the organization. Organizational goals and objectives are communicated to all levels so that departments and work areas can use them as a foundation to develop their internal goals and objectives. Goals and objectives are written

Figure 2.1.   Example of SWOT in healthcare

Prior to the implementation of ICD-10-CM/PCS, all HIM departments needed to develop a plan for switching from ICD-9-CM to ICD-10-CM. This was not a project that could be completed quickly; most HIM departments began their planning two to three years prior to the implementation date. In this example, Ruth is the HIM director at Memorial Hospital, a 400-bed community teaching hospital. Ruth and her manager, the chief financial officer, began discussing the transition to ICD-10-CM and he requested that Ruth put together an implementation plan for her department. Ruth knows that one of the first steps is to do an environmental scan so she and her staff can focus their planning efforts appropriately. Ruth meets with supervisors and lead personnel to perform a SWOT analysis. Some of their results are listed as follows.

Strengths: the internal elements (specific to Memorial Hospital) in place over which the HIM department has control and that will help with the ICD-10-CM transition

- All coders are HIM-credentialed and complete continuing education requirements to maintain their credentials
- The inpatient and outpatient coding accuracy rates are greater than 96 percent
- The coding manager and lead coder are seasoned employees with coding expertise and strong supervisory skills
- The electronic health record (EHR) is in place and all coders are proficient at working with the EHR
- There is a positive working relationship with the information technology (IT) department

Weaknesses: the internal elements (specific to Memorial Hospital) in place over which the HIM department has some control, and need to be addressed prior to the ICD-10-CM transition

- Four of the best coders are over the age of 60 and may choose to retire rather than learn a new classification system
- The working relationship between HIM and the business office is not great—neither area feels that the other area understands or appreciates them
- Training costs for ICD-10-CM will be more than what was budgeted
- Physician documentation is not at the level needed for accurate ICD-10-CM coding

Opportunities: the external elements (outside of Memorial Hospital) in place over which the HIM department has little, if any, control, but should help with the ICD-10-CM transition

- There is a local community college with an RHIT program that could be a source of new coders for future open positions
- The American Health Information Management Association (AHIMA) has published ICD-10-CM training material that is available at little or no cost to the organization
- Computer-assisted coding technology is improving

Threats: the external elements (outside of Memorial Hospital) in place over which the HIM department has little, if any, control, and could affect the ICD-10-CM transition in a negative way

- There is a national qualified coder shortage that will impact recruiting and coding outsourcing efforts if coding vendors have trouble recruiting coders
- Nationwide implementation of ICD-10-CM has been delayed at least twice and may be delayed again
- Third party payers may not be ready to accept claims with ICD-10-CM

© AHIMA

using the SMART method, which is detailed in chapter 8. Once the goals and objectives are written, it becomes the manager's responsibility to create plans to meet them. Tools used by managers to set plans in action are policies, procedures, and budgets.

Policies

Policies and procedures are introduced and defined in chapter 5. Policies translate goals into comprehensible and practical terms. They are intended to be overall guidelines that set the boundaries for action. The limits at either end of these actions are stated, defined, or at least clearly implied. Policies pre-decide issues so that situations that occur repeatedly are handled the same way. The language found in policies is broad to allow for flexibility to adapt to changing conditions. Policies should also consider legal, accrediting, and certification mandates as well as any other requirements imposed by external and internal authorities or sources. When creating policies, an HIM manager should examine the daily decisions that he or she makes on a repeated basis, and translate the decisions into policies. For example, if employees are repeatedly coming to work dressed inappropriately, a dress code policy is needed. Technological advances will also be a source for needed policies. If a newly implemented EHR has a copy-and-paste function, a policy will be necessary to address the use and consequences for abuse of this function. Each organization will have its own format for writing policies. The human resources (HR) department generally maintains the policy format for an organization. See figures 2.2 and 2.3 for the format of a policy and a sample policy. Some benefits of policies are that they:

- Guide thinking and actions throughout the organization or department
- Allow for consistent decision making or standardized actions
- Require, prohibit, or suggest detailed courses of action
- Reinforce goals and objectives
- Permit interpretation, especially in regards to unexpected or isolated circumstances

Procedures

A **procedure** is a series of related steps given in chronological order that details the prescribed manner of performing work. Job procedures should not be confused with job descriptions (chapter 6). A job description details the duties, reporting relationships, and job specifications for a specific position. A job description is created for a coder, a data analyst, or a cancer registrar. Job procedures are very specific and bring departmental plans down to the level of how and by whom the actual task is carried out. They detail the work that is done by the individuals named in the job descriptions. Procedures are developed for repetitive work in order to provide uniformity of practice, to facilitate personnel training,

Figure 2.2. Format of a policy

Policy No.:	All policies should be numbered via a system determined by the organization
Subject:	Title [what the policy is about]
Purpose:	Why the policy is required or necessitated. Example may be: OSHA or Joint Commission requirement
Division or Department:	Such as Health Information Management
Original Issue Date:	Date policy was originally written
Effective Date:	Date policy will go into effect. Original issue date and effective date may not be the same date. A span of time is usually allowed for those affected to read and understand a policy prior to it becoming effective.
Revision Date(s):	The same as the original issue date unless the policy is actually under revision
Approval Date:	Date policy is approved by the facility. This may be the responsibility of the HR department or a policy committee.
Policy:	Include a policy statement as necessary to cover: • Parameters • Required, prohibited, or suggested courses of action • State, define, or clearly imply the limits at either end of these actions • Pre-decide issues • Allow for repeated situations to be handled consistently • Use broad, flexible language • Allow for changing conditions • Conform to any known legal, accrediting, or registration mandates • Define terms where necessary in order for consistency to occur

Figure 2.3.   Sample policy

Policy Number:	1.1		
Department:	Health Information Management		
Original Issue Date:	12/1/12	Effective Date:	1/1/13
Revision Dates:	12/1/13, 12/1/15	Approval Date:	12/1/12

Subject:	Food and drink in the HIM department
Purpose:	The purpose of this policy is to outline when and where employees may have food and drink in the HIM department.
Policy:	Due to the increasing presence of technical equipment as well as health department regulations, it has become necessary to limit the presence of food and drink in the HIM department.
	No food items are allowed outside of the break room. Inside the break room, food items will be confined to the refrigerator and employee cubbies unless being eaten at a table or prepared in the microwave oven. Food must be in a closed container or package and disposed of in the labeled trash cans.
	No drink items are allowed outside of the break room unless they are in spill proof containers. Employees may have drinks at their desks, but they must be in spill proof containers. This means no pop cans, lidless coffee cups, or cups with snap-on plastic lids that may come off if the cup is knocked over. Questions about spill proof containers should be directed to the second-shift supervisor.
	Exception: When department events such as birthdays or special meals are scheduled, additional food items may be brought in (cakes, pizza, and so on) and left on the counter in the break room so employees may enjoy the food throughout their shift. Any and all remaining food must be disposed of at the end of the shift.
	Any questions about this policy should be directed to the second-shift supervisor.

and to permit the development of checks and controls in the workflow. Job procedures are revised more often than new ones are written. They are revised as jobs change, new technology is acquired, and work processes improve. An HIM manager should consider the repetitive job tasks when deciding when to write a job procedure, such as establishing what tasks need to be done by someone else when coverage for vacation or illness is needed. Examples would be how to prepare a health record in answer to a court order, how to abstract a record into a cancer registry, or how to review a health record for completeness. When writing job procedures, information about the processes or workflows should be gathered from individuals who actually do the work since they have the most insight into how the procedure operates.

Information for job procedures can be collected using some of the same methods described in chapter 6 for completing a job analysis. Observation, interviews, and task diaries track the actual processes that make up a job procedure. Results from these methods are used to create a step-by-step outline of how each task is performed. Use verb statements to begin each step, but do not make the step more complex than it needs to be. A list of verbs is provided in figure 2.4. It is not intended to be an exhaustive list, but an example of the types of verbs used. When finished, give the procedure to someone unfamiliar with the job to see if they can perform the procedure without questions. Similar to policies, procedures are formatted according to the preferences of the organization or department. The HR department generally maintains the procedure format for an organization. For a further look at job procedures, see figures 2.5 and 2.6. Some benefits of procedures are that they:

- Provide consistency of practice and results
- Help with new employee orientation and on-the-job training
- Reduce errors by eliminating some degree of decision making

Figure 2.4. List of verbs to be used when writing job procedures

The following list of verbs may be used when writing job procedures. This list is not meant to be exhaustive. It is to be used to find appropriate verbs for a procedure. Use the verbs correctly; do not use a more complex verb when a simpler one will do. Verbs should begin the procedure statement as per the example in figure 2.6.

abstract	create	extrapolate	locate	repeat
analyze	criticize	find	map	replace
apply	deduce	form	match	represent
approximate	define	generalize	measure	reproduce
associate	demonstrate	generate	name	round
balance	describe	group	observe	separate
build	design	guess	order	show
calculate	develop	identify	pair	simulate
cause	differentiate	illustrate	partition	solve
change	discover	imitate	perform	state
clarify	discriminate	infer	plan	structure
classify	distinguish	initiate	practice	substitute
collect	effect	inquire	predict	summarize
combine	eliminate	integrate	prepare	supply
compare	enumerate	interpolate	produce	support
complete	estimate	interpret	propose	symbolize
compute	evaluate	invent	prove	synthesize
conceptualize	examine	investigate	recall	tabulate
connect	exemplify	iterate	recite	tally
construct	exhibit	join	recognize	test
contrast	experiment	judge	reconstruct	theorize
convert	explain	justify	record	translate
copy	express	label	relate	unite
count	extend	list	reorganize	write

© AHIMA

Figure 2.5. Format of a job procedure

Title of the Procedure:	Name of the procedure to be followed
Summary:	A one or two sentence statement as to why the procedure exists. For example: This procedure describes the steps to correctly and accurately respond to a subpoena.
Responsible Person:	Title of the individual(s) who performs this job. The person's name is not used so the procedure does not have to be changed whenever someone leaves the position.
Materials Needed:	List any and all materials needed to perform the task.
Procedure:	A list of the steps in numbered order. Use verb statements to begin each step, but do not make the step more complex than it needs to be. If sub-steps are needed, use the numbering or lettering pattern seen in figure 2.6. Do not use sub-steps unless they are needed. If the procedure involves a process on a desktop or laptop computer, a good practice is to include screen shots with each step, providing a visual description of the process as well.

© AHIMA

Figure 2.6.   Sample job procedure

Title:	Printing the course manual
Summary:	This procedure follows the start of each new course taken in the HIM program. The course manual provides all due dates for assignments and quizzes for each course.
Responsible Person:	Student
Materials Needed:	Laptop Printer with full paper tray CLASSES binder Highlighter

Procedure:

1. Open the Blackboard application via Canopy.

2. Open the course in which you are currently enrolled.

3. Locate the Start Here menu tab on left side of screen on the course home page.
   a. Click the Start Here tab to open a new screen.

4. Scroll down the page to locate the Course Manual link in blue.
   a. Click Course Manual blue link to open the document.

5. Click the printer icon in the upper-right corner of the screen to open the print screen.
   a. Check that the printer name is correct.
   b. Check that the Print Range radial button is set to All.
   c. Click OK to print the document.

6. Gather sheets off printer tray.

7. Read through the entire course manual.
   a. Highlight all assignment and quiz due dates.

8. File course manual in CLASSES binder.

© AHIMA

Budgets

A **budget** is a plan that converts the organization's goals and objectives into targets for revenue and spending. A budget describes, in dollars and cents, what fiscal resources will be necessary to meet the goals and objectives. The budget gives the HIM manager a fiscal path to follow when it comes to accessing the organization's resources. Most budget procedures require that departments submit an annual budget to senior administration for approval. Budget preparation should be done with input from all employees involved so that all work areas' needs are represented. Needs will be prioritized, both at the department and organizational level, and some requests may be denied outright or delayed until a future budget cycle. Once approved, the budget becomes less of a plan and more of a control tool. This function is examined later in this chapter.

Organizing

Once the planning function is complete, the HIM manager becomes responsible for organizing the resources to meet the goals and objectives. **Organizing** is the coordinating of the activities of multiple people to achieve a common purpose or goal. An organization decides how best to accomplish its work and divides labor accordingly. A common division of labor in healthcare is departmentalization by function: nursing, emergency room, respiratory services, HIM, housekeeping, maintenance, and patient financial services. Division of labor by function allows for specialization among employees, which leads to efficiency and quality of patient care. Traditionally, HIM departments are also structured by function (coding, release of information, transcription, chart completion), although chapter 10 discusses the emerging concept of "HIM without walls."

Organizational structure is determined by senior management and illustrated by an **organizational chart**, which is a visual representation of an organization's formal reporting structure. Departmental structure is based on the overall organizational chart, but is more detailed. Sample departmental organizational charts are shown in figures 10.1 and 10.2 in chapter 10. Organizational charts also show the reporting lines in a department. They give a visual description of to whom each employee directly reports, and the chain of command that should be followed when questions or grievances arise (chapter 5). An HIM department's organizational chart should list job titles without employee names. Employee names are not used so the organizational chart does not have to be changed whenever someone leaves a position.

An organizational chart also helps to illustrate the span of control for an HIM manager. Chapter 10 defines span of control that is used to determine how many employees report to a single manager. There is no ideal number of direct reports for an HIM manager, but there are factors that should be taken into consideration when determining an appropriate span of control:

- Skills and abilities of the manager and his or her employees. When a manager demonstrates greater competence in their role, they are able to take on a larger span of control. In addition, when employees are more competent or have specialized skills, this allows a manager to have a larger span of control. Employees with specialized skills know more about their jobs and require less intervention from a manager.

- Geographical proximity of employees to each other and the manager. When employees are located in close proximity to one another, it is easier for the manager to oversee the work being done. Employees that are physically close to each other can ask questions and rely on each other, and less on the manager. This allows the manager to have a greater span of control. Geographical proximity becomes an issue when dealing with remote employees. The ability for a manager to be in contact with remote employees will impact the size of the span of control.

- Presence of procedures, rules, and guidelines. When there are up-to-date policy and procedure manuals, rules, and clear guidelines for employees to follow, they are less likely to need the help of a manager. This allows the manager to have a larger span of control.

- Similarity of supervised tasks. When employees are all performing similar tasks such as scanning or coding, it is easier for a manager to oversee more employees. The problems associated with work processes will be the same, requiring less of the manager's time.

- Complexity of supervised tasks. Conversely, when the tasks being performed by employees are complex or varied, it requires more of the manager's time, and they cannot manage as many employees at one time. The span of control is smaller.

- Frequency of interaction between managers and their employees. When a manager must interact frequently with employees, they are more limited in the number of employees they can oversee. This leads to a smaller span of control. However, if technology is available to aid in the communication process, the span of control may increase.

Span of control is linked to the concept of delegation. **Delegation** is the process by which managers distribute work to others along with the authority to make decisions and take action. Delegation is a skill that managers must develop, or they will end up doing most of the work of the department by themselves. Managers over-delegate when their time management skills are weak or when they are unsure of their own ability to complete a task; managers under-delegate when they do not trust their employees to complete a task because of lack of ability or lack of time; and managers improperly delegate when they choose the wrong person, time, or reason for delegating a task (Greenberg 2011). When delegating a task or project, an HIM manager must be careful to also delegate the authority that accompanies the task. **Authority** is the right to make decisions and take actions necessary to carry out assigned tasks. An individual cannot be expected to complete a task without having the correct level of authority. Granting authority is important regardless of whether the employee is working alone, or must enlist the help of others in completing the job. Five steps to effective delegation are:

1. Select the right person: Match the person to the job, not the job to the person. The individual must have the correct skill set and desire to perform the task.

2. Specify the desired result: Communicate clearly whether in person, email, or other media. The outcomes must be specific, so that there is no question as to whether the job was carried out correctly.

3. Set a deadline: A time frame is necessary so everyone knows when the project is due. If priorities change, it must be communicated to everyone involved. It may be helpful for both parties to determine a realistic schedule.

4. Determine authority: The manager decides what level of authority is given to the employee. However, once authority is granted, the manager must step back and let the individual proceed.

5. Track progress and results: Even though authority has been granted, the manager should monitor the progress of the task and provide guidance if necessary or requested (Boomer 2013).

Organizing consists of other activities that are sometimes considered to be a subset of organizing called staffing. **Staffing** is a managerial function concerned with determining the most appropriate and cost-effective mix of individuals necessary to complete the job functions in a department. Staffing includes recruiting, selection, compensation (chapter 7), evaluation of employees (chapter 8), and training and development (chapter 9). Committees (chapter 10) and teams (chapter 3) also are part of the organizing function.

Leading

Following planning and organizing is leading. **Leading** influences others to meet the goals and objectives of the organization by motivating subordinates, communicating effectively, and effectively using power (Helms 2009). Leading is sometimes referred to as actuating, directing, or influencing. Key concepts of the leading function are change management (chapter 4), conflict resolution (chapter 4), motivation and morale (chapter 3), disciplinary action (chapter 5), and leadership styles (chapter 1). An HIM manager must understand the leading function in order to influence employees to accomplish the goals and objectives created during planning and coordinated during organizing. Managers must address leadership power, communication, and barriers to communication.

Leadership Power

Leaders have the power to influence their employees and should know the source of their power. This is referred to as **social power**, which is "the potential or ability of an agent [in this case, a manager] to bring change in attitudes, behavior, or belief by using resources available to him or her" (Pierro et al. 2013). Six sources of social power can be found in an organization:

- Legitimate power: This is a type of formal power that is granted to an individual based on the position they hold in an organization. For example, the director of an HIM department has the power to influence the behavior and tasks of the people that report to her because she is their boss. Her employees will do as she requests because her position requires it, and their positions require they listen to her. If she should leave the position, she no longer has legitimate power over the members of the HIM department.

- Reward power: This is another type of formal power granted to an individual who has the ability to reward employees for doing what is requested of them. Reward may come in the form of a raise, promotion, time off, or other positive measure. For example, an HIM supervisor may implement an "employee of the month" award that comes with a small financial reward and public recognition in the organization's newsletter. The supervisor decides each month who will receive the award. Although positive in nature, this type of power may weaken over time if the rewards lose their appeal.

- Coercive power: This is almost the opposite of reward power. This type of formal power is granted to an individual who has the ability to punish employees for not doing what was requested of them. Punishment may come in the form of a demotion, poor performance appraisal, or an undesirable work assignment. A transcription supervisor may threaten a transcriptionist with losing remote working privileges if productivity does not improve. Coercive power is negative, and usually leads to other problems such as low morale and increased turnover.

- Expert power: This is a type of personal power in which, regardless of their position, power is perceived in an individual, who is a subject matter expert. Others recognize his knowledge, skills, and experience in a particular field, and look to him to be a leader. For example, a coder with many years of experience and continuing education may be consulted by other coders about difficult charts. His knowledge is respected, and he may be an informal leader with a degree of influence in the coding section.

- Referent power: This is another type of personal power. These leaders possess personal characteristics that make others want to be like them, to follow them, to want to be associated with them. Leaders who have referent power do not necessarily do anything to earn their power; it is more about personality traits. The leader may be smart, fair, trustworthy, kind, or have other qualities that make co-workers want to be around him or her. For example, an HIM manager may have a reputation for always being fair with employees, and this respect influences employees to follow the manager's lead.

- Informational power: This type of power is based on the leader possessing information. The information may be about a project, future plan, or new development in the organization. Informational power is based on the content of the message; once the information has been shared, the power is gone. This is short-term power and does not allow for continuing influence (Pierro et al. 2013).

Legitimate, reward, and coercive power all depend on the manager's position. Once they leave the position, the power disappears. Expert and referent power are personal in nature; neither depends on the person's position within an organization. Informational power is entirely based on content, with no position or personality traits involved as the power rests with the information. If information is desired, the owner of the information has power; if no one wants information, the owner has no power. An HIM manager may possess multiple types of power at one time. A manager may have been an expert coder or audit technician and been promoted to a management position. In this case the expert power combines with legitimate power. A manager should be able to examine a situation and apply the type of power base that is needed. For example, when speaking to a group of physicians regarding documentation issues, an HIM director must apply expert power as a subject matter expert with more knowledge on this topic than anyone else in the room. An HIM director must apply coercive power when dealing with an employee who has caused a breach of patient confidentiality. The most effective managers are those who demonstrate expert and referent power in their leadership positions.

Communication

Power and leadership influence others to accomplish the goals and objectives set forth by an organization or department, but another skill needed for effective leading is communication. Communication used in change management is defined in chapter 4, but effective communication is "the ability to both send and receive information, as well as convey and understand thoughts, feelings, and attitudes" (Anderson and Pulich 2002). Communication is always two-way, with both a sender and a receiver. Even if it appears that communication is one-way (a lecture, a voice message left on a phone), there must be someone on the other end to receive the information for communication to take place. Communication consists of oral, written, and visual information.

Oral (or verbal) communication can be in person or over the telephone. An HIM manager uses oral communication to give directions, complete performance appraisals, and deliver disciplinary action. The benefits to oral communication include receiving immediate feedback, the ability to read nonverbal cues such as voice tone and body language, and using the cues to adjust the message if necessary. If a sender notices the puzzled look on the receiver's face, he automatically knows the message was not understood. Oral communication, especially face-to-face contact, is faster and more efficient than writing a memo or email, but there is no permanent record kept of the communication. When speaking to others, the speaker should be upbeat and confident, honest and sincere, and follow these suggested best practices:

- Speak loudly enough so all can hear, especially when addressing a group.
- The message should be clear and concise. Do not add words simply to add length to the message.
- Make use of hands and facial expressions to emphasize key points in the message.
- Use eye contact to capture the attention of listeners.
- Stand up straight and erect to put force behind the message.
- Be careful not to use sounds such as "um" and "er" that distract from the message. It is best to pause when speaking for time to gather your thoughts.
- Keep the focus on finding solutions when discussing problems (Brounstein 2002).

Written communication is another skill that an HIM manager needs to develop in order to effectively communicate in the workplace. Written communication may be a memo or an email, a policy or procedure, an employee performance appraisal, or a budget justification. Written communication lacks the immediate feedback of oral communication, but does leave a permanent record that can be referred to later. This is especially helpful when using procedures to train new employees. Initial training may be verbal, but when a written procedure is also provided, an employee can study it later, and refer to it as a quick reference for questions. There are best practices for written communication that an HIM manager should follow:

- Be concise—try to keep emails to no more than five or six sentences and memos to no more than one page.
- Maintain a friendly, yet professional tone when writing emails and memos.
- Proofread carefully—all word processing applications have grammar and spell checking features.
- Use simple language to convey meaning instead of impressive or flowery words.
- Explain all abbreviations and unfamiliar terms the first time you use them; for example, not everyone knows CMS stands for the Centers for Medicare and Medicaid or HIM means health information management.
- Do not send an email or memo when angry or upset—let it sit until emotions have cooled.
- If a document is especially important (a budget justification or a report to the board of trustees), check for understanding by reading it out loud or letting is sit for a day or two and then re-reading it with fresh eyes; if possible, have someone else read the document.

Visual communication consists of PowerPoint presentations or the use of graphs and charts in written reports. HIM managers may present to a local HIM association meeting or give a career talk to an HIM class at a local community college. Visual aids enhance a presentation by making it more interesting and helping the visual learners in the group to understand the material better. A report with appropriate graphs or charts helps the reader to visualize statistics or data that may be difficult to put into words. Visual communication uses many of the same best practices as oral and written communication—be concise, proofread for spelling or grammar errors, and use plain language. The use of color and labeling the data displays are important to enhancing meaning.

An HIM manager will communicate daily with bosses, peers, and employees. There are two components to communicating with the boss:

- Understand the boss's expectations
- Upward communication (Anderson and Pulich 2002)

It is the HIM manager's job to meet the boss's expectations by making sure the organization's goals and objectives are met through the activity of the HIM department so that time is not wasted on unnecessary tasks. Priorities must be understood so that all parties involved are working toward the same goal. Effective communication with the boss is enhanced when the manager practices proactive listening (chapter 4) by asking questions for clarification and gathering the correct data for future use in meeting goals and objectives. **Upward communication** occurs when information moves from the lower levels in an organization to the upper levels (Business Dictionary 2015). An example is communication from the HIM manager to the chief financial officer, initiated by the HIM manager. Successful managers are "able to make judgments about what the boss *needs* to know, what the boss *should* know, *when* information should be communicated, and *what* is the most appropriate medium for communication" (Anderson and Pulich 2002).

The boss needs to know about issues that could escalate into bigger problems. It is better to be open and honest with a boss about a problem than to wait for the boss to be blindsided with the problem and subsequently ask for clarification. When presenting a need-to-know situation, it helps if the manager has a solution or two prepared for consideration. Even if the solutions are not acted on, the boss will appreciate the problem-solving process started at the manager's level.

What the boss should know is more difficult to judge. If the boss made expectations clear, regular updates or progress reports are part of what a boss should know. When receiving verbal updates or reading reports, most bosses are not interested in long conversations or multiple-page memos or reports. The best practice is to be concise with both written and oral communication unless your boss indicates otherwise.

When information should be communicated to the boss concerns timing. Most managers have regular weekly, bi-weekly, or monthly meetings with their boss to cover routine organizational and departmental matters. If an issue has the potential to escalate into a problem, a manager should not delay in communicating the situation. A manager should respect their boss's schedule, and not present issues on the day before he is to leave on vacation or at four o'clock on a Friday afternoon unless it is unavoidable.

The decision about what medium to use (face-to-face, email, or phone) will depend on the nature of the situation. Routine updates can be accomplished by email, while more complex issues require a face-to-face meeting or telephone call. Again, if expectations have been communicated clearly, it is easier to know what medium to use. It is always good practice to ask a boss what the preferred method of communication is for specific situations.

Communication with peers or others happens either laterally (horizontally) or diagonally as depicted on the organizational chart (chapter 10). The director of HIM communicates laterally with the director of IT over new scheduled down-time procedures, or with the HR director over missing employee performance appraisals. Lateral communication occurs when there is a need to coordinate activity between departments or to work on committees (chapter 10) or cross-functional teams (chapter 3). Diagonal communication occurs when the director of HIM communicates with the vice president of nursing services about a possible security breach, or with the chief financial officer about new reimbursement regulations for Medicaid patients. Diagonal communication does not follow the traditional top–down, bottom–up, or horizontal lines of organizational structure. An HIM director must be careful to avoid the appearance of neglecting the traditional lines of communication. This can be done by including those not directly involved with copies or courtesy calls. Regardless, effective communication needs to occur so problems can be solved.

From the HIM manager's perspective, communication with employees is downward. From the employee's perspective, communication with the manager is upward if initiated by the employee. **Downward communication** occurs when information moves from the upper levels of an organization to the lower levels (Business Dictionary 2015). This happens in situations such as when the HIM manager meets with coders to review annual coding updates, or with the entire HIM department to review an implementation strategy for an EHR upgrade. Downward communication is also training and mentoring (chapter 9). Sharing information with employees helps to ensure all levels of the organization know and understand the goals and objectives, and necessary policies and procedures. Rumors can be addressed and put to rest, and problems can be solved at a lower level before they grow to include upper levels of management.

Communication Barriers

An HIM manager must also deal with barriers to communication. There are physical barriers to communication such as geography, noise, and office layout. Managers who have employees who work remotely must deal with communication occurring via phone, text messaging, or email. This means there is a loss of the nonverbal cues present in face-to-face communication. Even using video conference technology (chapter 9) can be a problem if connections are not ideal. Diversity and cultural differences can be barriers to communication. People who speak English as a second language may have trouble finding the right word, or understanding what someone else is saying. Cultural issues such as personal space and gender roles can impact transmission from sender to receiver. Status within an organization can lead to barriers when different positions communicate with each other. Employees may feel uncomfortable with those on a higher level or lower level than themselves. Feelings of inequality may be present and hinder the ability to both send and receive messages.

Finally, the words themselves can be barriers to communication. Healthcare as a field has unique terminology that not everyone understands. Pronunciation for certain words differs depending on the region of the country, and those that work in dermatology may be unfamiliar with terms related to obstetrics and gynecology. Poor word choices, wrong word choices, and using a complex word when a simple one will do can also lead to confusion and misunderstanding between senders and receivers.

Controlling

Planning and organizing lead directly to the controlling, or evaluating function of management. **Controlling** is the monitoring and correcting of organizational, departmental, and individual performance so goals and objectives are met. Controlling is dependent on goals, objectives, and key indicators being set during the planning phase. **Key indicators** are quantifiable measures used over time to determine whether some structure, process, or outcome supports high-quality performance measured against best practice criteria. On an organizational or departmental level the progress toward a goal is monitored with key indicators to make sure tasks and activities necessary to meet the goal stay on course. Should performance slip, corrective action is taken to adjust and even change performance standards. For example, during the planning phase, the HIM department set an internal department goal to increase customer satisfaction by 3 percent by the year's end. Key indicators are determined to be the number of telephone courtesy complaints, release of information request turnaround time, and the number of completed physician queries. A plan is devised to improve telephone skills, reduce turnaround time for record requests, and have coders spend one-on-one time with physicians answering queries. Throughout the year, random customers (patients, physicians, patient accounts employees) are given customer satisfaction surveys, and each month the results are tallied and shared with employees in the department. Progress (or lack thereof) on the key indicators can be measured each month, and corrections can be made if necessary. For example, telephone training can be extended to all employees rather than just those in the reception area, changes to policies allowing for documents to be sent by email improved the turnaround time even more than anticipated, and physicians continue to avoid coders with queries. At the end of the year, final customer satisfaction surveys showed an improvement of 3.2 percent. The department goal was met, and it will be addressed during the planning phase whether to try to improve more or to monitor the gains.

Methods for Controlling Performance

Performance appraisals are a method of controlling individual performance and are discussed in chapter 8. Part of the performance appraisal process is setting individual job performance standards. Examples of key quality and quantity indicators are provided in chapter 8. The performance appraisal process requires the key job performance indicators be monitored throughout the appraisal period, and correction of any deviations occurs during the review.

Benchmarking, also defined in chapter 8, is another method for controlling performance. Managers obtain benchmark data for key indicators from other similar or professional organizations, and compare their performance against the benchmarked data. Areas that are either significantly higher or lower than the benchmarked data are reviewed. It is important to not just compare the benchmarked data, but to dig deeper to examine the processes that account for the data. For example, a children's hospital benchmarks coding volume data against coding volume data from other children's hospitals around the country. The coding manager is pleased to see that their inpatient records coded per hour compares favorably to the benchmark data. However, the coding manager notices their outpatient records coded per hour is significantly lower than the national norm. Further investigation with the professional association indicates that greater than 50 percent of hospitals report using a computer-assisted coding (CAC) product for outpatient coding, while the coding manager's hospital has yet to install CAC. In this case, further investigation supported the current outpatient coding volumes even though they did not compare favorably to benchmarked data.

Another control method used by managers to monitor performance is the department budget. Budgeting was discussed as a planning tool earlier in the chapter, but once completed it is used as a control tool. The annual budget is approved prior to the start of the fiscal year. Once the fiscal year begins a budget report is generated each month for the department manager's review. Each healthcare organization creates its own budget report, but common items show the budgeted amount for each budget category (salaries and wages, supplies, travel, training) and the actual amount spent in each budget category, along with the budget variance. If less than the budgeted amount was spent, it is a positive variance; if more than the budgeted amount was spent, it is a negative variance. A key indicator for a budget variance is set at plus or minus 2 percent, plus or minus 3 percent, or even plus or minus 5 percent. Assuming the key indicator is plus or minus 2 percent, if the actual budget variance is greater than 2 percent or less than 2 percent variance, the department director must explain the variance, usually in a written report. The department director should request input from supervisors and lead personnel in justifying any budget variances.

Monthly reviews of each budget category allow the HIM manager to see whether they are spending too much or have budgeted too much money for any one item. There may be acceptable reasons for the budget variances such as unplanned employee absences requiring overtime or contract workers, a delay in obtaining a piece of equipment that results in lower supply costs, or cancellation of a planned seminar resulting in saved travel dollars. Regardless, the HIM manager monitors the budget and can make course corrections prior to the budget getting out of control by the end of the fiscal year.

Other Controlling Function Tools

Other tools for carrying out the controlling function are dashboards and scorecards. Some organizations use the terms interchangeably, but there is a difference. A **dashboard** is a report of process measures to help leaders follow progress to assist with strategic planning. Dashboards are quick snapshots of the status of key performance indicators. A dashboard functions much the same as the dashboard in a car. With a quick glance, the driver can tell the speed, gas level, and mileage. Detailed information is provided, just enough so the driver knows the status of the car at one point in time. A healthcare organization dashboard pulls key indicators from various systems: accounting, payroll, time and attendance, accounts receivable, and other productivity reports into one visual report. Dashboards are used at all levels in an organization, reporting the key metrics important to a specific level of management or department. A chief executive officer's dashboard will report different items than an HIM director's dashboard. The benefits of a dashboard are:

- Visibility: visual presentation is easy to read and understand at a glance
- Ongoing improvements: allows measuring and monitoring of trends
- Time savings: everything presented in one place so no need to review many different reports
- Judge performance against the plan: shows progress of goals and objectives
- Employee performance improvements: improvements can be easily shared with employees so they can monitor their own performance (Lavinsky 2013)

A **scorecard** is a report of outcome measures to help leaders know what they have accomplished. Rather than reporting ongoing process measures, a scorecard looks at outcomes. A scorecard is a long-term report of how the organization is meeting its strategic goals. Both scorecards and dashboards monitor key performance indicators, and in many organizations the distinction is negligible.

Check Your **Understanding**

1. Name the four functions of management and how an HIM manager applies each to day-to-day operations.
2. Explain the difference between strategic, tactical, and operational plans.
3. What are the possible sources for creating policies?
4. What are the influences in determining managerial span of control?
5. What are the six types of power an HIM manager might possess and how would he or she use them?
6. What are some tools for use in the controlling management function?

Levels of Management

The four management functions are practiced at all levels of management. Typically, there are three levels of management within a healthcare organization: top, middle, and lower. Variations of these levels and positions will exist at each organization, as each organization determines its own structure. Some organizations will have more levels, some will have fewer levels. Chapter 10 discusses the differences between hierarchical and nonhierarchical organizations, and while the concept of levels of management would seem to support the hierarchical style of structure, nonhierarchical organizations generally have at least a few levels of management to provide structure and responsibility for decision making. The board of trustees or board of directors are the top level of senior management. The board is ultimately responsible for the entire organization and determines the structure of the organization. Immediately below the board is the senior management team. Position titles at this level are chief executive officer (CEO), chief operating officer (COO), chief financial officer (CFO), chief information officer (CIO), chief medical officer (CMO), and chief nursing officer (CNO). Because the abbreviations for these positions all begin with the letter c, this level is often referred to as the **c-suite**. The c-suite level of management is responsible for decisions that affect the entire organization; they do not generally get involved with the day-to-day operations, but focus on the big picture and the long-term success of the organization. This level spends most of the time in the planning and organizing functions of management. They determine the strategic plan for the organization and organize the overall structure of the organization. This level is sometimes broken down into another layer of management; position titles in this next level are vice-presidents or assistant administrators.

The middle level of management sits right below the top level on the organizational chart. Position titles at this level are director of HIM, department head, corporate director of HIM (which may be a senior level position at some organizations), senior manager of HIM, or manager of HIM. This level is responsible for meeting the organizational goals and objectives at the department level. As the name suggests, this level is in the middle, dealing with both senior management and lower levels of management. They are more involved in the day-to-day operations of their areas than the c-suite, and provide advice and data to senior management to assist their planning. This level spends most of their time performing the organizing and leading functions of management; managers organize their areas, recruit, and select employees while motivating and ensuring effective communication throughout their departments. This level may also be broken down into a second level, with position titles such as assistant director of HIM and assistant manager of HIM.

The lower level of management is at the bottom of the organizational chart. This level is also referred to as first-level, or frontline management. Position titles at this level are supervisor of HIM, shift supervisor, or office manager. This level is most involved with their direct reports and day-to-day operations of their assigned department. This level spends the majority of their time on the leading and controlling functions of management. They motivate, increase morale, schedule, and complete performance appraisals of their employees.

Check Your **Understanding**

1. Explain the three levels of management found in most healthcare organizations.
2. How are the four functions of management carried out at each level of management?

Ethics in Health Information Management

In most organizations, the individuals who hold management positions in the HIM department also have HIM credentials. These managers oversee employees in the HIM department who also have HIM credentials. An HIM credential carries an obligation to follow the credentialing body's code of ethics, such as the AHIMA Code of Ethics (appendix C). **Ethics** is a field of study that deals with moral principles, theories, and values. A code of ethics is a statement of ethical principles regarding business practices and professional behavior. In the workplace, HIM-credentialed individuals have a professional responsibility to uphold the code of ethics, which is in place to guide their conduct. An HIM manager who has an AHIMA HIM credential must adhere to the AHIMA Code of Ethics and also make sure their employees adhere to the same. The AHIMA Code of Ethics proposes 11 principles:

- Advocate, uphold, and defend the individual's right to privacy and the doctrine of confidentiality in the use and disclosure of information.
- Put service and the health and welfare of persons before self-interest and conduct oneself in the practice of the profession so as to bring honor to oneself, their peers, and to the HIM profession.
- Preserve, protect, and secure personal health information in any form or medium and hold in the highest regards health information and other information of a confidential nature obtained in an official capacity, taking into account the applicable statutes and regulations.
- Refuse to participate in or conceal unethical practices or procedures and report such practices.
- Advance HIM knowledge and practice through continuing education, research, publications, and presentations.
- Recruit and mentor students, peers, and colleagues to develop and strengthen professional workforce.
- Represent the profession to the public in a positive manner.

- Perform honorably HIM association responsibilities, either appointed or elected, and preserve the confidentiality of any privileged information made known in any official capacity.
- State truthfully and accurately one's credentials, professional education, and experiences.
- Facilitate interdisciplinary collaboration in situations supporting health information practice.
- Respect the inherent dignity and worth of every person (AHIMA House of Delegates 2011).

The code of ethics is a tool that HIM managers have to hold employees accountable for their actions and to support the manager's ethical decision making. An HIM manager will deal with each of these principles in their workplace. A manager arranges and participates in continuing education, recruits other credentialed individuals to open positions, adheres to release of information policies and procedures that protect health information, and collaborates daily with other healthcare professionals to support health information practice.

In addition to the code of ethics, there are ethical standards of practice for both coding professionals and clinical documentation improvement (CDI) professionals. HIM managers should be aware of these guiding principles and require that coding and data abstraction professionals, whether HIM credentialed or not, follow a standard of ethical coding, such as the AHIMA Standards of Ethical Coding (appendix D). Coding is a core HIM function, and "due to the complex regulatory requirements affecting the health information coding process, coding professionals are frequently faced with ethical challenges" (AHIMA House of Delegates 2013). Standards of ethical coding provide guidance for ethical decision making during the coding process, regardless of the purpose for which the codes are being reported. "They are relevant to all coding professionals and those who manage the coding function, regardless of the healthcare setting in which they work or whether they are AHIMA members or nonmembers" (AHIMA House of Delegates 2013). The same statement is found in the AHIMA Ethical Standards for Clinical Documentation Improvement Professionals (AHIMA House of Delegates 2010). In most HIM departments, all employees are asked to sign a confidentiality statement based on a code of ethics, and HIM-credentialed employees are expected to sign a confidentiality statement that includes a code of ethics and the ethical standards for coding and CDI, if applicable to their position.

Check Your **Understanding**

1. What is the purpose of the AHIMA Code of Ethics and ethical standards for coding and CDI?
2. Explain how an HIM manager might use the AHIMA Code of Ethics to guide behavior and decision making in an HIM department.

Case Study

Objectives

- Research best practices for dashboard presentation
- Create a dashboard to monitor key performance indicators
- Prepare a memo explaining the dashboard and implementation plan for the dashboard to present to the chief clinical officer

Instructions

Read the scenario that follows, perform research as indicated and create an HIM dashboard and memo to present to the chief clinical officer.

Scenario

Karen White, RHIA, was recently hired as the new HIM director at a 450-bed suburban teaching hospital. Karen has been in the HIM field for approximately three years. Her past experience includes being the data quality specialist for the HIM coding area at a large teaching facility. She is familiar with the functions of coding and data reporting, but not as familiar with the other functions within the HIM department. Her boss, the chief clinical officer, wants her to create a department dashboard for monitoring key performance indicators within the department. He would like the dashboard sent to him on the first day of each month. The HIM department is comprised of the following functions and staff to support the functions:

- *Coding:* Inpatient, outpatient, emergency department, and physician hospital-based coding
  - *Staff:* 1 coding manager, 1 data quality coder, 15 remote-based coders
- *Electronic Record Management (ERM):* Document imaging and file retrieval
  - *Staff:* 1 ERM lead, 2 document imaging technicians, 3 file retrieval clerks
- *Record Processing (RP):* ROI, electronic chart completion, and transcription (all outsourced)
  - *Staff:* 1 RP lead, 2 ROI coordinators, 1 chart analyst, 1 transcription coordinator
- *Administrative Support:* Phone support for ROI and file retrieval, administrative support for director
  - *Staff:* 1 lead support specialist (director support position), 2 support specialists
- *Technical Support:* Maintain hardware and software, computer upgrades, interface issues, workflow errors, perform duplicate master patient index clean up and health record merges
  - *Staff:* 1 application specialist, 2 application analysts

Assumptions

- Each functional area within the HIM department maintains productivity and quality performance data for the activities performed but none of the data is aggregated or shared on a regular basis, and there are no benchmarks in place for the activities.
- The dashboard will be basic: two indicators from each of the five functional areas (coding, ERM, RP, administrative support, technical support), and two indicators for the overall HIM department.
- The hospital does not offer a specific dashboard product.
- Additional research is needed in order to create a dashboard.
- The chief clinical officer requested a draft and implementation plan for the dashboard.
- Actual numbers for each key performance indicator should not be included on the dashboard; it should be a representation of what the dashboard will look like.

Deliverables

Create a user-friendly dashboard including key performance indicators from each functional area and the HIM department. Make sure a benchmark is included for each key performance indicator. Create a memo to the chief clinical officer to accompany the dashboard using these parameters:

1. There is no template provided. Part of the assignment requires the student to perform research on effective dashboards and create their own dashboard.
2. The dashboard should be created in Excel.
3. The memo to the chief clinical officer should include at least the following regarding implementation: data collection method, communication plan for the managers and leads, and the HIM department timeline.
4. An APA-formatted reference must be provided to support the dashboard research. This should not be part of the memo, but be provided following the memo.

Review Questions

1. One of the first steps in this managerial function is to perform an environmental scan of the internal organization and external industry. This is which managerial function?

   a. Planning
   b. Organizing
   c. Leading
   d. Controlling

2. Natalie is a lead coder hoping to move into a supervisory position. She is reading articles on how to motivate employees and improve department morale. These topics fall under what managerial function?

   a. Planning
   b. Organizing
   c. Leading
   d. Controlling

3. Elizabeth prepares a weekly dashboard report with key performance indicators of the HIM department to send to the chief executive officer. Preparation of this report falls under what managerial function?

   a. Planning
   b. Organizing
   c. Leading
   d. Controlling

4. Delegation is a skill that managers must develop to show employees that they trust them with the authority to perform certain projects on their own. Delegation falls under what managerial function?

   a. Planning
   b. Organizing
   c. Leading
   d. Controlling

5. Helen is the HIM department head, and has been asked to share a SWOT analysis of her department with her new boss. One aspect of Helen's SWOT analysis indicates that the chart tracking software is over 10 years old and is not compatible with the digital dictation system. In a SWOT analysis, this would be a(n):

   a. Strength
   b. Weakness
   c. Opportunity
   d. Threat

6. Another element of Helen's SWOT analysis mentions the hospital across town recently sent all their coders home to code remotely. Currently all coding done at Helen's hospital is done in-house. In a SWOT analysis, remote coding done by the other hospital would be a(n):

   a. Strength
   b. Weakness
   c. Opportunity
   d. Threat

7. Anna is the newly hired assistant director of HIM. By virtue of her position, she leads all HIM employees in the department, assigns work, and sets expectations. Anna has what type of power?

    a. Coercive
    b. Expert
    c. Legitimate
    d. Referent

8. Chloe has been a transcriptionist at University Hospital for 18 years. She is familiar with all types of dictation, and seems to be able to understand any accent she hears. Many of the transcriptionists call on her for help, and recognize her as the unofficial leader of the transcription area. Chloe has what type of power?

    a. Coercive
    b. Expert
    c. Informational
    d. Referent

9. As the director of HIM services, Mitch receives a weekly report from his coding supervisor. The report graphically displays inpatient and outpatient coding volume data, employee turnover rates, and the number of claim denials due to coding errors. This snapshot report is called a:

    a. Benchmark report
    b. Budget
    c. Dashboard
    d. Performance appraisal

10. Department heads and department directors comprise which level of management?

    a. Top level
    b. Middle level
    c. Lower level
    d. First level

References

AHIMA House of Delegates. 2013. AHIMA Standards of Ethical Coding. http://library.ahima.org/xpedio/groups/public/documents/ahima/bok2_001166.hcsp?dDocName=bok2_001166.

AHIMA House of Delegates. 2011. American Health Information Management Association Code of Ethics. http://library.ahima.org/xpedio/groups/public/documents/ahima/bok1_024277.hcsp?dDocName=bok1_024277.

AHIMA House of Delegates. 2010. Ethical Standards for Clinical Documentation Improvement (CDI) Professionals. http://library.ahima.org/xpedio/groups/public/documents/ahima/bok1_047843.pdf

Anderson, P. and M. Pulich. 2002. Managerial competencies necessary in today's dynamic health care environment. *Health Care Manager* 21(2):1–11.

Boomer, J. 2013 (May 27). Five Steps to Effective Delegation. *CPA Practice Advisor.* http://www.cpapracticeadvisor.com/article/10928740/five-steps-to-effective-delegation.

Brounstein, M. 2002. *Communicating Effectively for Dummies.* New York: Wiley Publishing.

Business Dictionary. 2015. http://www.businessdictionary.com/.

Helms, M.M., ed. 2009. *Encyclopedia of Management,* 6th edition. Detroit: Gale.

Greenberg, M.J. 2011. Delegation. Chapter in *Nursing Leadership,* 4th ed. Edited by Harriet R. Feldman. New York: Springer Publishing Company.

Lavinsky, D. 2013 (September 6). Executive Dashboards: What They Are and Why Every Business Needs One. *Forbes.* http://www.forbes.com/sites/davelavinsky/2013/09/06/executive-dashboards-what-they-are-why-every-business-needs-one/.

Pierro, A., Raven, B.H., Amato, C., and J.J. Bélanger. 2013. Bases of social power, leadership styles, and organizational commitment. *International Journal of Psychology* 48(6):1122–1134.

3

Leadership Concepts in Health Information Management

Learning Objectives

- Examine how cultural diversity impacts the health information management (HIM) workforce
- Assess the impact of changing workforce demographics on the HIM profession
- Identify the roles and responsibilities of team membership
- Discuss the attributes of virtual teams
- Explain common motivation theories
- Identify methods that HIM managers can use to motivate employees
- Explain how workplace morale contributes to the sustainability of the HIM department

Key Terms

Affinity groups	Hygiene factors	Motivation	Team charter
Bridge employment	Inclusion	Motivators	Team facilitator
Cross-functional teams	Informal teams	Operant conditioning	Team leader
Equity theory	Intrinsic	Recorder	Team members
Extrinsic	Job design changes	Reinforcement theory	Team sponsor
Formal teams	Job enlargement	Similarity-attraction	Timekeeper
Goal-setting theory	Job enrichment	Social identity	Virtual teams
Herzberg's two-factor	Job rotation	Stereotyping	Work-life balance
theory	Morale	Team	Workplace diversity

Effective health information management (HIM) professionals keep abreast of emerging concepts in management practice. It is not enough to understand changes to coding guidelines or privacy matters; an HIM manager is aware of developing concepts in the business world and their potential impact on healthcare in general and HIM specifically. Concepts discussed in this chapter are diversity in the workforce, the use of teams in healthcare, and the importance of motivation and morale in the workplace.

Diversity

Workplace diversity is the set of individual, group, and cultural differences employees bring to an organization (Konrad 2006). Individual differences refer to the abilities, skills, and qualifications people bring to the workplace and are represented by demographic elements such as race, age, and gender. Physical ability and sexual orientation are also individual differences. They make us unique, but also place us into groups. For example, age might place one into an "over 50" group, and gender might place one into a "women in healthcare management" group. Cultural differences are found in an individual's or group's values, beliefs, religion, language, and behaviors.

Healthcare organizations are no different than other organizations when it comes to managing workplace diversity. A 2011 survey on healthcare diversity leadership indicates that healthcare organizations value workplace diversity. Respondents report that diverse leadership is an important business tool for their organizations: 62 percent believe that cultural diversity improves patient satisfaction, 57 percent believe that it supports successful decision making, and 54 percent believe that diversity in recruiting contributes to reaching organizational strategic goals (Witt/Kieffer 2011). However, a 2013 survey completed by the Institute for Diversity in Health Management (an affiliate of the American Hospital Association) reports that while minorities represent 31 percent of the patient population in the United States, minorities comprise only 14 percent of hospital board members, 12 percent of healthcare executive leadership positions, and 17 percent of first- and mid-level management positions (Institute for Diversity in Health Management 2013). Results from these surveys indicate there is a disconnect between the perceived value of diversity in the workplace and the actual presence of diversity in the workplace in healthcare. Leaders in healthcare may believe that diversity leads to patient satisfaction and improves successful decision making, but the lack of minorities on hospital boards and in management positions indicates that there is little minority representation in decision-making positions in hospitals.

The following sections examine cultural diversity, barriers to diversity, diversity management, and issues surrounding an aging workforce. An understanding of cultural diversity and current barriers to increasing diversity in the healthcare environment lead to a discussion of how diversity management can improve workforce demographics in healthcare. The issues of one specific type of workplace diversity, age, are discussed in an attempt to create a positive mindset when it comes to working with an aging population.

Cultural Diversity

A culturally diverse workplace offers many benefits to a healthcare organization. Patient satisfaction is impacted when patients see their community represented in the workforce of the local hospitals and healthcare facilities. Professional interpreters and multilingual staff are used to enhance patient and family communication. Interpreters are tested to ensure their translation competency of medical and clinical terminology is sufficient. Healthcare documents are translated into languages that are common among patients and visitors. Patient satisfaction surveys collect feedback on improving language needs and other services that affect the care of diverse patients. All of these elements contribute to increased satisfaction among culturally diverse patients.

A multicultural organization is attractive to a diverse talent pool of individuals. Employees with different backgrounds and beliefs provide added value to organizational decision making and, as such, impact overall performance and idea generation. Diverse employees bring their own perspective to an organization, and offer different viewpoints, experiences, and insights into management discussions.

Barriers to Increasing Diversity in the Healthcare Environment

Despite the benefits, minorities are underrepresented in healthcare organization board rooms and executive offices (Institute for Diversity in Health Management 2013). Barriers to improving workplace diversity are both psychological and organizational (Konrad 2006). Psychological barriers are similarity-attraction, social identity, stereotyping, and cognitive biases. **Similarity-attraction** means that, overall, people prefer to interact with others who are similar to themselves. When given a choice, people prefer to spend time with others whose attitudes and values are like their own. Interacting with homogeneous others validates a person's ideas and beliefs. **Social identity** is a person's sense of belonging to a social group. People identify with more than one social group. Examples of social groups are gender (women), occupation (lawyers), or age ("baby boomers"). People will strive to improve the status of the social group with which they identify. Membership in a social group maintains an individual's self-image. As a result, a person belonging to a particular social group is more likely to discriminate against someone belonging to a different social group. Social groups also practice **stereotyping** and exhibit cultural bias. Stereotypes are generalizations about individuals based on their identity, group membership, or affiliations (Fried and Fottler 2008).

Traditional human resource management methods of recruiting, motivation, and retention can be organizational barriers to diversity and include the following:

- Lack of commitment to achieving diversity by the board of directors
- Lack of commitment to achieving diversity by top management
- Lack of commitment to achieving diversity by the human resource department
- Lack of access to a diverse candidate pool of applicants
- Lack of diverse candidates within an organization available for promotion
- Perception that serious consideration for promotion would not be given to diverse candidates
- Limited resources for diversity initiatives in recruiting and retention (Witt/Kieffer 2011)

Traditional recruiting channels may not target a diverse population. For example, newspaper advertising may not reach minority populations if those populations do not subscribe to newspapers. Social groups rely on locating new members that represent their current social group. Motivation techniques (addressed later in the chapter) may also not work outside existing social groups. New ideas presented by employees with different values and beliefs may not be accepted by the organization and, therefore, the employees are reluctant to present them. Promotion opportunities may not be as available to members of a minority social group if they do not traditionally have the necessary education or training for higher positions. For the same reasons, retention can be a barrier to diversity. Employees that do not feel connected to a social work group may leave the organization. Conversely, minority employees who feel accepted and valued by an organization are more committed to that organization.

Work-life balance issues may also be barriers to creating a diverse workforce. Employees at all levels of an organization strive to maintain a balance between their work and personal life. This is especially difficult for single-parent and dual-income families. For example, a single mother may need to juggle a request for overtime from her employer and her commitment to coaching her son's soccer team. A dual-income family may be unable to schedule vacations that allow everyone to enjoy time off together. Work-life balance issues can be addressed by offering a variety of benefits to employees. Flexible scheduling allows for flextime (adjusting arrival and departure times) and compressed work weeks. Compressed work weeks allow employees to work a 40-hour week in three or four longer days rather than over five straight days. Job sharing among employees creates options for part-time work. Technological advancements open the door to remote work being done from almost any location the employee may choose.

The extent to which an organization tolerates harassment and exclusion is another barrier to diversity. First and foremost, employee harassment is outlawed by the Civil Rights Act. The Civil Rights Act of 1964 (addressed in chapter 5) specifically prohibits discrimination in hiring, compensation, and training on the basis of race, religion, gender, national origin, disability, or sexual orientation. Harassment and exclusion promote a hostile work environment that leads to employee dissatisfaction, decreased performance, and increased turnover. Employees who are in the minority due to racial, cultural, religious, or physical differences may be fearful of the dominant group. Minority employees may remain silent for fear of rejection or ridicule; their creativity is stifled and performance is hampered.

Diversity Management

As the diversity in the healthcare workforce continues to increase, there are many ways for an organization to create and improve their diverse environment. A hospital with a diversity improvement plan:

- Has a nondiscrimination policy that includes ethnic, racial, lesbian, gay, bisexual, transgender, and transsexual communities

[handwritten margin note: Diversity Imp. plan ☆]

- Educates all clinical staff during orientation about how to address the unique cultural and linguistic factors affecting the care of diverse patients and communities
- Collaborates with other healthcare organizations to improve professional and allied healthcare workforce training and educational programs in the communities served
- Requires all employees to attend diversity training
- Has implemented a program that identifies diverse, talented employees within the organization for promotion
- Has a documented plan to recruit and retain a diverse workforce that reflects the organization's patient population
- Hiring managers have a diversity goal in their performance expectations (Institute for Diversity in Health Management 2013)

Mentoring and leadership training programs develop high-potential minority candidates (as well as majority candidates) and contribute to increased motivation and retention.

Employee **affinity groups** are a way for social groups to come together in the workplace. Affinity groups are formed by employees with common interests. They come together for a specific purpose such as mentoring, continuing education, or participation in a service project. For example, Microsoft supports Resource Groups for employee groups such as Asians; Blacks; people with disabilities; members of the lesbian, gay, bisexual, and transgender (LGBT) community; Hispanics or Latinos; parents; and women (Microsoft 2015).

Workplace harassment must be taken seriously at all levels of an organization. Allegations of harassment must be investigated, from both a legal perspective and from a diversity awareness perspective. Anti-harassment and sensitivity training should be offered to all employees, including members of the board of directors.

The following are best practices that contribute to the advancement of cultural competence at healthcare organizations.

[handwritten margin note: Best Practices]

- Create mentoring programs
- Create programs or opportunities to expose young people to healthcare careers
- Sensitize management to diversity needs
- Develop cultural sensitivity initiatives and strategies
- Communicate diversity initiatives to all employees (Witt/Kieffer 2011)

Cultural sensitivity should be practiced at all levels of a healthcare organization. Here are straightforward ways to promote effective behavior in a diverse work group:

[handwritten margin note: Promote effective behavior]

- Explain acronyms prior to using them. An individual's socioeconomic or job status may limit his or her knowledge of acronyms.
- Use idioms sparingly. Many idioms are used as metaphors to make an idea or a point more vivid, however, they may not be universally understood by all ethnic groups and may be insulting.
- Expect employees not to use slang in the workplace. Slang is multicultural. Each group has its own words.
- Ask individuals to speak more slowly if it will help others better understand what they are saying.
- Identify motives for criticizing employees and choose words carefully. Criticize the behavior, not the person. The key is to criticize without crippling.
- If it is necessary to correct an employee's grammar, do it privately and kindly.
- Use friendly tones when talking to all ethnic groups; don't talk down to anyone.
- Pay attention to body language. Respect others' personal space and keep an appropriate distance (four to 12 feet).
- Listen for what is not being said, especially in staff meetings.
- Encourage and invite people to talk in group settings. The results may be surprising (Smothers and Stelter 2001).

Aging Workforce

With the post-WWII baby boom generation aging, workers age 55 and older are expected to make up a larger share of the labor force than in the past (BLS 2014). The actual and projected statistics indicate that at the same time the older workforce is growing, the younger workforce is declining (refer to figure 3.1). Workers over the age of 55 are not only more plentiful in number, but are choosing to stay in the workplace longer, mostly due to financial reasons such as the need for money or health insurance as people discover that their personal assets and savings will not last long in an extended retirement (Stanford Center on Longevity 2013). The competition for newer, younger employees will be strong. The lack of younger workers to replace retiring workers may also cause older workers to remain in the workplace for a longer period of time.

Healthcare organizations can foster a positive mindset within the organization about an age-diverse workforce (Voelpel 2010). Actionable areas include focusing on human resource services, combating stereotyping, improving transfer of knowledge from seasoned workers to new workers, and creating solutions for retirement options.

A positive organizational mindset recognizes that human resource management practices might need to be adjusted to incorporate the needs of an aging population. Consideration should be given to tools such as recruitment when examining human resource practices. The expected decline in the labor force of younger workers will result in fewer such workers available for hire and so persons over the age of 50 may present a labor pool from which to draw experienced and motivated workers.

Figure 3.1. Percentage distribution of civilian labor force, by age, 1992, 2002, 2012, and projected 2022

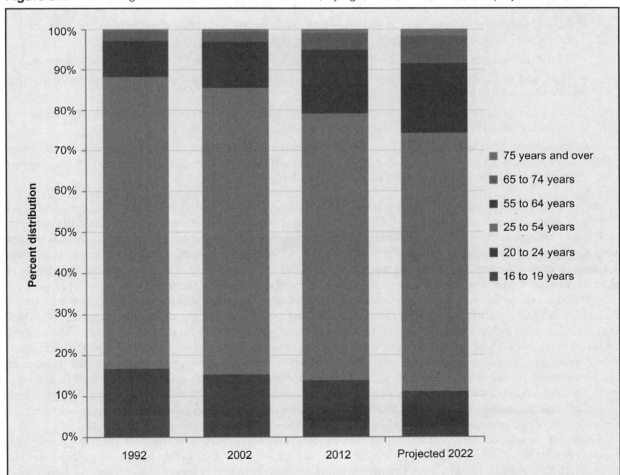

Source: Bureau of Labor Statistics, U.S. Department of Labor. 2014. Share of Labor Force Projected to Rise for People Age 55 and Over and Fall for Younger Age Groups. *The Economics Daily*. http://www.bls.gov/opub/ted/2014/ted_20140124.htm.

Implementing flexible work practices such as staggered start times and job sharing improves retention of older employees who might be struggling with issues related to care of elderly parents or young grandchildren. Human resources services encompass health management actions that deal with the physical aspects of aging. Organizations should offer health and wellness education tailored to an aging workforce. Physical and mental health issues are addressed through routine health checks and wellness training. The physical work environment should be assessed for safety as well as ergonomic features that benefit all employees, but have particular appeal to older individuals. Examples of such features include adequate lighting, slip-resistant flooring, removal of tripping hazards, and height-adjustable workstations. Adjustable workstations allow each individual using the workstation to make the necessary changes in seat height, computer monitor position, and keyboard placement for maximum comfort and prevention of repetitive motion injuries and illnesses such as carpal tunnel syndrome, eye strain, and back pain. This capability is especially important if multiple employees share the same workstation over different shifts. The following basic principles of good sitting posture should be practiced by anyone sitting at a workstation all day, regardless of age:

- Feet should rest flat on the floor or footrest.
- A fist-width space should be measurable between the back of the knees and the edge of the seat pan of the chair.
- The hips should be at a 90-degree angle (or slightly greater) in relation to the body. To help ensure this angle, the knees should be at or below hip height.
- The lower back (lumbar region) should be supported.
- Shoulders should be relaxed, not shrugged, slouched, or rolled forward.
- Elbows should rest comfortably at the side or on armrests. When typing, elbows should be at 90-degree angles and preferably supported by an adjustable armrest at an appropriate height.
- Wrists should be maintained in a neutral (straight) position while typing or using any variety of keyboard.
- Head and neck should be in an upright position. To confirm this, the ears should be directly over the shoulders, which are directly over the hips.
- Computer monitors should be positioned directly in front of the worker. The top line of print should be horizontal with the eyes when looking directly forward.
- Ergonomic aids should be used to help maintain comfortable posture. Examples include footrests, wrist rests for keyboard and mouse, antiglare screens for computer monitors, copy stands, and adjustable chair height for those working at a multitask station. (Oachs 2013)

Stereotyping accompanies age diversity in the workplace. Typical negative stereotypes related to older workers are that they are not as productive as younger workers, they have more health issues, and they are not as flexible or receptive to change as younger workers. Repeated research has shown the negative stereotypes in regard to productivity, flexibility, and receptiveness to change are not true. Evidence does demonstrate that older workers do not call in sick more often, but do need more time to recover from illness (Streb et al. 2008). A positive mindset to appreciate the experiences of older workers must exist in an organization and be reinforced at all levels in order to combat these stereotypes.

Knowledge management applies to the learning environment in an organization as well as the transfer of knowledge and skills from one generation of workers to the next. Offering continuing training and learning opportunities to all employees, regardless of age, helps to debunk the stereotype that "you can't teach an old dog new tricks." Rather than assuming senior coders will not be interested in learning new versions of coding such as ICD-10-CM/PCS, education should be offered to all coders. Recognition of their expertise in reviewing charts, knowledge obtained in anatomy and physiology, and understanding of individual physician documentation patterns should be highlighted and ways to transfer this knowledge to newer coders developed. One example might be mentoring programs that pair more experienced coders with new coders, which in addition to allowing senior coders to impart their knowledge, has the added benefit of allowing new coders to update senior coders on recent coding changes.

A positive organizational mindset allows for changes in policies and procedures related to retirement. Employees nearing retirement age may have been busy focusing on careers, or caring for elderly parents, and not given much thought to what to expect in retirement. Therefore, retirement issues become greater in importance and programs designed to help employees with retirement decisions can be offered. For example, older employees may be allowed to phase into retirement with reduced work hours. While this might appear to negatively influence productivity, a phased approach allows time for older workers to impart their knowledge gained from experience to younger workers. The concept of **bridge employment** should be examined as well. Bridge employment is a job that an individual takes between leaving their full-time position and beginning full-time retirement. The job could be part-time in the same organization or in the same field, part-time in a new field, self-employment, or even temporary work. Bridge employment allows a new retiree to transition mentally and physically into full-time retirement status. Bridge employment also provides an economic cushion for those individuals worried about their financial situation in retirement.

Inclusion

All organizations are diverse, but not all organizations are inclusive. Diversity encompasses all the differences that individuals exhibit in the workplace. **Inclusion** means that the differences between individuals are truly respected and valued in the workplace. Inclusion is the result of successful diversity management and enables all employees, regardless of aspects like age, gender, race, or religion, to be as productive as possible. Accepting diversity and valuing the contributions of all employees is necessary for an organization to reach its potential.

Check Your **Understanding**

1. List at least five different elements of diversity.
2. Discuss the benefits of a diverse healthcare organization.
3. Explain the psychological barriers to having a diverse organization.
4. What is the impact of stereotyping on creating a diverse workplace?
5. Explain how work-life balance issues can be barriers to diversity.
6. What are the components of a diversity improvement plan?
7. What are the best practices for encouraging a culturally diverse workforce at a healthcare organization?
8. What are some solutions to the problem of an aging workforce?
9. Explain the difference between diversity and inclusion.

Teams

The evidence of diversity is no more apparent in an organization than in teams. With the proliferation of quality improvement projects in healthcare, teams have become a popular way to improve outcomes and reduce costs. Teams may offer employees an opportunity for job enrichment or autonomy. It may make sense to create a team when the proposed work is too cumbersome or complex for an individual. Teams can also reduce the workload of a department supervisor. A **team** is a group of people working together to achieve a common goal for which they hold themselves accountable (Scholtes et al. 2010). In a team:

- Members work toward a common purpose
- The end product could not be completed without people working together; the tasks depend on a team effort
- Members share responsibility for the end product
- Members respect the necessity of working together to accomplish the common goal
- Members engage in team activities that cross departmental boundaries within an organization (Scholtes et al. 2010)

When forming a team, it is important to first have a clear sense of the team's purpose or goal. Ideally, a team's goal or output is clearly connected to the organization's strategic plan, mission, and vision. Linking to the strategic plan puts everyone on the same page. Without this connection, there is little hope for support from administration, funding, or successful outcomes. There is no point in moving a team forward if the outcomes have no impact on the organization's strategic plan.

Teams also need sufficient resources to function. This generally means that team members must be granted the time and technology necessary to serve on a team. A team member cannot contribute completely to a team effort if he must miss team meetings or deadlines due to work commitments in his originating department. Team members need to know that their routine work responsibilities will be covered in their absence, or the thought of the work piling up and waiting can be a distraction. Teams need access to the right communication tools to function. Team members in remote locations need access to the right technology to attend meetings in a virtual environment. Data-sharing technology allows all team members to have simultaneous access to the same documents. This ensures everyone is working from the most recent version of a document. Resources might include the money needed to meet goals. If communication technology is not already in place or sufficient, it may need to be purchased or updated. Teams may need to travel to inspect a product or attend a conference. Any necessary data gathering may require the creation of surveys or questionnaires. Teams may be responsible for purchasing new equipment or upgrades. A budget provided to the team at the beginning of their project helps to ensure financial resources are adequate and managed wisely.

The team's statement of purpose must be clear as to their authority and access so that all people involved in the team's efforts understand the limits placed on the team. Team members must be confident that they have enough decision-making power to accomplish their goals. Does the team have the appropriate level of authority to make necessary decisions? A team needs to understand the impact of their decisions on individuals as well as on the organization. Most likely, decisions will cross department lines and a team must have the confidence that their decisions will be supported by all parties involved in the process. In addition, a team needs access to data to make decisions. Team members need to spend sufficient time with the necessary people to become informed, and be granted access to the necessary data to aid in decision making.

The following sections discuss the creation of teams as well as the different types of teams found in the healthcare workplace. Each team member has a role to play in the success of the team operation. There are formal and informal teams, cross-functional teams, and virtual teams; the purpose of each type of team is defined so managers understand when teams are appropriate for use in the healthcare workplace.

Members of the Team

Team roles are assigned so that the work of the team can get done in a timely and effective manner. The **team sponsor** is the individual who initially brings the team together and assigns their charter. The **team charter** clearly defines the expectations of the team, details the mission and vision of the team, provides the scope, sets the boundaries, names the leader and members, and identifies the key outcomes. The team sponsor is usually a member of the executive or management level and does not participate in actual team meetings. The sponsor oversees the work of the team: selecting members, making sure the team moves in the right direction and has the resources they need to function, and supports team efforts across the organization.

On a formal team, the **team leader** is usually selected by the sponsor, although team members may have input. The team leader is responsible for the administrative aspects of team management like setting and running meetings, assigning tasks, keeping the team focused, resolving conflicts among members, communicating with the team sponsor, and making sure that the resources are being used efficiently.

Team members do the work of the team such as participating in discussions, putting forth ideas, sharing solutions, carrying out assigned tasks, and supporting team actions in their individual work areas. Team members may also perform the additional roles of recorder and timekeeper. The **recorder** creates a meeting agenda, takes and distributes meeting minutes, helps to create charts, and sends out necessary correspondence. The **timekeeper** is responsible for keeping meetings on track by managing time. The timekeeper tells all members how much time has been spent on a topic and if too much time is being spent on a particular agenda item. Many formal teams also have a **team facilitator**, or coach, who is present at meetings but is neither the leader nor a member. The facilitator understands the team process, and is available to assist with the mechanics of the team process, but he or she is not as concerned with the outcome of the project as much as they are concerned that the team functions productively. The facilitator provides coaching on how to run a meeting, assign tasks, and make decisions.

Selecting team members is a crucial step in the team process. It is important to get the right mix of people together so the work can be done with as little disruption as possible. The following are suggestions for how to form a successful team:

- Ensure there is representation from all areas of the organization that are affected by the problem
- Allow for diversity of perspectives
- Pay attention to positive personal chemistry among team members
- Create a team with a manageable size (for example, no more than 8 to 10 members)
- Enlist members with a desire or interest to serve the purpose of the team
- Choose a leader who collaborates, not dominates

Once team members are chosen, it is important to remember that as work progresses it is possible to change the membership composition. Certain team members may no longer be relevant to the task, or it may be necessary to invite others with specific knowledge or insight to join the team, if only for a few meetings.

Teams come together to perform the necessary work to meet their assigned outcomes. There are four stages of team growth:

1. Forming: Team members are established, tasks defined, and behaviors and ground rules are outlined
2. Storming: Team members work together to learn to effectively manage differences of opinions and outright conflict so collaboration can occur and move the project forward
3. Norming: Team members make progress on their work, overcoming differences and accepting the established ground rules
4. Performing: Team members perform consistently to get the work done, choosing and implementing changes and working through group problems (Scholtes et al. 2010)

Team membership and selection occurs with the creation of any type of team in the healthcare workplace. There are different kinds of teams: formal and informal, cross-functional, and virtual. Each type of team has its useful place in a work setting and has a specific purpose.

Formal vs. Informal Teams

Up to this point, the discussion has been about formal teams. **Formal teams** are structured, assigned a charter, and usually proceed with meetings, minutes, and agendas. Members are assigned by the team sponsor. Formal teams can be short term, as in the case of planning for a department relocation; or long term, as evidenced by a hospital infection control committee. Additional examples of reasons for the creation of formal teams are preparation for an upcoming survey, implementing a new employee appraisal process, or a discovered performance improvement opportunity.

Informal teams are part of the workplace too. **Informal teams** are employees who develop groups around shared interests that may or may not pertain to organizational business. Managers need to be aware of such teams, as they can have a positive or negative impact on morale, or lead to union activity. For example, some members of an HIM department may organize a "biggest loser" weight management team. This may improve morale as team members support each other in weight-loss efforts or backfire if the weight loss program does not work or becomes too much of a focus and negatively impacts productivity. Other members of the coding section may informally gather to help one another study for the Certified Coding Specialist (CCS) exam. There is no team sponsor; in fact, informal teams usually exist outside of traditional organizational charts. Informal teams do have leaders, either self-appointed or appointed by the group.

Cross-Functional Teams

Cross-functional teams (or interdisciplinary teams) are made up of members from different departments. Cross-functional teams work best when the problem to be addressed requires input from different sources. In some cases, it is unlikely that one department would have the knowledge and resources necessary to resolve all issues. For example, implementation of a clinical documentation improvement plan would require representation from various departments throughout a healthcare organization including HIM, nursing, case management, compliance, information technology, and the business office.

Cross-functional teams are not without challenges. Keep in mind that members of an interdisciplinary team still have responsibilities and work to do in their home department. This might lead to loyalty and prioritization issues. It may also mean that team members are not happy to be assigned to a team when they know they have work waiting for them when they return to their departments. In a cross-functional setting, the team leader will not have direct authority over all team members, so care must be used in assigning tasks, motivating members to perform, and making decisions.

Virtual Teams

Virtual teams are teams whose members are geographically distributed, requiring them to work together through electronic means with minimal face-to-face contact (Malhotra et al. 2007). They operate across time zones and are cross-functional in nature. Geographic differences may mean an increase in the diversity of team members. In extreme cases, team members have never met and will never meet. Virtual teams rely on information sharing (shared websites, intranets) and communication technology (email, video conferencing or teleconferencing, webinars, which are addressed in chapter 9) to accomplish their work. Success factors for virtual teams include the following:

- Establish trust. Trust develops over time in face-to-face interactions, but this is not an option for virtual teams. Trust in virtual teams is developed through the actions and demonstrated abilities of team members.

- Support diversity. Geographic differences mean that language and cultural differences may be more present than in the traditional workplace. Diversity in work styles and decision-making styles is another obstacle for virtual teams to overcome.

- Communicate. Virtual teams need technology tools to communicate. Training may be necessary so all members know how and when to use technology. Interpersonal communication skills must also be in place. Simple things such as greeting members by name and checking in with silent members might be taken for granted in a face-to-face setting, but need to be consciously managed in a virtual setting. "Netiquette" rules (etiquette for virtual communication) for both email and video or teleconferencing should be reviewed so there is no confusion or offense in regular communication.

- Create clear goals. This is an important success factor for any team, but the unique issue of asynchronous communication may lead to confusion or misunderstanding of stated goals and their intent. Progress toward meeting goals should be highlighted on a regular basis so that all team members remain focused and knowledgeable about the process.

- Recognize team members. Periodic reports to each individual team member's supervisor recognize contributions made by individuals. Virtual team members need to feel that their input is important to the success of the outcomes. Virtual reward ceremonies can be held as recognition at the conclusion of a team's tenure.

The increase in virtual teams in healthcare require those involved with leading and facilitating teams to develop new expertise in managing virtual teams. In general, team leaders must possess excellent written and oral communication skills. The lack of face-to-face interaction requires all team members to rely heavily on written communication methods such as email and texting. Oral communication skills are hampered when remote dialogue does not allow for facial expressions and body language. The practices of effective virtual team leaders are to establish and maintain trust through the appropriate use of communication methods, ensure diverse knowledge and opinions of team members are understood and leveraged, manage virtual work meetings; monitor team progress using appropriate technology, enhance visibility of the team and its members throughout the organization, and ensure individuals are recognized and rewarded for participating in virtual teams (Malhotra et al. 2007).

Check Your **Understanding**

1. What are the benefits of using teams in the workplace?
2. Identify team roles and responsibilities.
3. What factors contribute to the formation of a successful team?
4. Explain the four stages of team growth.
5. Differentiate between formal and informal teams.
6. What are the challenges presented by cross-functional teams?
7. Discuss the five factors exhibited by successful virtual teams.

Motivation

Motivational theory is a topic health information managers need to be familiar with in order to begin to understand what makes employees behave and act as they do. **Motivation** is "the forces acting on or within a person that cause the person to behave in a specific, goal-directed manner" (Hellreigel and Slocum 2004). Understanding employee behavior helps the manager to influence and improve performance using motivation techniques. We examined how the workplace is increasingly more diverse. Technological advances make remote employees a reality. Technology allows for the rise of virtual teams, although traditional workplace teams continue to grow in number and effectiveness. All of the previous examples require employees to successfully complete their work tasks, and motivation is the individual drive that leads to task accomplishment. An explanation of work motivation theories is followed by a discussion of strategies used to improve employee motivation in individuals as well as in teams.

Work Motivation Theories

An explanation of work motivation theories contributes to the manager's understanding of employee behavior. Positively motivated employees perform on a higher level and produce higher quality work. Motivation is based on both intrinsic and extrinsic elements. **Intrinsic** (or internal) motivating factors come from within the individual. There may be an inner drive to succeed, or an intangible feeling of accomplishment in a job done well. **Extrinsic** (or external) motivating factors are tangible and obvious to others. Extrinsic factors might include a promotion or a salary increase. At the same time, motivation is a highly personal topic. What motivates an employee at the start of their career does not necessarily continue to motivate after 20 years on the job. What motivates one employee may not motivate a different employee doing the same type of work. A newly credentialed coder might be more intrinsically motivated to perform well in an effort to showcase coding skills and knowledge. A new coder may be excited to work in a teaching hospital coding difficult charts, learning from co-workers, and navigating the ups and downs of a first professional job. Conversely, a coder with 10 years of experience may be more extrinsically motivated by job security or the possibility of a promotion to a supervisory or even managerial position. An effective HIM manager will work to understand the motivating factors for each individual employee. HIM managers need to communicate with employees to know which elements matter most to the individual. Work motivation theories are not a one-size-fits-all solution to performance and productivity issues. The following are some tools that HIM managers can use to better understand employee behavior and work to improve employee motivation.

Maslow's Hierarchy of Needs

Addressed in chapter 1, Abraham Maslow's theory puts forth the idea that individuals are motivated based on a hierarchy of needs. As each need is met, the individual moves to the next level in an attempt to satisfy the next need. When represented as a pyramid (figure 3.2 on the next page), the foundational base represents *physiological needs* of food, water, and shelter. An individual is motivated to satisfy these needs before moving to the next level, *safety needs* of security, health, and employment. A new HIM graduate may take a position in an HIM department for which they are overqualified simply to gain employment in the field and satisfy this second level. Once employed, the graduate

Figure 3.2. Maslow's hierarchy of needs

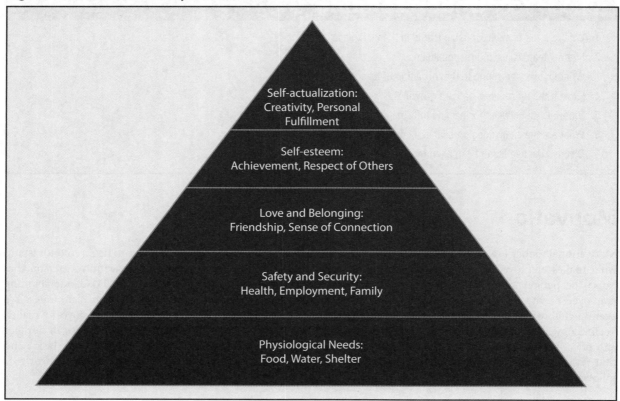

Self-actualization:
Creativity, Personal
Fulfillment

Self-esteem:
Achievement, Respect of Others

Love and Belonging:
Friendship, Sense of Connection

Safety and Security:
Health, Employment, Family

Physiological Needs:
Food, Water, Shelter

© AHIMA

may then move up the pyramid as they search for their next job. The third level is the *belonging and love need,* which consists of the need for family and friends, and a sense of connection to a group. A newly credentialed HIM professional is motivated to satisfy this need when accepting a first supervisory job, even if the pay is less than expected or the shift is not desired. The fourth level, *self-esteem needs,* represents the highly personal needs of recognition and respect by others, achievement, and confidence. An HIM professional that begins to get involved in their local or state professional organization may be looking to satisfy this need. The final and highest level is that of *self-actualization.* The needs at this level center on creativity and personal fulfillment. At this level, an HIM professional has reached their full potential, confident that they are working to their maximum level of capability. Their job is personally satisfying and they are giving back to the profession in ways that also provide for personal fulfillment.

Herzberg's Two-Factor Theory

Fredrick Herzberg (1923–2000) was a clinical psychologist interested in the effects of motivation on the workplace. His original studies were done with engineers and accountants in the late 1950s and led to the creation of the two-factor theory. **Herzberg's two-factor theory** is also known as the *motivation-hygiene theory.* Herzberg identified two motivational elements—motivators (satisfiers) and hygiene factors (dissatisfiers). **Motivators** are elements that can provide job satisfaction to employees and consist of achievement, recognition, the work itself, advancement, and responsibility. **Hygiene factors** are elements that can provide job dissatisfaction to employees and consist of company policies, supervision, working conditions, and financial rewards. These items are not motivators, but rather indicate whether an employee is happy or unhappy, and can act as de-motivators. Herzberg's research found that the two factors did not correlate with each other. In other words, improving working conditions might satisfy employees, but if there remains no opportunity for career advancement, they will not be motivated. To apply this theory, managers must address both factors. They must meet the satisfiers and eliminate the dissatisfiers. Figure 3.3 depicts the hygiene factors that if *not met* can cause job dissatisfaction and the motivation factors that if *met* can create job satisfaction.

Figure 3.3. Herzberg's motivators and hygiene factors

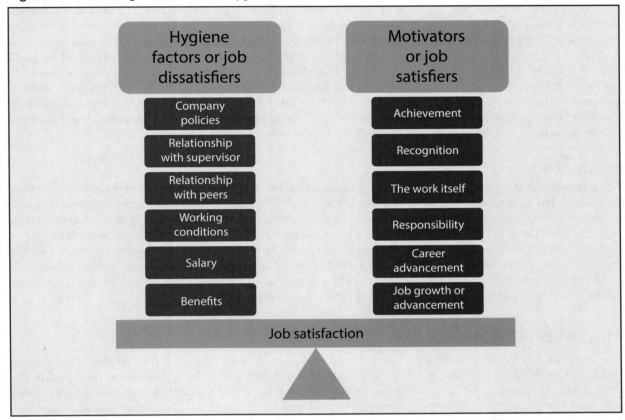

© AHIMA

Goal-setting Theory

Edwin Locke (1938–) is an organizational psychologist interested in the effects of goal setting on workplace motivation. His research in the late 1960s led to the creation of the goal-setting theory. The **goal-setting theory** is based on the premise that employees respond best when goals are clearly defined and feedback is provided about goal progress. The positive impact of the goal-setting theory on employee motivation is found in the employee's commitment to the goals that have been set. Goals must be challenging yet attainable. Goals must be specific rather than vague. For example, to set a goal to "code as accurately as possible" is not specific. A goal of "an abstracting accuracy rate of 80 percent" is specific and attainable, but hardly challenging to a clinical data abstractor with minimal experience. A goal of "100 percent abstracting accuracy" is both challenging and specific, but not attainable for anyone over time. Positive work performance results when goals are developed by the employee or assigned by a supervisor. Regular feedback on the progress toward achieving goals is also an important component of the goal-setting theory.

smart goals

Reinforcement Theory

Burrhus Frederic (B. F.) Skinner (1904–1990) was a psychologist interested in the effect of positive and negative reinforcement on human behavior. His research from the late 1930s on the effects of reinforcement led to the development of the reinforcement theory. The **reinforcement theory** of motivation is built on the incentive and reward concept. Employees are motivated to perform in relation to incentives or positive reinforcement as well as disincentives or negative reinforcement. Reinforcement theory also introduces the concept of operant conditioning. In **operant conditioning**, behavior is associated with a positive or negative reward, and is modified or learned over time. For example, when an employee exhibits a desired behavior and positive reinforcement is given for that behavior, over time the employee is more likely to repeat the desired behavior as she learns to associate the behavior with the positive reinforcement. Conversely, behaviors that are associated with negative reinforcement will not be repeated.

Examples of positive reinforcement can be expensive: promotions, bonuses, paid trips, or other tangible rewards. However, positive reinforcement can be used and is as simple as praise from a supervisor, a handwritten thank you note, or a public performance recognition award. Negative reinforcement most often takes the form of criticism or punishment. Punishment might be docked pay or assignment of a menial task. It is important to note that for the reward (or punishment) to be effective as a motivator, the employee must see value in the reward or punishment. It also helps for the reinforcement to be given as close to the desired behavior as possible. A performance bonus will not be as effective if given at the end of the year as it would be if the bonus appeared on the next paycheck. Incentive pay programs are a type of positive reinforcement and in HIM are most popular in transcription and coding. Transcriptionists are paid by the line or report, and coders are paid by the number of records coded. There must be a quality indicator as well, or increased quantity will be at the expense of quality outcomes.

Equity Theory

J. Stacey Adams was a behavioral psychologist interested in the impact of fair treatment of employees on workplace motivation. His research done in the mid 1960s led to the development of the equity theory of motivation. The **equity theory** of motivation suggests that employees are motivated by the balance of their inputs in relation to their outputs as compared to both their employer and other workers. In other words, an employee is motivated to do well when they believe what they contribute (inputs) to a job in the way of effort, skills, loyalty, and trust is equally matched by what they receive (outputs) from a job in the way of salary, benefits, recognition, and job security. An employee who perceives an inequity between inputs and outputs will try to correct the imbalance by reducing productivity, increasing absenteeism, or even separating from the organization.

Motivation Strategies

Knowledge of motivational theories is applied in the workplace by managers when they develop strategies and techniques to influence employee behavior. One motivational theory cannot be applied across the board in any department. A manager must know which theory to apply, to whom to apply it, and in what situations the theory will work best. The key to developing motivational strategies for the workplace is communication. Since each individual is motivated in a different way, a manager must learn what methods will work with what employee, and communication is the necessary means. A manager can spend time with an employee discussing his or her individual motivating factors, or a written survey or questionnaire might be used to gather the same information.

The following 10 factors affect employee motivation:

- Interesting work
- Good wages
- Full appreciation of work done
- Job security
- Good working conditions
- Promotions and growth in the organization
- Feeling of being in on things
- Personal loyalty to employees
- Tactful discipline
- Sympathetic help with personal problems (Lindner 1998)

Motivation strategies that use these 10 factors as their focus will be more successful. Strategies that link to a specific motivational theory will also be more successful. For employees who respond to the reinforcement theory of motivation, consider incentive pay programs as a motivating strategy. Programs such as profit sharing and stock ownership by employees, even though initiated by senior management and offered to the entire organization, also tie compensation directly to company performance and give employees positive reinforcement for their efforts. A strategy for employees who respond to the goal-setting theory of motivation involves the employee both in setting goals and determining the actions necessary for completing the goals. In other words, the employees should have a say in how the goals will be met.

Other motivational strategies center on redesigning job descriptions. **Job design changes** are used to motivate employees by making their jobs more interesting and increasing an individual's usefulness throughout the organization. **Job enlargement** is a horizontal expansion of an employee's duties. Tasks are added to the current job, but employees have the same degree of autonomy and responsibility. An example of job enlargement would be adding outpatient coding to an inpatient coding position; no new skill sets are required, but additional training in Current Procedural Terminology (CPT) would be provided. **Job enrichment** is a vertical expansion of a person's duties. Generally, a new skill set is required and responsibility and autonomy are increased. An example of job enrichment would be requiring clinical documentation specialists to prepare and present documentation tips and query examples to physicians at monthly medical and surgical department meetings. Clinical documentation specialists will need to develop both verbal and display presentation skills as they communicate directly with physicians. **Job rotation** requires employees to rotate among different tasks or jobs, usually at the same level. Employees learn new job tasks and job rotation offers a break from the monotony of a repetitive job. It may be possible that one day a week a transcriptionist is rotated to the job of delivering and mailing transcribed reports. This allows the transcriptionist to stand, walk around, and perform other tasks beyond that of routine transcription.

Motivating Teams

What motivates an individual to improve performance is different than what motivates a team. Teams must work together to achieve common rather than individual goals. In fact, individual goals may conflict with group goals.

Managers should consider the impact of social identity when motivating teams. From a positive perspective, an individual may regard herself as a "data analyst" or "cancer registrar" but when put on a team to plan HIM week activities, the individual is now identified as an "HIM professional." The individual identity is not lost, nor does it conflict with the goal of the new team. The cancer registrar may adopt this new social identity and work hard to help her new team make HIM week a success. However, a negative perspective is illustrated when a merger of departments takes place. A person who identifies as a member of the HIM department may not adapt well when the department is merged with the patient accounts department to form a new patient information department. Employees may not want to surrender their previous identity and their performance could decline as a result.

When motivating virtual teams, it is necessary to create a social identity for the team. This gives people who do not normally work together, or even know each other, a sense of commonality and lessens their reliance on their identity as an individual. The idea of social identity also applies to choosing a team leader. Team members are more apt to be motivated by a leader who shares their perceived social identity. The team leader should be seen as part of the group rather than a separate entity.

Another way to motivate teams is to compare the performance of teams to one another. The idea that a particular team may not be performing as well as other teams brings the nonperforming group together to improve their outcomes.

Aging Workforce Motivation

What motivates the younger worker may not motivate the older worker. For example, early in a career the possibility of a promotion and more money may motivate an individual to high performance. Later in a career, extrinsic rewards such as promotion and pay increases may not be as attractive and may be replaced by intrinsic desires for job security or positive interpersonal relationships in the workplace. More mature workers may respond to the opportunity to share their accumulated knowledge and experience with younger workers in the form of mentoring or team building. Communication with the older employee will help determine what motivation factors work for the individual.

Morale

Morale is "the feelings of enthusiasm and loyalty that a person or group has about a task or job" (Merriam-Webster 2015). There is a positive relationship between morale and productivity, although the effects diminish as morale increases. Increasing low morale to a moderate or high level can increase productivity. However, employees that already exhibit high levels of morale probably cannot increase their productivity measurably.

Many elements affect an employee's enthusiasm for their job. As the degree of autonomy present in a job increases, so does morale. In addition, morale is higher when there are positive feelings about an organization and management. An example would be when an organization introduces changes to the workplace. When there is low morale, employees are more likely to distrust changes and treat them as threats to their job security or pay. When there is high morale, employees are more likely to view changes as benefits to both their job and the organization.

Workplace safety is another component of employee morale. Healthcare organizations implement safety programs for all employees. Universal precautions protect against disease transmission, education on body mechanics prevents back injuries, and lifestyle programs support smoking cessation, healthy eating, and weight loss. The degree to which employees are encouraged to participate in safety programs can be perceived as a measure of how much an organization values their workforce. When employees see that managers care about their health and safety and are not simply paying lip service to meet required safety standards, enthusiasm and loyalty for a job increases. Workplace safety is also affected when employees themselves create an unsafe environment. Employees with low morale may go so far as to sabotage the workplace, creating safety hazards for everyone.

Morale-boosting efforts should focus on creating a positive atmosphere in the workplace. Managers can show genuine appreciation for their employees in many ways. Department social gatherings such as picnics and recognition dinners held off-site can boost morale. Routine efforts such as handwritten thank you notes, public recognition of professional achievements, and afternoon treats can be less expensive ways to help build positive feelings about the workplace. As managers develop morale-boosting programs, it is important to remember that expensive measures to impact morale come at a cost to the organization and can negate any productivity gains.

Check Your **Understanding**

1. Why do managers need to understand motivational theory?
2. Identify the key factors in each of the five motivational theories presented in this chapter.
3. How does motivation of teams differ from motivation of individuals?
4. Differentiate between motivation and morale.

Case Study

Objectives

- Explain the reasons for creation of a virtual team
- Evaluate the assignment of a team leader based on employee characteristics
- Investigate communication technology used for virtual team meetings
- Assess motivation theories and strategies to identify solutions for motivation concerns
- Assess diversity statistics in regards to developing a diversity improvement plan
- Create a written report

Instructions

Review the following case study and answer the questions for the scenario by creating a written report to the president of the company.

Scenario

Jennifer is the vice-president of coding operations of a company that offers remote coding services. The company is located in the Midwest, but has client sites nationwide and in India. Jennifer oversees five regional managers and to this point each region has operated fairly autonomously. With the recent expansion to India, Jennifer saw her time spent in communication with the regional managers grow. She finds herself answering the same question multiple times and puts out the same fires across the country. Jennifer hired each regional manager and knows their capabilities well. She is confident that given the opportunity they can come together as a team and self-manage in areas such as recruitment, training, compliance, and customer satisfaction. Jennifer would be kept in the communication loop, but would not be a member of the team.

The regional managers are the following individuals.

- *Northeast:* Devon, a 31-year-old single African-American male. He has a bachelor's degree in biology and the Certified Coding Specialist (CCS) and Certified Coding Specialist–Physician-based (CCS-P) credentials. He has been with the company for two years. He came from a consulting company where he was a remote coder for eight years. He has been vocal about the lack of minority representation and lack of a diversity plan in the company.
- *Midwest:* Sarah, a 36-year-old married white female. She has a bachelor's degree in business and the Registered Health Information Technician (RHIT) and CCS credentials. She has been with the company for five years and has worked her way up from a temporary coder to regional manager. Sarah is concerned about the decreasing motivation among the coders in her region.
- *South:* Alice, a 62-year-old divorced white female, has a masters degree in business administration (MBA), and the Registered Health Information Administrator (RHIA), CCS, and CCS-P credentials. She has been with the company from day one, almost 11 years. She came to the company from a management position at a large teaching hospital, and relocated to the South in order to care for her elderly mother. Alice is worried that the younger managers will perceive her need to care for her mother as a lack of commitment to the organization.
- *West:* Maria, a 32-year-old married white female. She has a bachelor's degree in HIM and the RHIA credential. She has been with the company for four years and worked her way up from a temporary coder to a regional manager. Maria echoes Sarah's concerns about decreasing motivation.
- *India:* Pavan, a 40-year-old single Indian male. He is a medical doctor (MD) with no coding credentials. He has less than one year with the company. Pavan has not vocalized any personal concerns with either Jennifer or other regional managers.

Assumptions

- Jennifer is the team sponsor. She expects to be kept in the communication loop.
- All of the US employees have met face-to-face at least once. Pavan has not met any employee in the United States face-to-face.
- There are no immediate plans to bring the regional managers together for face-to-face meetings.
- All coders go through an intensive orientation, but once they are on their own, there is no formal quality check plan. There are no written policies and procedures for recruitment, training (other than a coding orientation program), or logging of customer feedback.
- Current company statistics indicate that upper level management is 100 percent white female, middle level management is 87 percent white female, and coding professionals are 83 percent white female.

Deliverables

Create a report to send to the president of the company. The report should include the following components:

- Recommendation for creating a self-managing team including the rationale for creating the team
- Outline of communication technology to be used for meetings
- Suggest a person for appointment of a team leader and provide a rationale for the choice
- Recommendations for frequency and time for meetings
- Assessment of the need for a diversity plan
- Description of three strategies to address motivation concerns

Review Questions

1. When given a choice, people prefer to spend time with others whose values are like their own. This is referred to as:

   a. Cultural bias
   b. Similarity-attraction
   c. Social identity
   d. Stereotyping

2. The US Bureau of Labor statistics indicates that over the next 10 years which of the following will occur?

   a. Both the age 55 and older as well as the ages 16 to 22 labor force will increase
   b. Both the age 55 and older as well as the ages 16 to 22 labor force will decrease
   c. The age 55 and older labor force will increase and the ages 16 to 22 labor force will decrease
   d. The age 55 and older labor force will decrease and the ages 16 to 22 labor force will increase

3. This team member has responsibility for all administrative aspects of the team functions of assigning tasks, calling meetings, running meetings, and resolving conflicts.

   a. Coach
   b. Facilitator
   c. Leader
   d. Sponsor

4. During this last stage of team growth, team members complete the goals assigned to them working together consistently and effectively.

   a. Forming
   b. Norming
   c. Performing
   d. Storming

5. A group of HIM employees gather each day for one week at lunch to plan a baby shower for their supervisor. This is an example of what kind of team?

   a. Cross-functional
   b. Formal
   c. Informal
   d. Virtual

6. After retiring from University Hospital, Mark is hired back as a temporary cancer registrar to help reduce occasional abstracting backlogs. This is an example of:

   a. Age-related stereotyping
   b. Bridge employment
   c. Phased retirement
   d. Temporary retirement

7. As the newest EHR implementation specialist in the department, Sarah brings a homemade treat to share with her co-workers every Friday. This is an example of which level of Maslow's hierarchy of needs?

   a. Belonging and love
   b. Physiological
   c. Self-actualization
   d. Self-esteem

8. Which of the following is an example of an intrinsic element of motivation?

   a. Incentive pay
   b. Pay raise
   c. Personal feeling of satisfaction
   d. Promotion

9. This motivational theory supports the idea that employees are motivated when they feel that what they contribute to an organization is matched by what they receive in the way of salary, benefits, and job security.

   a. Equity theory
   b. Goal-setting theory
   c. Herzberg's two-factor theory
   d. Reinforcement theory

10. Which of the following has little to no impact on an employee's job morale?

   a. Autonomy
   b. Positive feelings about management
   c. Size of the organization
   d. Workplace safety

References

Bureau of Labor Statistics, U.S. Department of Labor. 2014. Share of Labor Force Projected to Rise for People Age 55 and Over and Fall for Younger Age Groups. *The Economics Daily.* http://www.bls.gov/opub/ted/2014/ted_20140124.htm.

Fried, B.J. and M.D. Fottler, eds. 2008. Workforce Diversity. Chapter 6 in *Human Resources in Healthcare: Managing for Success*, 3rd ed. Chicago: Health Administration Press.

Hellriegel, D. and J.W. Slocum, Jr. 2004. Achieving Motivation in the Workplace. Chapter 5 in *Organizational Behavior*, 10th ed. Mason, OH: Thompson South-Western.

Institute for Diversity in Health Management. 2013. The State of Health Care Diversity and Disparities: A Benchmarking Study of U.S. Hospitals. http://www.diversityconnection.org/diversityconnection/leadership-conferences/Benchmarking-Survey.jsp?fll=S8.

Konrad, A.M. 2006. Leveraging workplace diversity in organizations. *Organization Management Journal* 3(3):164–189.

Oachs, P. K. 2013. Work Design and Process Improvement. Chapter 26 in *Health Information Management: Concepts, Principles, and Practice.* 4th ed. Edited by LaTour, K. M., S. E. Maki, and P. Oachs. Chicago: AHIMA.

Lindner, J.R. 1998. Understanding employee motivation. *Journal of Extension.* 36(3).

Malhotra, A. Majchrzak, and B. Rosen. 2007. Leading virtual teams. *Academy of Management Perspectives* 21(1):60–70.

Merriam-Webster. 2015. http://www.merriam-webster.com.

Microsoft. 2015. Microsoft Resource Groups. http://www.microsoft.com/en-us/diversity/inside-microsoft/default.aspx#fbid=tQwOu68QUxW.

Scholtes, P.R., B.L. Joiner, and B.J. Streibel. 2010. *The TEAM Handbook*, 3rd ed. Edison, NJ: Oriel STAT A MATRIX.

Smothers, G. and A. Stelter. 2001. Diversity challenge: Understanding cultural differences and communication. *Journal of AHIMA* 72(3):42–45.

Stanford Center on Longevity. 2013. The Aging Workforce: A Chartbook of Demographic Shifts. http://longevity3.stanford.edu/wp-content/uploads/2014/01/The_Aging_U.S.-Workforce.pdf.

Streb, C.K., S.C. Voelpel, and M. Leibold. 2008. Managing the aging workforce: Status quo and implications for the advancement of theory and practice. *European Management Journal* 26(1):1–10.

Voelpel, S.C. and C.K. Streb. 2010. A balanced scorecard for managing the aging workforce. *Organizational Dynamics* 39(1):84–90.

Witt/Kieffer. 2011. Healthcare Diversity Leadership: A National Survey Report. http://www.wittkieffer.com/file/thought-leadership/practice/Diversity%20as%20a%20business%20builder_2011.pdf.

Change Management in Health Information Management

Learning Objectives

- Outline strategic planning in healthcare
- Define organizational development in terms of strategic planning
- Explain the techniques used to promote change
- Identify the stages associated with the adoption of innovation or change
- Differentiate between internal and external change agents
- Contrast the impact of differing conflict management styles required for managing resistance and conflict associated within change

Key Terms

Active listening
ADKAR model
Adoption of innovation
Anchoring
Bridges' transition model
Change
Change agent
Change initiatives
Change management
Collaboration
Communication
Conflict
Conflict management

Diffusion of innovation
    theory
Early adopters
Early majority
Emergent change
External change agent
Innovation
Innovators
Input-output process
    model
Internal change agent
John Kotter's change
    management model

Kurt Lewin's three-stage
    change management
    model
Laggards
Late majority
Learning organization
Mission statement
Negotiation
Organizational culture
Organizational
    development (OD)
Phases of grief
Planned change

Power in negotiation
Refreezing
Resistance to change
Senge's theory of change
Strategic change
Strategic planning
Thomas Kilmann conflict
    mode instrument
Transitioning
Unfreezing
Vision statement
Work environment scale
    (WES)

The ability to successfully manage change is a skill necessary for all health information management (HIM) professionals. **Change** is "to make or become different" (Merriam-Webster 2015). Change cannot be discussed in a vacuum as change within a healthcare organization usually is a direct result of strategic planning and the need for organizational development to meet strategic initiatives. The first section of this chapter addresses strategic planning in healthcare organizations and how developing new strategic initiatives results in organizational development to meet the changing needs of today's healthcare environment. This section also specifically addresses the role the HIM department plays in meeting strategic initiatives through change initiatives. The second section of this chapter outlines theories of change management and notable change management techniques. The third section of the chapter delineates the critical conversations and conflict management skills required to overcome the resistance evident within a changing environment. This section outlines negotiation techniques, conflict management, and collaborative skills needed to manage change in a healthcare organization.

Strategic Planning and Organizational Development

Strategic planning evolves in healthcare organizations when drivers such as rising healthcare costs, major regulatory and policy reform, implementation of new technologies, and a competitive market for new services emerge (Goes 2011). **Strategic planning** is the process in which the leadership of a healthcare organization develops the organization's overall mission, vision, and goals to help guide the direction of the organization as a business entity. Strategic planning includes all the measures taken to provide a broad picture of what must be achieved and in what order, including how to organize within a healthcare organization to achieve the goals of the plan. Figure 4.1 reflects a typical strategic planning process within an organization. Strategic planning is a production process where the output is a new or revised strategic plan. The overall strategic planning process is to outline steps designed for the entire organization as whole, rather than development of goals for a specific division or department (Strategic planning 2014).

Figure 4.1. Strategic planning process

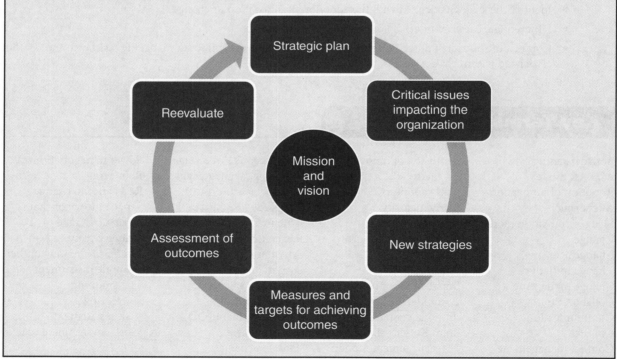

Best practices in healthcare strategic planning applying the model outlined in figure 4.1 are to:

- Review the organization's strategic plan in relation to the organization's mission and vision and make sure the plan is congruent with the organization's mission and vision.

- Assess the critical issues impacting the organization and evaluate how these issues may change the strategic plan of the organization.

- Establish new strategic goals based on the issues impacting the organization in the previous step. Develop focused and clear strategies that will differentiate the organization from its competition.

- Achieve real benefits of a strategic plan by creating targets and measures for assessing the efficacy of new strategic goals.

- Manage implementation of the strategic plan by assessing the outcomes of the plan.

- Manage the plan strategically by reevaluating the plan whenever critical issues impact the organization (Zuckerman 2006).

Healthcare organizations, as in other industries, are able to develop strategic plans that provide direction and focus for the organization. Healthcare organizations can learn from other successful industries that have implemented effective strategic plans. Healthcare organizations often employ experienced outside consultants to facilitate the strategic planning process. The request for proposal for obtaining an external consultant should contain a comprehensive outline of the exact expectations from the consultant. The goal of the external consultant would be the same as if the strategic planning process was performed internally by management. At the end of the strategic planning process there would be clear planning objectives and deliverables described within a final comprehensive report that management would use for implementing the new strategic plan.

The strategic plan revolves around the healthcare organization's mission and vision statement. A **mission statement** is a written statement that sets forth the core purpose and philosophies of an organization or group; it defines the organization or group's general purpose for existing. A **vision statement** is the prescription for carrying out the mission and is a short description of an organization's ideal future state. The critical success of any healthcare organization requires development of a meaningful mission statement that is transparent throughout all levels of the organization. The mission statement is considered a strategic tool for most organizations and it is critical to the ongoing success of the organization's development. The two most important elements of an effective mission statement are (1) the content is relevant to the healthcare organization and (2) the mission statement is clearly communicated throughout the entire organization. There are three factors that enhance the quality of the communication regarding the mission statement and strengthen the effectiveness of the mission statement overall:

- Communication channels must be used that are appropriate for the audience. For example, if the main mode of communication within a healthcare organization is an email announcement, the mission statement along with any other additional communications regarding the mission statement should be shared via email.

- All levels of management should be included in how to communicate the mission statement appropriately.

- The mission statement should align closely to the actual vision of the healthcare organization so as to add strength to the statement (Deschmidt and Prinzie 2011).

Healthcare organizations can revise their mission and vision statements during the strategic planning process when the organization needs to achieve significant changes in performance or when the organization is in need of a facelift in terms of branding. Branding is a marketing strategy that helps to define a healthcare organization's image and that helps the entity differentiate itself from others within the healthcare arena. After a healthcare organization completes the strategic planning process, the branding communication that occurs can increase the awareness and enhance the image of the organization within the healthcare market place.

The preplanning stage prior to the actual creation of a new strategic plan is very important because this sets the organizational structure for the strategic plan. The mission and vision statement of the organization are assessed along with organization's values. A plan for communicating the goals and strategies of the plan are developed within this preplanning phase (Sollenberger 2006).

Decision making is an important aspect of strategic planning. Decision makers within an organization must be able to prioritize organizational needs in order to optimize organizational performance. A standardized method for evaluating critical issues (as in figure 4.1, for example) should be used to assist upper management in the evaluation and prioritization of organizational issues during the strategic planning process (Akdere and Altman 2009). The strategic planning process often results in organizational development that impacts all departments and employees within the organization.

Organizational Development

Organizational development (OD) is the application of behavioral science research and practices (as discussed in chapter 1) to planned organizational change. In addition, organizational development is a "systemwide application and transfer of behavioral knowledge to the planned development, improvement, and reinforcement of the strategies, structures, and process that lead to organization effectiveness" (Akdere and Altman 2009). Organizations develop through change management techniques (as explained later in this chapter). OD is a blueprint for an adaptive process for planning and implementing change within an organization. Within this text the assumption is made that OD is associated with strategic planning and change. **Strategic change** involves improving the alignment of an organization's strategy, culture, and design (Waddell et al. 2011).

Health Information Management Roles in Strategic Planning

Strategic planning must be initiated from the top down and the process must be embraced by the management team in order for the process to be effective. Strategic planning requires ownership within the organization and the ownership needs to start with the chief executive officer (CEO) and the board of directors (who are ultimately responsible for setting the strategy and direction for the organization). Health information managers and directors fall into the middle manager role in terms of healthcare innovation and change that result from strategic planning and OD. The roles that middle managers play in healthcare innovation are to:

- Diffuse information about the implementation or plan: Middle managers must provide the necessary information regarding the change implementation from a middle management perspective.
- Synthesize information: Middle managers must culminate all information particular to the healthcare innovation or change in an understandable manner and make it useable within their own departments or units.
- Mediate between strategy and day-to-day operations: Middle managers put into work the flexibility and adaptability needed to translate the broad strategy into concrete tasks.
- Encourage employees to consistently and effectively use the technology or change in order to implement the change or innovation successfully (Birken et al. 2012).

HIM professionals must be knowledgeable in terms of understanding the roles individuals play within the strategic planning process, how these individuals will help drive changes necessary to successfully implement strategic goals, and also identify the behaviors associated with change experienced throughout the process. These individuals are often called change agents or change leaders and both of these terms are used interchangeably throughout the next section of the text as they are defined. The typical behaviors associated with the adoption of change and innovation are outlined as well as how resistance to change is often exhibited in organizations.

Change Agents

Change strategies must be guided by change agents who are invested in improving the organizational culture. The individual (or individuals) selected to lead change in the organization depends on the significance of the change to the organization, span of control or power within the organization, and the change skills expertise of the individual. The individual or group that undertakes the task of initiating and managing change in an organization is known as a **change agent** (Lunenburg 2010). A change agent is an individual who voluntarily undertakes extraordinary interest in the adoption, implementation, and success of a cause, policy, program, project, or product. A change agent's role can either be internal or external to an organization and the goal of the change agent is to facilitate the transformation needed by people within the organization to accept changes in technologies, structure, and tasks

(Business Dictionary 2015). An **internal change agent** is someone who is employed within the organization and is familiar with the inner workings of the organization. An **external change agent** is an individual such as an external consultant who is employed by the organization temporarily to escort the organization through the change.

There are four competencies that make an effective change agent:

- Broad knowledge. The change agent should have broad multidisciplinary knowledge of healthcare operations.
- Operational and relational knowledge. The change agent should be familiar with the operations and the relationships within the organization.
- Sensitivity and maturity. The change agent should be sensitive to the needs and emotions of all individuals associated with the change process. The change agent should also be able to handle the inevitable conflicts that occur within a change initiative with maturity.
- Authenticity. The change agent should be actively involved and vested in the change initiative to understand the dynamics occurring throughout the process (Livne-Tarandach and Bartunek 2009).

In addition to the competencies listed, there are different types of change agents based on the characteristics and methods utilized for implementing change.

- Outside pressure. The change agent in this model works to change systems from outside of the organization. An example of this would be a union representative who stages picketing for a contract negotiation.
- People-change-technology. The change agent in this model focuses on the individuals within the organization and is concerned with employee morale and motivation as technology is implemented. The premise behind this type of change is if individuals change their behavior in regards to embracing rather than fighting new technologies, the entire organization can move forward faster with the technology changes.
- Analysis from the top. In this model, the change agent focuses on changing the organizational structure and improving the output and efficiency of the organization.
- Organization development. The focus of this change activity is associated with a cultural change approach, as the change agent strives to work on intergroup relations, communication, and decision making. *final project*

Depending on the change required by the organization, any one of these models may be used or a combination of the models can be employed to ensure that the change process is appropriately implemented (Lunenburg 2010).

An effective change agent stays focused on the tasks that need to be completed throughout the change initiative. There are four tactics that he or she uses to overcome obstacles to change as well to create a culture accepting of change. A change agent must focus on:

- Identifying the problem, framing the problem, then solving the problem
- Waiting for a solution rather than forcing a solution to the problem
- Leading through collaboration
- Learning rather than the ultimate outcome (Foley 2013)

When a change is introduced in an organization there will be a significant drop in organizational performance before the change is adopted. An effective change agent or change leader needs to know how to minimize the drop in performance, minimize the time needed to achieve the desired performance levels, and improve the organization's capacity to initiate, implement, and sustain successful change. Effective change leaders also need to know when change is necessary by comparing what is happening now within an organization and what the actual optimal performance level should be for the organization (Blanchard 2010).

Within healthcare organizations, change at the organizational level often is disbursed to the managers of departments. Two different models can be deployed to enable change within the healthcare organization and within each department. In one model, change responsibility is deployed by a change agent who works alongside the manager of a department where the change is occurring. In a second model, the change responsibility is delegated entirely to the manager of a department and this manager must serve as the change agent for the department.

2 Models for Δ

In the first model, a change agent will work closely with the department manager or director to ensure change occurs. When the change agent works closely with the manager, the manager needs to provide open, positive support to the change agent as well as for the employees. The manager can provide the change agent with insight into employee relationships and values that will be essential to the acceptance of the change by the employees. The manager can also assist the change agent when employee resistance to the change is observed. The manager must not lose sight of the vital role of managing the department when a change agent is being utilized to facilitate change. He or she must continue to support and assist employees in a positive manner to overcome the employee resistance to change (Stonehouse 2013).

When the manager of a department is assigned the role as the change agent of the department, it benefits the manager greatly to work with someone in the healthcare organization who can assist the manager in developing change management skills. Communication is essential to the change management process and the manager should communicate the future desired state or change to employees using appropriate communication methods. It is important for the manager to involve employees in the change process and create a sense of ownership for the change for each individual as well as for the entire team, and to systematically use the change experience from existing systems including people as well as technology. The manager needs to be clear about the rationale for improvements associated with the change and who benefits from the change. He or she should always strive to introduce change that aims to improve productivity for employees and continuously manage the expectations of employees regarding the change.

Adoption of Change

The human behaviors associated within change management initiatives are often explained in terms of the diffusion of innovation theory, which was introduced in 1962 by Everett M. Rogers, PhD (Boston University School of Public Health 2013). Rogers was a professor at the University of Mexico and scholar who researched how farmers adopt agricultural innovations; his writings were based on his research that embraced topics related to the diffusion of innovation. The **diffusion of innovation theory** explains how a typical population embraces the adoption of innovation or adoption of change. **Innovation** is the act or process of introducing new ideas, devices, or methods (Merriam-Webster.com 2015). **Adoption of innovation** or change relates to how individuals adapt to the situations presented to them. The five established categories noted within the adoption of innovation or change model are innovators, early adopters, early majority, late majority, and laggards. The following are detailed descriptions of these categories and what percentage of the group within a change initiative fall into these categories. These percentages are well established and are based on significant studies performed in relation to adoption of change or innovation (Boston University School of Public Health 2013).

- **Innovators** are individuals willing to step up to try the innovation or process first. These individuals are risk takers and not afraid of change. Innovators are the individuals who buy into the change immediately and persuade others to come along. Innovators are usually a small percentage of the individuals involved in the process and are essential to engaging others while leading the change (Law 2009). In general, about two and a half percent of the population involved in the change initiative will fall into this category.

- **Early adopters** are a little more cautious than the innovators but these individuals are the change leaders within the organization. These individuals do not require information to change but they like to have how-to-manuals and information sheets on how to participate within the change, which can be provided by the change agents. Approximately 13.5 percent of the individuals participating within a change initiative or innovation fall into the category of early adopters.

- The **early majority** are those individuals within the organization who tend to adopt change quicker than the average person. The individuals who fall into the early majority require evidence or proof of the effectiveness of the change initiative or innovation in terms of success stories and statistics from early adopters. Approximately 34 percent of the individuals fall into this category during a change initiative or innovation.

- The **late majority** are individuals who are skeptical of change and will only participate in the change or innovation after it has been tried by the majority of the people involved in the change initiative or innovation. The typical percentage of individuals that fall into this category is about 34 percent of the population involved.

- **Laggards** are those individuals who resist change; they are bound by tradition and are very skeptical of change. Often these individuals only participate in the change process when there are adverse outcomes outlined such as job loss or lower pay scales for not participating within the change. About 16 percent of the population associated within a change initiative or innovation fall into this category (Boston University School of Public Health 2013).

Figure 4.2 reflects the typical adoption of innovation curve. This curve reflects the percentage of people that typically fall into each of these categories based on many research studies. The use of this curve can assist change agents in understanding the typical behaviors that will be experienced throughout the change initiative. For an HIM department implementing an electronic health record (EHR), this typical adoption of change or innovation curve will mostly likely be demonstrated by the entire HIM team. The HIM manager (as the change agent) should:

- Communicate advantages of the change or innovation
- Communicate commonalities between current record processes workflows and the new technology
- Minimize the complexity of learning the new technology through hands-on-training
- Allow HIM staff time to practice operating the new technology before the technology becomes part of the routine work processes
- Provide feedback on tangible improvements associated with implementation of the technology (Boston University School of Public Health 2013)

Resistance to change is a force that slows or stops the motion of change efforts, which then increases the amount of work and energy needed to propel the efforts forward. Individuals within organizations acquire reputations based on their resistance behaviors and often, accommodations are made by others to accept this behavior. For example, Dr. Smith, a surgeon, was recently assigned to the HIM committee and he is always late for the committee meetings.

Figure 4.2.   Typical adoption of change or innovation curve

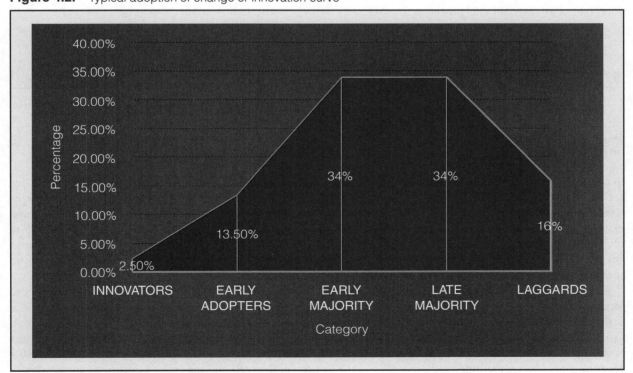

Adapted from: Boston University School of Public Health 2013

The healthcare organization feels that physicians should serve on hospital committees but Dr. Smith does not feel this is a reasonable expectation. The committee members within the team accept his behavior and go over the missed conversations when he eventually arrives at the meeting. Dr. Smith is always complaining about the fact that physicians are always being pulled away from patient care roles to participate in "useless committees." Examples of resistance by employees that impede organizational operations on a day-to-day basis are being late, missing meetings, complaining, and not following directions; these are often magnified during a change initiative.

Knowing that resistance is often a byproduct of the interjection of change, change agents are effective in reducing everyday resistance by applying methods that neutralize resistance to the change (Ford and Ford 2009). In the previous example, the change agent would be able to run interference for the committee and communicate with Dr. Smith explaining how his lateness impacts the committee. Also, the change agent would communicate the importance of Dr. Smith's input to the overall operations of the HIM committee and will assist the committee in creating guidelines for more effective meetings by outlining the responsibilities of each committee member. Some examples would be outlining the committee's adherence to starting meetings on time, and if a member is late it is his or her responsibility to follow up on missed items rather than the committee repeating the missed minutes. The change agent can assist the committee in upholding the guidelines and not allowing members to backslide when resistance to the process is evident. Resistance is not always detrimental to the change process and it can identify issues that need to be handled early in the process. Internal change agents may have an advantage in overcoming resistance as they may already have existing relationships with the individuals involved and may know how these individuals react to change in terms of resistance (Ford and Ford 2009).

Check Your **Understanding**

1. Identify when a healthcare organization initiates development of a new or revised strategic plan.
2. Explain how strategic planning results in organizational development.
3. Delineate the role of the health information manager in strategic planning and organizational development.
4. Differentiate between a mission and vision statement.
5. Differentiate between an internal and external change agent.
6. Outline four strategies employed by change agents to facilitate and mitigate resistance to change.
7. Explain the adoption of innovation or change theory.

Change Management

Healthcare organizations undergoing strategic planning and organizational development to meet the fluctuating healthcare environment and to improve the organization's performance by reaching a future state results in change. Changes do not happen on their own; they happen when change management techniques are employed. **Change management** can best be described as the formal process of introducing change (becoming different), getting it adopted, and diffusing it throughout the organization. It is the process, tools, and techniques to manage the people side of change to achieve the required business outcome (Creasey 2009). Constant change is a way of life in most healthcare organizations today.

Change can occur singularly among individuals within the organization or simultaneously within teams, units, departments, or the entire healthcare organization. In order for change to occur in healthcare organizations, a large number of individuals need to adapt their behaviors in order for performance to be improved or enhanced. A structured approach to change needs to be employed to ensure the individuals, teams, units, departments, healthcare organization, or healthcare delivery system transition from a current state to the desired future state (Garde 2010). An example of change that impacts how work is done by both individuals and the entire healthcare organization is the implementation of an EHR.

project

Planned change dominates the theory and practice of change management but emergent change is another aspect of change that evolves within organizations as well. **Planned change** is a formal process that is introduced methodically and is actively influenced by managers or change agents. **Emergent change** is a continuous, open-ended process of adaptation to changing circumstances and conditions. Emergent change is managed through a more informal process and sometimes not really managed at all. Because of the multitude of factors that impact healthcare organizations, both planned and emergent changes need to be assessed and managed (Livne-Tarandach and Bartunek 2009). Health information managers need to be cognizant of the emergent changes that may occur within an HIM department based on other change initiatives occurring throughout the healthcare organization.

Internal and External Change Initiatives

Change initiatives can be external or internal to the healthcare organization. For example, internal change initiatives such as implementation of EHRs and clinical documentation improvement programs as well as external change initiatives such as new governmental reimbursement systems will all result in major changes for a healthcare organization. Strategic planning frequently occurs when external factors impact the need for change. Healthcare organizations must also realize that human dynamics within an organization continually shift so internal factors may necessitate change as well. Other clues that might indicate a need for internal change would be an increase in the formation of workgroup silos and a decrease in the communication and collaboration between workgroups or units. Another factor would be if the organization functions the same way for an extended period of time with no new initiatives for improvement and then in turn the organization becomes very inefficient in allocating resources within the organization. Every change within the organization does not have to be a major initiative and the more often an organization undergoes varying and periodic change initiatives, the better the organization will manage change (Vermeulen et al. 2010). HIM professionals typically do not embrace change and the longer a process is in place, the more difficult the transition to another process is, such as updating from ICD-9-CM coding to ICD-10-CM/PCS. Adaptability to change is an essential attribute for all health information professionals. *oh no*

Contemporary Change Management Models and Techniques

As discussed, the adoption of innovation or change is a typical reaction to change management initiatives. Research performed by notable scholars and professors attempts to describe change and provide models or techniques for enabling change to occur within organizations. These contemporary change management models and techniques are described in detail.

Lewin's Three-stage Change Management Model

Kurt Lewin's three-stage change management model was developed over 50 years ago but still provides practical guidance for change initiatives. Kurt Lewin, PhD, was a German-American psychologist who is best known for his research on experiential learning and group dynamics. His studies of group dynamics in relation to change initiatives resulted in the creation of a three-stage change management model (Darity 2008). The three stages of this model are unfreezing, changing or transitioning, and freezing.

psychological safety.

- **Unfreezing.** This first stage of change management requires employees to discard and let go of existing old behaviors or processes to prepare for change. The change agent must identify and communicate the need for change as well as mobilize others to see the need for change. The employees experiencing the change need to feel safe in this environment in order to let go of current behaviors. The change leader or change agent needs to provide psychological safety by listening to employees' concerns and supporting the employees' feelings while continuing to communicate the need for change.

- **Transitioning** or moving. In this second stage, Lewin's theory relates to change as a process rather than one single event. This is the inner movement employees make in reaction to change. The change leader or change agent needs to communicate the expected behaviors and model these behaviors. The change agent or leader needs to make sure employees understand and embrace the mission and vision of the organization so new behaviors are ingrained into daily operations rather than as temporary adjustments (Dannar 2011).

- **Refreezing**. This final stage requires that change stabilizes so that it is embedded into the organization's culture and daily practices. The change leader or agent needs to ensure implementation and follow through is inherent to all employees and employees do not regress to former behaviors. Organizational transformation occurs as the change has moved from an initial state to the desired state. In this stage, it is important the change is locked in so the organization can sustain this higher level of desired performance (Shirey 2013).

In a change process using Lewin's model, the change agent should ask what significant events need to happen from both the managers and employees so that that the change will occur. The fundamental principle of effective change management within this model is that the individuals experiencing the change participate in the change and support the changes occurring.

A demonstrative HIM example using Lewin's model is the implementation of a computer-assisted coding (CAC) product. Most change initiatives related to implementation of new technology fail because of lack of effective communication at the beginning of the change process. The coding manager should include the coding staff in strategic planning for work processes, which should include introduction of new coding technologies that may be purchased by the healthcare organization for the HIM department. Coding staff should be involved in the selection of an appropriate CAC process and not be surprised when management purchases the technology. Allowing coding staff to be involved from the start is an excellent way to enter the unfreezing stage for this change. If coders understand the strategic plan and vision for purchasing such a product and see the benefits this product will provide to their work processes, unfreezing will start to occur.

The second stage of Lewin's model is reflected in the actual change process when the CAC product is implemented. The coding manager should actively participate with coding staff during the implementation process to increase acceptance to the change process. Even though coding staff were involved in the selection process and received regular communication about its implementation, the actual transition or move to use the CAC product still may not be an easy transition.

The third stage of Lewin's model requires commitment by the coding manager and the coding staff to remain actively involved in the effective use of the CAC product. Lewin's model does not offer an estimated amount of time needed to move through each stage, but the greater the impact to work process and how far individual's comfort levels are moved will be equivalent to the time that it takes an individual, department, or healthcare organization to move through the stage of the change (Shirey 2013).

Kubler-Ross Phases of Grief

The **phases of grief** coined by Elisabeth Kubler-Ross in 1969 have been closely related to how individuals experience change within organizations. She was a psychiatrist who spent much of her career studying the phases of grief in terminally ill individuals (Smaldone and Uzzo 2013). Kubler-Ross describes an emotional framework for grief in her book *Death and Dying* and that same construct has been noted in relation to how employees experience change within organizations. The five grief stages are denial, anger, bargaining, depression, and acceptance. The initial defense mechanism most employees exhibit when a change is initiated is to deny the action and refuse to listen to any of the change initiatives. The second emotion that employees who are the target of change may exhibit is anger, which is projected resentment of the change. Employees may then bargain by trying to postpone the change. Depression happens when employees start letting go of old behaviors and realizing there is no turning back. The last emotion is acceptance; employees accept the change is occurring and start to embrace the positive elements of the change. It is important that individuals work through all of these emotions during change initiatives so the change can be sustained long term (Boerner 2008).

Using the example of implementation of a CAC product within an HIM department, the phases of grief could be experienced by the coding manager or coding staff during this change process. Some coding staff will take longer than others to move through each stage of grief, but involving everyone at the beginning of the change initiative may assist these individuals to move through the stages faster than if they were not involved from the start.

Kotter's Change Management Model

John Kotter's change management model, an eight-step process, was introduced in 1995 by John P. Kotter, researcher and Harvard Business School professor, in an article in the *Harvard Business Review* and again in his book

Leading Change (Appelbaum et al. 2012). Kotter outlines eight steps that management needs to perform in order to transform an organization through change. Leadership needs to:

1. Create a sense of urgency encouraging others that the change is necessary.
2. Form a coalition, a group of individuals who will assist the organization through the change process.
3. Determine a vision for the change and develop a strategy for the change process.
4. Communicate the vision and what the changes will look like to the organization.
5. Eliminate or dissolve the resistance to the change.
6. Share short-term wins that appear as a result of the change.
7. Build on each short-term win to capture all the positive components that are happening within the change process.
8. Adopt the changes as they occur so that the organization moves to its desired state of change (Thompson 2015).

Figure 4.3 depicts the eight steps of Kotter's model.

Kotter's model was developed to address fundamental changes within organizations but it may not be applicable to all scenarios without some modifications. Kotter asserts that all eight steps should be completed in sequence without overlap, but in some instances overlap of the steps may be required in order for the change to progress. Not all the steps may be relevant within certain change contexts and the steps do not specifically outline how to handle difficulties during a change situation. Kotter's model is an excellent starting point for embarking on change but it may need modifications in order to be applicable to all change management situations (Appelbaum et al. 2012).

By deploying a change management model such as Kotter's, a coding manager will have a solid framework when implementing a CAC program. Applying the steps outlined by Kotter will assist the coding manager and coding staff

Figure 4.3.   Kotter's change management model

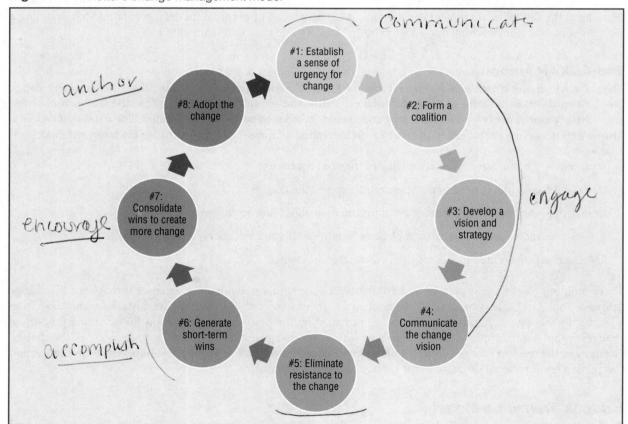

to move through the change management initiative in a systematic manner. The coding manager can create urgency to adopt CAC to improve employee productivity particularly with the implementation of new coding classification systems such as ICD-10-CM/PCS and eventually ICD-11. Kotter's steps two through four will engage the coding staff in the decision-making process and create a vision for the coding department. Step five will empower coding staff to provide recommendations for the best product for the workgroup, develop implementation and training plans, and collaborate as a team while improving work processes. Step six allows coding staff to feel accomplished as the team celebrates positive impacts of the coding product on workflow and work processes. Step seven encourages the coding manager and coding staff to incorporate efficiencies into the use of the CAC product thereby resulting in additional gains for the healthcare organization. Step eight anchors the change to the coding area as improvements and efficiencies gained are tangibly noted through increased productivity and adoption of the change by all coding staff.

Senge's Theory of Change

Peter Senge is the director of the center for organizational learning at the Massachusetts Institute of Technology and he studies how businesses and other organizations adapt to complex and rapid organizational changes (Capstone Encyclopedia of Business 2003). **Senge's theory of change** was introduced in 1990 in his book, *The Fifth Discipline*, where he highlights the concept of systems thinking in terms of a learning organization. A **learning organization** is an organization that quickly adapts to environmental changes and thus attains knowledge and skills that can be utilized in the future when experiencing change. Senge outlines disciplines that contribute toward a learning organization: personal mastery, mental models, building shared visions, and team learning. A discipline is an orderly or prescribed conduct or pattern of behavior (Merriam-Webster 2015). These disciplines revolve around organizational team collaboration that occurs as part of the organizational change process (Kazmi et al. 2014). This is a complex model that eventually results in the entire healthcare organization moving to a higher level of understanding as to the type of organizational learning that has occurred during a change initiative. The higher level of learning is noted to be systems thinking, which is coined as the fifth discipline within Senge's model. Systems thinking is the discipline that integrates the four other disciplines of personal mastery, mental models, building a shared vision, and team learning into a logical body of theory and practice (Senge 2006).

The ADKAR Model

The **ADKAR model** is a change management model that is used to assess individual change management issues. Five building blocks—**awareness**, **desire**, **knowledge**, **ability**, and **reinforcement** in regards to the change initiative— are necessary components for individuals to understand in order to participate in change. The building blocks are further defined as to what is needed in order for an individual to move through this change management model:

Awareness—An individual's understanding of the need for change

Desire—An individual's need to participate and support the change

Knowledge—An individual's acquisition of information about how to change

Ability—An individual's capacity to implement required skills and behaviors during the change

Reinforcement—An individual's capability to sustain the change

These building blocks are sequential and are the typical steps that individuals experience throughout the change process (Cook 2013). This process can be applied to any change initiative within a healthcare organization from a change in the type of health insurance being provided by the healthcare organization to individual procedural changes within a job. Employees need to engage within the change initiatives by being made aware of the change, engaging in the need to change (desire), gaining knowledge and abilities to acquire and implement the change, and then giving reinforcement throughout the change so that it is sustainable.

Bridges' Transition Model

Bridges' transition model was developed by William Bridges, an American speaker, author, and recognized organizational consultant on managing change in the workplace, and was published in his 1991 book *Managing*

Transitions. This model provides a guide for how individuals experience change by transitioning through different phases. The three phases noted by Bridges are:

Stage 1: Ending, losing, and letting go. This is the first stage of transition after you present employees with a change initiative. Employees may reflect many emotions such as fear, anger, denial, frustration, uncertainty, and a sense of loss. These emotions may be exhibited as a resistance to the change but managers must understand these emotions and accept that resistance to change is expected. Managers should listen to employee concerns but also try to mitigate some of these fears by educating and communicating positive outcomes of the change.

Stage 2: The neutral zone. The neutral zone is the second stage of transition employees experience when confronted with a change. In this stage the emotions exhibited by employees most likely will be resentment toward the change, low morale and low productivity, anxiety about future job roles, and general skepticism toward the change. Managers should meet with employees on a regular basis to improve morale and curb productivity loss. Managers should provide positive feedback on each employee's performance and how his or her role is important to the change initiative.

Stage 3: The new beginning. This is the third stage of transition employees experience when confronted with a change. In this stage employees usually exhibit acceptance to the change and a high energy level in regards to learning. Employees begin to adopt the change and managers need to make sure this positive adoption of the change is sustainable. Managers should work with employees to set realistic performance goals and celebrate the goals achieved thus far through the change process (Manktelow 2015b).

Bridges' transition model provides a very clear and concise way for assisting employees through the transition stages associated with change initiatives. HIM managers can easily outline the stages of emotions exhibited by employees throughout the change initiative and develop ways to move employees through each stage of the change.

Check Your **Understanding**

1. Differentiate between planned and emergent change.
2. Outline the three stages of Lewin's model that are experienced during change.
3. Identify the stages of grief individuals may experience during a change process.
4. Outline the steps of Kotter's change management model and how these steps can be exhibited within an HIM department change initiative.

Organizational Culture and Change

Organizational culture plays a big role in an organization's performance and, in particular, how organizational development evolves over time. **Organizational culture** is shared values and beliefs that guide behavior within organizations. HIM organizational culture is often difficult to define but usually plays a part in whether or not successful changes such as mergers, acquisitions, and joint ventures occur within healthcare. Assessing the need for change based on the internal factors of an organization is often measured by employee surveys, a tool used by healthcare organizations to assess the culture of the organization. It is essential during an employee survey that employees understand the structure of the questions within the survey, their role in the survey process, and that the results of the survey are shared (Wiley 2012). The results of the employee survey, particularly negative results, prompt management to focus on changes that are required to improve future survey results. Positive survey results should be shared with all employees and management. The overall culture of a department or entire healthcare organization can be improved by engaging employees and management in performance improvement initiatives directly related to the employee survey. The following sections of this chapter describe two methods—surveys and the work environment scale—used to assess organization culture.

Surveys

Sound survey methodology should be employed by healthcare organizations when deploying employee surveys. The survey questions should demonstrate reliability and validity as tested within a formal research setting or by using standardized questions created by a company or organization experienced in employee survey development. The same survey should be administered to all employees in the organization although management levels may have additional questions within the survey that deal with topics specifically related to management issues. The process of administering the survey should be standardized throughout the organization and provide for unbiased selection and results. Manager–employee reporting relationships should be clear as statistics are aggregated by work team, department, and service lines within the organization. Prior to taking the survey, employees will be educated on the importance of selecting their appropriate manager (to whom they directly report) when taking the survey. Specific results from each employee will remain anonymous but aggregated information for each manager will be collected. In order for results to be meaningful to a particular work team or department, the data must be collected from the appropriate employees within that work area. Results of the survey should be calculated using descriptive and analytical statistics and a report should be shared with all employees that have completed the survey (Pellegrin and Currey 2011). As noted earlier in this chapter, if performance improvement initiatives are deployed in direct relation to employee survey results, survey data can be a powerful tool for change (Wiley 2012).

The Work Environment Scale

The **work environment scale (WES)** is one of the most rigorous and validated measures for assessing healthcare organizational culture. The WES was developed by Rudolph Moos, PhD, and professor emeritus of psychiatry and behavioral science at Stanford University, based on his research of development of a conceptual framework that assesses the interplay of individuals and their work environment. The WES was designed to measure the social environments of different types of work settings through completion of a questionnaire. The WES assists organizations to evaluate employee productivity, assess employee satisfaction, and clarify employee expectations to ensure a healthy work environment. The three dimensions assessed using the WES questionnaire are:

- Relationships in terms of involvement, coworker cohesion, and supervisor support
- Personal growth or orientation relating to autonomy, task orientation, and work pressure
- System maintenance and change addressing clarity, control, innovation, and physical comfort

Aggregated scores from completion of the WES questionnaires are used to describe the workgroup's perception of the social functioning of its work environment. Results of a WES can assist in evaluating problems and risks within the organization; can be performed before a change, to promote change, and after change to evaluate the organization's culture; can evaluate and improve leadership within the organization; and may help build teams within the organization (Moos 1987).

Values and Change Management

In chapter 1, values-based leadership was discussed as a basic leadership style and it is important to note the impact that values make on healthcare organizational change initiatives. Value-based leadership is an approach that emphasizes values, ethics, and stewardship as central to effective leadership. In leading change, the values of the individuals within the organization must be considered; and depending on the incongruence or congruence with the change to the values, the transition or transformation to change will be impacted (Amis et al. 2002).

Check Your **Understanding**

1. Describe organizational culture and how it can impact employee's perception of change.
2. Outline how WES can assess a healthcare organization's culture.

Communication and Change Management

Communication is an essential component while managing change. **Communication** is a "process of using words, sounds, signs, or behaviors to exchange or share information" (Merriam-Webster 2015). Change communication is a key element for an organization undergoing transformation. The manner in which internal messages are conveyed to the individuals experiencing the change greatly impact individual behaviors and the overall perception of the change process. The design and execution of effective change communication requires the same diligence as any other strategic organizational process.

Internal communications for change initiatives should have proactive plans in place to support anticipated events and reactions to the messages. Internal change communications should be assessed for all organizational levels in which change occurs:

- Among and between people in small group meetings
- One-on-one between the manager and employee
- Within large group meetings with organizational leadership

Change messages should be consistent no matter the level to which the information is communicated. Fundamental communication methods should be promoted in the change communication process that includes sharing the change message multiple times and exercising different channels of communication to share the change message. It is important to assess the message source and medium used to convey the change communication. The three modes for communication within organizations are face-to-face interactions (such as one-on-one meetings, group meetings), print media (such as flyers, newsletters, and monthly reports) and electronic media (such as a healthcare organization's intranet, emails, and social media). All of these modes of communication should be utilized to support communications throughout the change initiative (Bjorkman 2009).

One-on-one exchanges between the manager or change agent and employees are an essential component of the change communication initiative. Communication is a two-way interchange of information in that the manager needs to communicate changes to employees but in turn the manager or change agent listens to how employees perceive the changes. The type of activity that needs to occur within the communication process is **active listening**. Active listening is when an individual makes a conscious effort to hear and understand the message being conveyed. Active listening engages both parties in the communication process with an intent to solve problems before they occur and also helps strengthen and maintain work relationships while facilitating change in a meaningful manner. The key steps to active listening are to show interest in what the employee has to say; ask questions to clarify, gather information, and focus on the conversation; and let the employee know you understand what he or she is trying to convey (Manktelow 2015a). Active listening is an important component of the communication process particularly when critical conversations, negotiations, and conflicts need to be managed during a change initiative.

Change Management and Negotiation

Within a change management cycle there may be a time when negotiation skills are required between different members of the team. **Negotiation** is a formal discussion between people who are trying to reach an agreement (Merriam-Webster 2015). The ability to negotiate is an important skill for all HIM professionals to learn to be successful change leaders. HIM professionals at any level may negotiate change in hours, salary, or working conditions. For example, at the health information manager level, negotiation skills are important when additional space is needed for the department, additional departmental resources are needed, adopting external contracts for transcription or outsourced coding, developing the annual budget, and requesting capital budget expenditures. A challenge to negotiation is negotiating parties often have differing interests or goals. Usually whenever a negotiation occurs at least one participating party is hoping for an optimal agreement.

When negotiating, there are three different values or points associated with the negotiation:

- Target value or point—the best possible outcome for the negotiation in which both parties are in agreement (referred to as a *win-win* situation)

- Reservation value or point—the lowest possible outcome for the negotiation in which neither party comes to an agreement
- Best alternative to a negotiated agreement—this may not be the target value of the negotiating parties, but it is an acceptable alternative to that ideal value (Berlin 2008)

The purpose of a successful negotiation is to resolve situations where the desired outcome conflicts between the parties involved. Two other concepts that must be considered within a negotiation are anchoring and understanding who has the power within the negotiation. **Anchoring** is making the first offer in a negotiation and this is the foundation upon which the rest of the negotiation builds. **Power in negotiation** refers to any unique attributes or position a particular negotiation party possesses (Berlin 2008). Power is the ability to make things happen and the individual who possesses the power within a negotiation setting is able to negotiate the situation within his or her direction. As noted previously, the aim of a negotiation is an optimal agreement, or a win-win situation within a negotiation. A win-win negotiation is a solution that is acceptable to both parties and leaves all involved feeling that they have won, in some way, when the negotiation is complete. Depending on the circumstances and the relationships between the parties, different negotiation styles may be required. A good change leader will know when negotiation needs to occur and where there is no negotiation option. An example of this is within an electronic health record design, build, and implementation—negotiations may take place for what type of electronic document tools will be employed, but negotiation will not take place about whether or not to remain in a paper environment.

Preparing for a negotiation situation is important. Figure 4.4 outlines the steps required to prepare for a negotiation. Prepare by prioritizing the issues, and noting which items are the most important versus which items are of least importance. Set goals for the negotiation, taking into account the prioritized list. Make a list of the items you are willing to trade or swap in order to come to an agreement. Outline a list of alternatives for the negotiation and name the reserve target or point for the negotiation. The negotiator should analyze the relationship with the other parties within the negotiation and ascertain who has the power within the relationship. The negotiator should describe projected outcomes and consequences when the agreement is reached. Determine the consequences for winning or losing the negotiation from both parties' perspectives. The negotiator should list the best alternative to the agreement (Berlin 2008).

During a change initiative, negotiation is a give and take discussion that requires preparation in order for positive outcomes to occur. Good negotiators are able to get what he or she wants from the negotiation while still allowing the other party to feel like he or she won as well.

Change Management and Collaboration

Collaboration is the relationships and interactions that occur between co-workers within an organization. Collaboration within healthcare involves the joining of two or more healthcare professionals to work on achieving similar goals (Merriam-Webster 2015). Collaboration between and within healthcare teams is a very complex dynamic process in most organizations.

Figure 4.4. Steps for preparing for a negotiation Dr Jones

> Checklist for preparing for a negotiation
>
> ☐ Prioritize the issues and outcomes
> ☐ Set goals
> ☐ List items to swap or trade
> ☐ List alternate outcomes
> ☐ Determine who has the power within the negotiating relationship
> ☐ Describe projected outcomes
> ☐ Describe consequences for winning and losing from both sides
> ☐ Create an alternative to the agreement

© AHIMA

Some of the collaborative attributes that are valued within a multidisciplinary healthcare team are shared power based on knowledge, lack of hierarchy (everyone is equal), open communication, cooperation, assertiveness, negotiation, and coordination (Vaughn 2009). Although the concept of teamwork is often synonymously used in place of collaboration, teamwork is actually an attribute of a collaborative relationship (Rahim 2002).

Collaboration within healthcare workgroups can be hindered when the specific expectations of individuals are not met relating to communication, professionalism, mutual respect, climate of collaboration, and quality of work. Communication should be clear and concise so ideas can be exchanged and information transparent to all team members. There should be a mutual respect or a balanced relationship within a collaborative workgroup, no matter what level of education or position the individuals hold within the organization. All workgroup members should be respected for their professional knowledge and the skills they bring to the collaboration. There needs to be a climate of collaboration for the workgroup in that everyone is working toward the same goal. The last essential facet of collaboration is that quality of work produced by the workgroup is enhanced rather than hindered by collaborative efforts (Leever et al. 2010).

The most commonly noted barriers to collaboration within healthcare workgroups include lack of time; gender, generational, and cultural differences; and lack of role clarification of team members. Whenever these barriers are experienced within a collaborative environment, conflict may result (Vaughn 2009).

A model developed in 1964 by researcher Joseph E. McGrath is the **input-output process model**, a seven-component model that evaluates the effectiveness of collaboration within teams. McGrath's research focused on the interaction between and among team members as well as the team as a single functional entity. Input refers to group composition and structure as well as the tasks required within a particular work environment. Processes are the group's activities based on the flow of events and interactions among team members. Outputs are the group's tasks and performance, group development, and the overall effect of the group dynamics on an individual team member's performance within a collaborative work situation (Gaboury et al. 2009). This model assesses the impact of collaboration or lack of collaboration within a particular workgroup and the resultant effects. This model could be used during a change management initiative to assess the inputs—group composition, tasks and environment, and group structure, along with how the group processes the changes. The resultant outputs—tasks and performance, effects on members, and actual group development—will provide a measurement if the change initiative was effective or if additional improvements need to be made.

The key foundation for building a collaborative work environment is to invest in healthy work relationships that avoid competition and circumvention of problems. HIM managers should adopt a collaborative perspective by attempting to see things from others' viewpoints and commit to problem solving as a way to building better relationships within the workgroup (Gunderman and Saravanan 2010). Being aware of the barriers that impact collaboration and the expectations of individuals within a workgroup can assist the HIM manager in creating and maintaining a collaborative work environment.

Conflict Management

The opposite of collaboration is conflict and as noted within the last section of this chapter, barriers within collaborative workgroups can cause conflicts. Change can also result in conflict as behaviors and paradigms within organizations evolve. **Conflict** is a clash between hostile or opposing elements, ideas, or forces (Merriam-Webster 2015). Conflict can also be described as any difference in opinion, value, need, want, and such that causes frustration in one or more interdependent people and blocks them from achieving their tasks or goals (Pearce 2005). Negative connotations usually surround the concept of conflict but if conflict is managed effectively, a negative situation can be turned into a positive outcome.

Emotions play a big role in conflict situations and how individuals manage conflict over time. The behavioral elements of emotion are how emotional experiences are expressed during a conflict situation. The type of behaviors that individuals demonstrate during a conflict situation can be expressed nonverbally, verbally, physiologically, and cognitively. The amount of emotional intensity an individual exhibits during a conflict situation can vary greatly depending on the level of stress the conflict causes each individual. There are five principles of conflict and emotion, listed as follows.

- Conflict is innately emotionally defined.
- Conflict is emotionally charged.

- Conflict invokes a moral stance in most individuals.
- Conflict is identity-based.
- Conflict is relationally-based (Bodtker and Jameson 2001).

A conflict manager should be aware of the emotions attached to conflict situations in order to manage the conflict appropriately and within the emotional context of the individuals involved (Bodtker and Jameson 2001).

Conflict management is a problem-solving technique that focuses on working with individuals to find a mutually acceptable solution. All healthcare organizations experience conflict at some level and the most frequently exercised tactics to mitigate conflict fall under the umbrella of reducing the conflict, resolving conflict, or minimizing conflict within collaborative workgroups. Conflict is inevitable because of human nature so the best way to manage conflict is through the use of effective conflict management strategies. Conflict management involves designing effective strategies to minimize the dysfunctions of conflict and enhance the constructive functions of conflict in order to enhance learning and effectiveness in an organization. Conflict managers are able to understand the dynamics of conflict and they can offer effective choices throughout the conflict situation. Healthcare organizations need to provide strategies to individuals within the organization that embrace conflict so that the organizational learning and effectiveness is maximized, the needs of all individuals are considered and all situations are handled ethically (Rahim 2002).

Whenever there are two or more people, conflict is inevitable. Conflict is about people, emotions, and negative energy or an atmosphere that blocks a group from doing its work successfully. Conflict occurs as naturally as cooperation and a workgroup should strive to constructively solve conflict when it occurs. Conflict has both benefits and risks (Pearce 2005).

Conflict in workgroups is very complex and can have detrimental effects on the health and morale of employees. Conflict in itself can undermine workgroup effectiveness and managers or supervisors of workgroups may spend a significant amount of time managing conflict so as to mitigate the actual impact of conflict on the workgroup. There are four ways that individuals usually respond to conflict. Individuals may:

- Collaborate with others through problem solving and make trade-offs or compromises within the conflict situation
- Yield to the other party, letting go of their own needs or wants within the situation
- Impose their will on others with the use of threats
- Withdraw from the situation by performing no action (Way et al. 2014)

The ways individuals approach conflict within a workgroup directly impacts individual job performance as well as the entire workgroup's performance (Way et al. 2014). The supervisor or manager is often brought in as a third party to the dispute to offer conflict management tactics. The job of a supervisor or manager includes role setting and monitoring employee behavior, which can encompass conflict situations. Conflict within workgroups and across workgroups can be very costly to organizations. Ensuring that supervisors and managers have the tools and intervention techniques necessitating conflict management skills is a key management training element for any organization. The supervisor or manager can turn negative conflict situations around by promoting fair and consistent conflict management processes such as the ones described in the following sections (Way et al. 2014).

Thomas Kilmann Conflict Mode Instrument

A questionnaire tool used to assess the manner in which individuals manage conflict is the **Thomas Kilmann conflict mode instrument**. The Thomas Kilmann instrument (TKI) was developed by Ken Thomas, PhD, and Ralph Kilmann, PhD, who were both professors of management at the University of Pittsburgh in the early 1970s (Brown 2012). This instrument is relevant to HIM assessment of conflict management styles as it has been applied in the majority of studies on conflict management in healthcare (Sportsman and Hamilton 2007). This tool assesses conflict management styles by using two parameters—assertiveness and cooperation—which manifest in five distinct styles. The five conflict styles (displayed in figure 4.5) are to avoid, compete, collaborate, accommodate,

Figure 4.5. Relationship of conflict management styles in the Thomas Kilmann conflict mode instrument

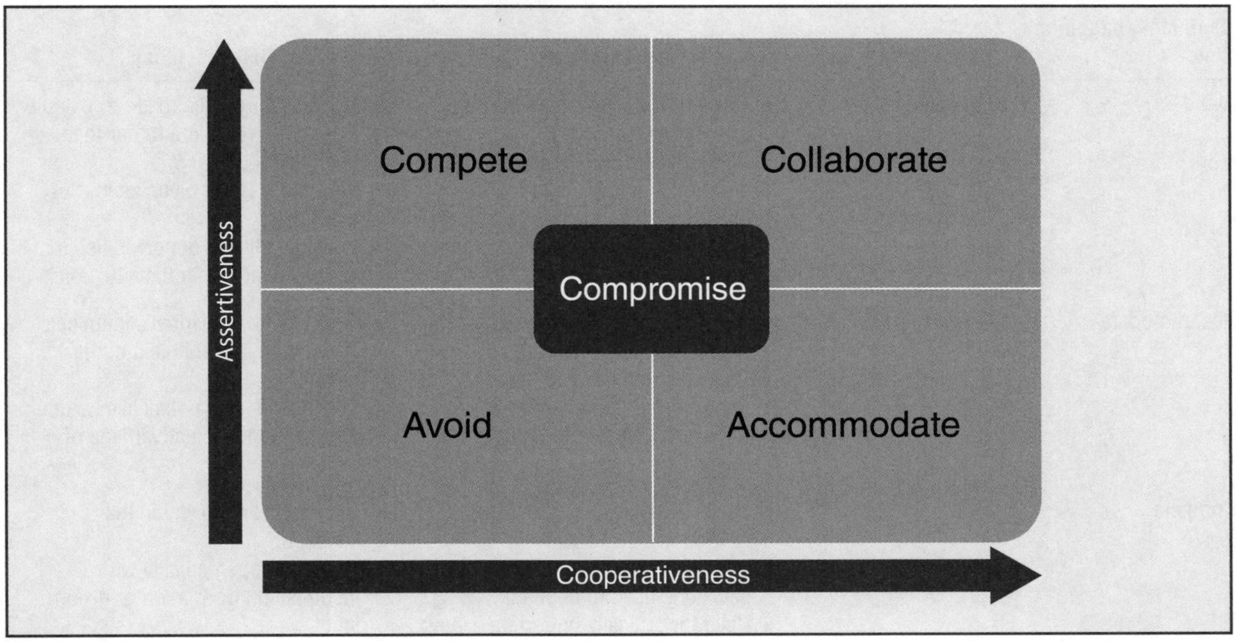

© AHIMA

and compromise (Slabbert 2004). Table 4.1 (on the following page) outlines each conflict management style and the advantages and disadvantages of each of the styles in managing conflict. The standard TKI uses a questionnaire that consists of 30 two-choice questions. Individuals respond to each question by selecting one of the two conflict reactions (assertiveness or cooperation) based how they would typically respond to a conflict situation within a superior and subordinate relationship. The results place the individual into one of five distinct styles. The five styles fall into the matrix and are determined by questionnaire scores on two axes (Slabbert 2004). This questionnaire can be used by anyone within an organization to assess the manner in which individuals are managing conflict and to develop strategies for negotiating the conflicts.

Once an individual's conflict management style is identified, the individual will tend to use the same pattern over and over again in conflict situations. In some situations the typical response will resolve the conflict but in other situations it will escalate the situation. The level of education of healthcare professionals does not make a difference in a choice of an individual's conflict management style (Sportsman and Hamilton 2007). It is important for HIM professionals to select a conflict management style that best matches the conflict situation occurring at the time.

Conflict Management Best Practices

Conflict management techniques can be used to mitigate or resolve a conflict. A seven-step problem-solving method can be used to get to the bottom of the conflict and find a solution. Often conflict is associated with emotions so employing a standardized method keeps everyone involved within the conflict focused on the issues at hand. The steps are outlined as follows.

1. Define the problem or the conflict—is it a relationship issue or a process issue?
2. Identify and clarify all possible options for a solution.
3. Evaluate options for the solution.
4. Decide on an acceptable solution.
5. Develop an implementation plan.
6. Develop a process for evaluating effectiveness of the solution.
7. Talk about the experience.

Table 4.1. Advantages and disadvantages of the five conflict management styles

Conflict Management Style	Goal	Advantages	Disadvantages
Avoid	To delay	• Use when issues are of low importance • Allows a cool-down time period and brings emotions to a lower level • Use when more data or information is needed	• Decisions are often made by default • Issues may escalate rather than cool down • Your input is not given as part of a group • Possible missed opportunities for engagement within the situation
Accommodate	To yield	• Use when peace is required for the situation • Use when the issue is more important to the other individual • Allows all involved to make mistakes	• Restricts an individual's influence • Perception is that little input is given • The individual may feel like he or she is being taken advantage of
Compete	To win	• Use when quick decisions are needed • Use when difficult or unpopular decisions need to be made • Used for critically important issues • Use when individual protection is needed	• Reduces learning within the situation • Actions happen quickly with insufficient information or group input • Individuals may tend to say "yes" to get their way
Compromise	To find a mutual ground	• Used for moderately important issues • Perceived as a temporary solution in order to buy time • Helps two strong individuals with opposing goals reach agreement	• The big picture can be lost • Low trust for the manager • Never truly makes a concrete decision
Collaborate	To find a win-win solution	• Used when both sides must agree • Mutual learning occurs • Consensus is sought • Improves difficult relationships	• Takes a lot of time for both situation and relationship building • Delegation is necessary • Perceived as pushing "peace" too far

Source: Pearce 2005.

This is a typical problem-solving methodology that can be used in many different ways within the workplace, but it is also effective in outlining the problems associated with conflict (Bolland 2012). Providing a constructive conflict management strategy such as the seven-step problem-solving method to HIM professionals is essential to creating a healthy working environment.

Managing Critical Conversations

While managing conflict, there are times when difficult or critical conversations need to take place in order for resolution to occur to move change to the next level. Poor communication creates obstacles for managing critical conversations in conflict situations. Critical or crucial conversations are about challenging issues where emotions are involved and the outcomes of the conversation have a large impact on relationships or workplace dynamics. Planning prior to entering a critical conversation will result in a better outcome to the situation (Clancy 2014). The planning steps for managing critical conversations are:

• Develop awareness of your own communication patterns and how you typically react to difficult conversations; for example, how you act or react to anger or withdrawal

- Identify and clarify what you want from the conversation; stay focused and keep a handle on your emotions
- Establish a mutual purpose or shared goal for the conversation
- Establish respect by demonstrating respect for the others' position even if you may not agree with their stance
- STATE your course:
  - S = Share your fact
  - T = Tell your story
  - A = Ask for others' input and viable compromise solutions
  - T = Talk about what is fact
  - E = Encourage differing views
- Let others STATE their course
- Finish clearly by recording commitments, developing measurable results, and set a follow-up time to meet (Smith 2006)

The end result of a critical conversation is that all individuals feel like their stance was heard and that some mutually agreeable solution evolved from the conversation. Critical conversations often happen spontaneously, which may not allow the individuals to be prepared for the conversation. If emotions are too high, it is best to delay the conversation until emotions subside and a productive conversation can take place.

Check Your **Understanding**

1. Evaluate the role of active listening when communicating change initiatives.
2. Explain two differences between negotiating change initiatives and collaborating within change initiatives.
3. Discuss the advantages and disadvantages of the five conflict management styles.
4. Create a plan for approaching a critical conversation that needs to take place as a result of conflict.

Case Study

Objectives

- Identify components of employee satisfaction requiring improvement based on parameters outlined by a healthcare organization
- Outline action steps for improving employee satisfaction that incorporate strategic planning and change management initiatives
- Identify the collaboration, negotiation, and conflict management skills required to deploy the performance improvement plans

Instructions

Review the following case study and create an action plan for improving employee job satisfaction scores within an HIM department.

Scenario

Mary Beth is the director of HIM at a large acute-care healthcare organization. Every three years the healthcare organization undertakes a hospital-wide employee survey in which information is collected from employees regarding job satisfaction and other components. The 2015 employee survey assessed the following components:

- Alignment of employee goals with healthcare organization's mission and vision—including questions reflecting employee awareness of the organization's mission and vision and how it impacts individual jobs within the organization
- Employee job satisfaction—Assessment of the employee's satisfaction with job tasks, peer group relationships, and employee–manager relationships in regard to overall job performance
- Work-life balance—Evaluation of the employee's perception of the balance between work and home life
- Communication within the healthcare organization—evaluated communication at the organizational level, departmental level, and work area level

The survey was deployed by an outside consulting agency that has experience with creating reliable and valid healthcare employee surveys. The management team from the healthcare organization was required to attend an initial training session regarding the goals of the survey and the managers were provided nonbiased ways to encourage their employees to complete the surveys. The surveys were web-based and employees received links within their email to complete the surveys. Employees (both management and nonmanagement) were allowed to complete the survey during work hours. The survey was deployed in a systematic manner. The questions within the survey were broken down into the four categories outlined previously and the options for each answer were scored on a five-point scale. The scale options were: 5 = Extremely satisfied, 4 = Satisfied, 3 = Neutral, 2 = Dissatisfied, 1 = Extremely dissatisfied.

Weekly, each department head received a report on the percentage of departmental employees that completed the survey but individual names and responses from the employees were anonymous. Results of the 2015 survey were calculated by the consulting company and standard reports were provided to all directors and managers within the healthcare organization. Mary Beth received the 2015 employee satisfaction survey results on January 5, 2016. The HIM department results are provided in figure 4.6. The organization's human resources department and the survey consultant met with all department directors to discuss the results of the survey and what the next steps were for the healthcare organization. Each department is required to complete an action plan for improving the five components that fall below a score of 3.5.

Assumptions

- The HIM director will meet with the HIM management team to discuss the survey results and the action plan for improvement will be completed collaboratively by the HIM management team.
- The HIM director will need to incorporate strategic planning and change initiatives as part of the action plan for improving the HIM department's overall employee satisfaction results.
- A follow-up employee satisfaction survey will be deployed by the healthcare organization at the end of calendar year 2016, which will allow departments time to initiate improvement action plans from January to November 2016.
- Management annual performance evaluations and incentives are partially based on the results of the employee satisfaction survey.
- Reasonable goals are set for score improvement as slight gains are perceived as a positive movement toward employee satisfaction.

Deliverables

1. Create an action plan (template provided in figure 4.7) for improving the results of the next employee satisfaction survey by identifying any components of the survey that fall below a score of 3.5 for the overall HIM department.

Figure 4.6. 2015 employee satisfaction survey results

2015 Employee Satisfaction Survey Results

Department: Health Information Management

Response rate: 95% Compliance, n = 74, HIM employees total = 78

Scale rating: 5 = Extremely satisfied, 4 = Satisfied, 3 = Neutral, 2 = Dissatisfied, 1 = Extremely dissatisfied,
0 = Not applicable

Section of survey	HIM manager 1 N = 20	HIM manager 2 N = 22	HIM manager 3 N = 26	HIM director N = 6	Overall department score
	Overall score	**Overall score**	**Overall score**	**Overall score**	
I. Mission and vision	4.0	3.8	3.7	4.2	3.9
II. Job satisfaction	3.2	2.9	2.2	4.0	3.1
III. Work-life balance	4.0	4.0	4.0	2.9	3.7
IV. Communication	2.8	2.6	2.5	3.5	2.9

Report legend

- HIM manager 1 area duties: Release of information, transcription, and chart completion
- HIM manager 2 area duties: Electronic record management and document imaging
- HIM manager 3 area duties: Coding (coding employees work remotely)
- HIM director: Three managers and three data quality specialists report to HIM director

© AHIMA

Figure 4.7. Employee satisfaction improvement plan

Employee Satisfaction Improvement Plan

Department:

Date:

Component requiring improvement from survey (Any area scoring <3.5)	Action items—Identify three action steps for each component	Identify collaboration, negotiation, or conflict management skills required to deploy each action step	Projected goal for score improvement (>3.5)

© AHIMA

2. Identify three action steps to improve each component of the survey by identifying appropriate change management skills and conflict resolution skills discussed within this chapter.

3. Outline the communication method for each of the action steps such as meetings, emails, online training, webinars, and such.

4. Provide the projected score for each component of the overall HIM department survey that requires an action plan.

Review Questions

1. Following a strategic planning retreat, the University Hospital board of trustees wrote this: "University Hospital exists to bring quality healthcare to the surrounding community and region and to educate future healthcare providers." This is an example of what kind of statement?

   a. Mission
   b. Value
   c. Vision
   d. Strategic

2. The HIM department at Memorial Hospital will install CAC next month. Meetings were held with all coders so they had input into the process and could address any concerns. HIM managers are working together to ensure the process is as smooth as possible. This is an example of what kind of change?

   a. Emergent
   b. Open-ended
   c. Planned
   d. Strategic

3. Emily, one of the coders at Memorial Hospital, has refused to attend any meetings on the CAC project, and when the other coders bring up the topic she quickly changes the subject saying she is sure it will never happen. Emily demonstrates what step in the grief process?

   a. Acceptance
   b. Bargaining
   c. Denial
   d. Depression

4. University Hospital made the decision to allow coders to code remotely from home. As preparations are made, some of the coders who were originally in favor of the idea are now reluctant to leave their workstations. This change phase is called:

   a. Changing
   b. Refreezing
   c. Transition
   d. Unfreezing

5. During remote coding implementation at University Hospital, the problem of how to keep a sense of community among the coders surfaced. The coders decided to create a group for themselves on a popular social media website to keep in touch. This change phase is called:

   a. Beginning
   b. Freezing
   c. Transition
   d. Unfreezing

6. Which of the following behaviors is an early indicator of resistance to change that an employee might exhibit when presented with a new project?

   a. Asking repeated questions during a department meeting about the new project
   b. Missing planning meetings to determine the implementation schedule for the new project
   c. Reading industry articles on the new project to gain knowledge prior to installation
   d. Volunteering to be on an implementation committee for the new project

7. Dr. Jones is the first physician in the practice to adopt the e-prescribing application. He says he likes to try out new technologies and to be a role model for other physicians. Dr. Jones is at what step in the innovation adoption life cycle?

   a. Early adopter
   b. Early majority
   c. Laggard
   d. Late majority

8. Caroline is an evening shift manager in the HIM department. When employees are arguing among themselves, she often delays intervening in the hopes that they will work out their problems and she will not have to get involved. Caroline exhibits which conflict style?

   a. Accommodating
   b. Avoiding
   c. Collaborating
   d. Compromising

9. Jacob is the assistant department head in the HIM department. When the director offers her opinion on how to handle a disciplinary problem, Jacob usually acts on her advice even if he disagrees with it. Jacob exhibits which conflict style?

   a. Accommodating
   b. Avoiding
   c. Collaborating
   d. Compromising

10. Which of the following items on Abigail's to do list is most likely to require a critical conversation?

    a. Ask Thomas to act as a coach for the new scanning clerk scheduled to start next week
    b. Meet with the director for a discussion on whether I should consider going back to school for my master's degree
    c. Tell Patricia she has been selected for promotion to lead transcriptionist to fill the vacancy left when Sara retired
    d. Place Daniel on probation due to continuing problems with decreasing coding productivity and coding accuracy

References

Akdere, M. and B.A. Altman. 2009. An organization development framework in decision making: Implications for practice. *Organization Development Journal* 27(4):47–56.

Amis, J., T. Slack and C.R. Hinings. 2002. Values and organizational change. *The Journal of Applied Behavioral Science* 38(4):436–465.

Appelbaum S.H., S. Habashy, J-L. Malo, and H. Shafiq. 2012. Back to the Future: Revisiting Kotter's 1996 change model. *Journal of Management Development* 31(8):764–782.

Berlin, J.W. 2008. The fundamentals of negotiation. *Canadian Association of Radiologists Journal* 59(1):13–15.

Birken, S.A., S-Y. D. Lee, and B.J. Weiner. 2012. Uncovering middle manager's Role in healthcare innovation implementation. *Implementation Science* 7(4):1–12.

Bjorkman, J.M. 2009. Change Communication: Enabling Individuals to Act. Chapter in *Research in Organizational Change and Development*. Edited by R. Woodman, W. Pasmore, A.B. (Rami) Shani. Bingley, UK: Emerald Group Publishing Limited.

Blanchard, K. 2010. Mastering the art of change: Ken Blanchard offers some strategies for successfully leading change. *Training Journal* 1(1):44–47.

Bodtker, A.M. and J. Katz Jameson. 2001. Emotion in conflict formation and its transformation: Application to organizational conflict management. *International Journal of Conflict Management* 12(3):259.

Boerner, C.M. 2008. Web site will help you explore your compliance culture in terms of Kubler-Ross' five stages of grief and other models. *Journal of Health Care Compliance* 10(2):37–38.

Bolland, E. and F. Fletcher, eds. 2012. *Solutions: Business Problem Solving*. Abingdon, UK: Ashgate Publishing Ltd.

Boston University School of Public Health. 2013. Diffusion of Innovation Theory. http://sphweb.bumc.bu.edu/otlt/MPH-Modules/SB/SB721-Models/SB721-Models4.html.

Brown, J.G. 2012. Empowering students to create and claim value through the Thomas Kilmann Conflict Mode Instrument. *Negotiation Journal* 28(1):79–91.

Business Dictionary. 2015. http://www.businessdictionary.com.

Capstone Encyclopedia of Business. 2003. CapstonePress. Hoboken: Wiley.

Clancy, C. 2014. *Critical Conversations: Scripts and Techniques for Effective Interprofessional and Patient Communication*. Indianapolis: Sigma Theta Tau International.

Cook, K. *The Power of Cooperation: How to Deploy a Contract Wide Task Management System through the Lens of ADKAR* [thesis]. Dominguez Hills, California. California State University; 2013.

Creasey, T. 2009. Defining Change Management: Helping Others Understand Change Management in Relation to Project Management and Organizational Change. http://www.change-management.com/Prosci-Defining-Change-Management-2009.pdf.

Dannar, P.R. 2011. Change starts with the heart: The emotional impact of Lewin's change model. *Strategic Leadership Review* 1(2):46–52.

Darity, W.A., ed. 2008. Lewin, Kurt. *International Encyclopedia of the Social Sciences,* 2nd ed. Vol. 4. Detroit: Macmillan.

Deschmidt, S. and A. Prinzie. 2011. The Organization's Mission Statement: Give Up Hope or Resuscitate? A Search for Evidence-Based Recommendations. Chapter in *Organization Development in Healthcare: Conversations on Research and Strategies*. Edited by J.A. Wolf, M.J. Moir, H. Hanson, L.H. Friedman, G.T. Savage, J. D. Blair, and M.D. Fottler. Bingley, UK: Emerald Group Publishing Limited.

Foley, N. 2013. Change Agents. *Leadership Excellence* 30(4):9.

Ford, J.D. and L.W. Ford. 2009. Resistance to Change: A Reexamination and Extension. Chapter in *Research in Organizational Change and Development*. Edited by R. Woodman, W. Pasmore, A.B. (Rami) Shani. Bingley, UK: Emerald Group Publishing Limited.

Gaboury, I., M. Bujold, H. Boon, and D. Moher. 2009. Interprofessional collaboration within Canadian integrative healthcare clinics: Key components. *Social Science and Medicine* 69(5):707–715.

Garde, S. 2010. Change Management—An overview. Chapter in *Studies in Health Technology and Informatics*. Edited by E.J.S. Hovenga, M.R. Kidd, S. Garde, C. Hullin, and L. Cossio. Amsterdam: IOS Press.

Goes, J. 2011. Achieving Organization Change in Health Care throughout People and Culture: A Commentary. Chapter in *Organization Development in Healthcare: Conversations on Research and Strategies*. Edited by J.A. Wolf, M.J. Moir, H. Hanson, L.H. Friedman, G.T. Savage, J.D. Blair, and M.D. Fottler. Bingley, UK: Emerald Group Publishing Limited.

Gunderman, R.B., and A. Saravanan. 2010. From conflict to collaboration. *Journal of the American College of Radiology* 7(11):831–834.

Kazmi, S., A. Zenab, and M. Naarananoja. 2014. Collection of change management models—An opportunity to make the best choice from the various organizational transformational techniques. *Global Science and Technology Forum Business Review* 3(3):1–14.

Law, J., ed. 2009. Adoption of Innovations. *A Dictionary of Business and Management*. Oxford: Oxford University Press.

Leever, A.M., Hulst, M.V.D., Berendsen, A.J., Boendemaker, P.M., Roodenburg, J.L.N., and J. Pols. 2010. Conflicts and conflict management in the collaboration between nurses and physicians—A qualitative study. *Journal of Interprofessional Care* 24(6):612–624.

Livne-Tarandach, R. and J.M. Bartunek. 2009. A New Horizon for Organizational Change and Development Scholarship: Connecting Planned and Emergent Change. Chapter in *Research in Organizational Change and Development*. Edited by R.W. Woodman, W.A. Pasmore, and A.B. (Rami) Shani. Bingley, UK: Emerald Group Publishing Limited.

Lunenburg F.C. 2010. Managing change: The role of the change agent. *International Journal of Management, Business and Administration* 13(1):2–6.

Manktelow, J. 2015a. Active Listening. Mind Tools.com. http://www.mindtools.com/CommSkll/ActiveListening.htm.

Manktelow, J. 2015b. Bridge's Transition Model. Mind Tools.com. http://www.mindtools.com/pages/article/bridges-transition-model.htm.

Moos, R.H. 1987. Person-environment congruence in work, school, and health care settings. *Journal of Vocational Behavior* 31(3):231–247.

Merriam-Webster. 2015. http://www.merriam-webster.com.

Pearce, D. 2005. How to Manage Inevitable Conflicts. *Presented as a management workshop at Cincinnati Children's Hospital Medical Center*, pp 1–26. Pearce Communications Group, LLC. Cincinnati, OH.

Pellegrin, K.L. and H.S. Currey. 2011. Demystifying and Improving Organizational Culture in Health Care. Chapter in *Organization Development in Healthcare: Conversations on Research and Strategies*. Edited by J.A. Wolf, H. Hanson, M.J. Moir, L. Friedman and G.T. Savage. Bingley, UK: Emerald Group Publishing Limited.

Rahim, M. Afzalur. 2002. Toward a theory of managing organizational conflict. *International Journal of Conflict Management* 13(3):206–235.

Senge, P. 2006. *The Fifth Discipline: The Art and Practice of the Learning Organisation*. London: Random House.

Shirey, M. 2013. Lewin's theory of planned change as a strategic resource. *Journal of Nursing Administration* 43(2):69–72.

Slabbert, A.D. 2004. Conflict management styles in traditional organisations. *The Social Science Journal* 41(1):83–92.

Smaldone, M. and R. Uzzo. 2013. The Kubler-Ross model, physician distress and performance reporting. *Nature Reviews Urology* 10:425–428.

Smith, E.L. 2006. Critical Conversations Made Easy. *E.L. Smith Consulting*. http://elsmithconsulting.com/critical-conversations

Sollenberger, D.K. 2006. Strategic planning healthcare: The experience of the University of Wisconsin Hospital and Clinics. *Frontiers of Health Services Management* 23(2):17–31.

Sportsman, S. and P. Hamilton. 2007. Conflict management styles in the health professions. *Journal of Professional Nursing* 23(3):157–166.

Stonehouse D. 2013. The change agent: The manager's role in change. *British Journal of Healthcare Management* 19(9):443–445.

Strategic Planning. 2014. *Scandinavian Journal of Public Health* 42(14):106–112.

Thompson, R. 2015. Kotter's 8-Step Change Model. http://www.mindtools.com/pages/article/newPPM_82.htm.

Vaughn, P. 2009. Collaboration and conflict management: A brief review of current thought. *The Oklahoma Nurse* 54(3):4.

Vermeulen, F., P. Puranam and R. Gulati. 2010. Change for change's sake. *Harvard Business Review* 88(6):70–76.

Waddell D., T. Cummings , and C. Worley. 2011. *Organisational Change Development and Transformation*, 4th edition. Australia: Cengage Learning.

Way, K.A., N.L. Jimmieson, and P. Bordia. 2014. Supervisor conflict management, justice, and strain: Multilevel relationships. *Journal of Managerial Psych* 29(8):1044–1063.

Wiley, J. 2012. Achieving change through a best practice employee survey. *Strategic HR Review* 11(5):265–271.

Zuckerman, A.M. 2006. Advancing the state of art in healthcare strategic planning. *Frontiers of Health Services Management* 23(2):1–15.

5

Legal Aspects of Healthcare Management

Learning Objectives

- Discuss federal equal employment opportunity legislation
- Discuss key components of the Americans with Disabilities Act
- Evaluate legal practices in relation to interviewing and hiring practices
- Explain the key components of dismissal for cause and due process
- Identify progressive disciplinary action procedures

Key Terms

Age Discrimination in
  Employment Act
  (ADEA)
Americans with
  Disabilities Act
  (ADA)
Arbitration
Bona fide occupational
  qualification (BFOQ)
Civil Rights Act of 1964
Civil Rights Act of 1991
Compensatory damages
Compressed workweek

Consolidated Omnibus
  Budget Reconciliation
  Act (COBRA)
Corrective action plan
Due process
Electronic PHI (ePHI)
Employment-at-will
Equal Employment
  Opportunity
  Commission
  (EEOC)
Fair Labor Standards
  Act (FLSA)

Family and Medical Leave
  Act (FMLA)
Flextime
Health Insurance
  Portability and
  Accountability Act
  (HIPAA)
Hostile work environment
Job sharing
Mediation
Office for Civil Rights
  (OCR)
Policy

Privacy Rule
Procedure
Progressive discipline
Protected health
  information (PHI)
Punitive damages
Quid pro quo
Reasonable
  accommodation
Retaliation
Security Rule
Sexual harassment
Undue hardship

Understanding the laws that affect the workplace is the responsibility of each health information management (HIM) manager. Traditionally, most organizations operated under the employment-at-will concept. **Employment-at-will** means that employees can be fired at any time and for almost any reason based on the idea that, in turn, employees can quit at any time and for almost any reason. Over time, aspects of the employment-at-will concept led to discriminatory practices by employers: companies would not hire persons of a particular religion or nationality, and persons were fired for non–work-related reasons such as refusing sexual advances or developing a disability. Consequently, federal legislation was passed to prohibit such discrimination. The employment-at-will concept remains the principle by which most organizations operate, however, regulation modified the concept to say that an employer cannot terminate an employee for a reason the law says is illegal. The resulting laws and implications for healthcare management are intended to promote fairness and equity in the workplace.

This chapter discusses major laws impacting the US workforce and the implications the laws have on interviewing, counseling, and progressive discipline practices in the healthcare workplace. Many provisions of the laws overlap one another. What is prohibited under one law may also be prohibited by other laws. Knowledge of employment law allows a manager to act with confidence and assurance, but should never be a substitute for advice and recommendation from a human resources (HR) department or legal counsel. When in doubt as to how to proceed on any legal matter in the workplace, consulting with an expert in employment law is the first step to take in making a decision. Enforcement of many employment laws is handled by the US **Equal Employment Opportunity Commission (EEOC)**. The Equal Employment Opportunity Commission is a federal agency with the authority to investigate discrimination claims, render decisions, and file lawsuits if necessary. The EEOC works to prevent discrimination through training and education on employment laws. All HIM managers should be familiar with the EEOC website and publications as well as their own organization's internal policies and procedures in regards to employment law.

Employment Laws Impacting Healthcare

Each of the following laws listed is a result of federal legislation. Some states enacted their own similar laws, but unless the state laws are more stringent, the federal laws take precedence. The Americans with Disabilities Act, the Civil Rights Acts, and the Age Discrimination in Employment Act all address employee discrimination. The Family and Medical Leave Act, Fair Labor Standards Act, Health Insurance Portability and Accountability Act, and the Consolidated Omnibus Budget Reconciliation Act deal with wage and benefit regulation.

Americans with Disabilities Act

The **Americans with Disabilities Act (ADA)** passed in 1990. The act was amended in 2008 with passage of the Americans with Disabilities Act Amendment Act (ADAAA). The ADA prohibits job discrimination against people with disabilities. According to the ADA, a disability is defined as "a physical or mental impairment that substantially limits one or more major life activities" (ADA 1990). To be covered under the law, an individual must currently have the impairment, have a record of the impairment, or have been affected by an action that is outlawed by the ADA because another person perceived them as having the impairment. In addition, the impairment must be either long term (lasting for six months or more) or permanent.

The definition also addresses the fact that the impairment must limit one or more major life activity. A major life activity includes, but is not limited to "caring for oneself, performing manual tasks, seeing, hearing, eating, sleeping, walking, standing, lifting, bending, speaking, breathing, learning, reading, concentrating, thinking, communicating, and working" (ADA 1990). Being confined to a wheelchair would be an impairment of the major life activity of walking, but wearing glasses for near-sightedness would not be considered to be an impairment of the major activity of seeing.

In order to be protected in the workplace by the ADA, an individual must have a disability as previously defined, and also be able to meet the job requirements of a position with respect to the necessary educational background, skills, licenses, and employment experience. An individual must be able to perform the basic job duties of a position with or without **reasonable accommodation**. Accommodation in this case means a change or adjustment to a work environment that allows a disabled employee to perform basic job duties (ADA 1990). Reasonable accommodation means the adjustment cannot place an **undue hardship** on the employer. In other words, the accommodation cannot be too disruptive or expensive for the employer to implement (ADA 1990). The concept of an undue hardship will vary among employers. An accommodation that is too expensive to implement for a small physician practice may not be too expensive for a large healthcare system. Examples of reasonable accommodations are:

- Job restructuring
- Part-time or modified work schedules
- Acquisition or modification of equipment or devices
- Adjustment or modification of examinations, training materials or policies
- Provision of qualified readers or interpreters (ADA 1990)

In most cases, identification of a reasonable accommodation will come from the impaired employee as they have the knowledge and experience to determine what accommodations will work best. If a reasonable accommodation is not readily apparent, a manager may ask an employee for suggestions as to what might assist the employee in performing the basic job duties required of a position.

The ADA prohibits discrimination against not only individuals with disabilities, but also prohibits discrimination against individuals because of a family, business, or social relationship with someone who has a disability (EEOC 2015a). Discrimination covers the following employment practices:

- Recruitment
- Pay
- Hiring
- Firing
- Promotion
- Job assignments
- Training
- Leave
- Lay-off
- Benefits (EEOC 2015a)

The ADA prohibits an employer from not hiring an applicant solely on the basis of his or her disability. To be clear, the ADA does not require an employer to hire someone with a disability over other qualified applicants. An employer should still hire the person most suited for the position. Enforcement of the ADA is provided by the EEOC.

Civil Rights Act of 1964

The **Civil Rights Act of 1964** is an antidiscrimination law that prohibits employment discrimination because of race, color, religion, sex, or national origin. Discrimination is not allowed in hiring, promotion, termination, compensation, training, benefits, or other privileges of employment (Title VII, Civil Rights Act 1964). Each of the elements of the Civil Rights Act of 1964 are further defined.

Race and Color

Race and color may appear to be the same thing, but according to the Civil Rights Act of 1964 they are different. Discrimination based on race includes skin color as well as other race-related characteristics such as hair texture or facial features. Skin color can vary among members of the same or different races or ethnicities. Discrimination is not allowed on the basis of the lightness or darkness of skin tone.

National Origin

National origin refers to the ancestry, birthplace, culture, or language characteristics of an individual. Language characteristics include accents and English-fluency. Accents and fluency may be considered in hiring practices if they interfere with job performance. For example, an accent may not affect the job performance of a clinical data analyst, but English-fluency may impact the job performance of an HIM professional hired by a vendor to give product demonstrations or provide customer training.

Sex

Discrimination on the basis of sex refers to gender, and is expanded to include pregnancy in women. Discrimination may not occur based on pregnancy, childbirth, or related obstetrical medical conditions. Discrimination on the basis of sexual orientation is not specifically covered by the Civil Rights Act of 1964. Laws regarding sexual-orientation discrimination are passed at the state and local levels of government.

Sexual harassment is also considered a type of sex discrimination. The EEOC defines sexual harassment as unwelcome sexual advances, requests for sexual favors, and other verbal or physical conduct of a sexual nature when:

- Submission to such conduct is made, either explicitly or implicitly, a term or condition of an individual's employment
- Submission to or rejection of such conduct by an individual is used as the basis for employment decisions affecting such an individual
- Such conduct has the purpose or effect of unreasonably interfering with an individual's work performance or creating an intimidating, hostile, or offensive working environment (EEOC 2014)

One type of sexual harassment is **quid pro quo**. Quid pro quo is about one person using their authority over another to demand some kind of sexual favor in return for job actions such as promotion, hiring, or continued employment. A supervisor may tell an employee that a promotion or pay raise is contingent on them dating or the employee performing sexual favors for the supervisor. Sexual harassment can occur between individuals of the same or opposite sex. The second type of sexual harassment is creation of a **hostile work environment**. This example of sexual harassment is less obvious than quid pro quo. A hostile work environment occurs when one employee's behavior is interpreted as being offensive by another employee. A hostile work environment may include unwanted touching, unwelcome jokes, language, emails, or texts. It may include sexually explicit pictures posted or circulated in the workplace. In general, there must be a pattern of unwelcome actions. A co-worker who makes one lewd comment about another is not perceived by most reasonable people as creating a hostile work environment. However, making continued comments, especially after being asked to stop, could result in a charge of sexual harassment.

A manager must be aware of the possibility of sexual harassment charges being made in the workplace. Any charge of sexual harassment must be taken seriously and investigated. The definition identifies three areas of consideration for a manager to use when trying to determine if sexual harassment has occurred: (1) the actions must be unwelcome, or uninvited; (2) the actions must be severe enough to interfere with the employee's performance; and (3) whether or not the employer knew, or should have known, about the actions. Managers must also be aware that harassment may occur on social media sites. An organization may be held liable for charges of sexual harassment if the employer knows of the action on social media, or if the harassing is being done on employer-owned devices (EEOC 2014).

The EEOC published guidelines for preventive and remedial action relating to sexual harassment. An effective preventive program should include an explicit policy against sexual harassment that is clearly and regularly communicated to all employees (EEOC 1990). The policy should detail a procedure for all employees to follow when reporting harassing behavior and be clear about the punishments for harassing behaviors. Corrective action should be prompt and thorough, following policies and procedures. The intent of the corrective action should be to stop the harassment, make appropriate amends to the victim, and prevent the behavior from recurring. Any punitive action should match the seriousness of the offense. For example, a series of off-color remarks may result in a formal reprimand and an apology, while a more serious offense may result in discharge of the offender and restoration of lost pay to the victim. Finally, the concept of harassment does not only apply to sexual harassment, but extends to behavior in cases of race, color, national origin, religion, and disability.

Religion

Religious discrimination refers to a person's religious beliefs, or lack of religious beliefs. In addition, the law requires employers to provide reasonable accommodation for religious practices. Examples of reasonable accommodations might be flexible scheduling to allow for time off for religious holidays, providing a place to pray, or accepting religious dress or grooming practices. Accommodations for dress or grooming might not be possible due to safety considerations in the workplace. For example, long hair, facial hair, footwear, or headdress may be a safety issue in certain environments where a sterile field is necessary or machinery is used. A manager should work with the employee to determine if an acceptable accommodation exists.

Retaliation

The Civil Rights Act of 1964 prohibits workplace discrimination against employees and applicants based on their race, color, sex, religion, or national origin. The law also prohibits discrimination against individuals because of their marriage or association with someone of a particular race, color, national origin, sex, or religion. The Civil Rights Act of 1964 protects an employee or applicant against **retaliation**. This means that if a person complains to their employer, files a claim of discrimination, or participates in an investigation of their employer charged with discrimination, the person cannot be fired, demoted, or otherwise penalized for their actions. An employee cannot have his or her pay cut, job reassigned, benefits reduced, or not be promoted because he or she made a charge of discrimination. Likewise, an applicant cannot be refused employment for the same reason. Enforcement of charges of discrimination and harassment are provided by the EEOC (Title VII, Civil Rights Act of 1964).

Civil Rights Act of 1991

The **Civil Rights Act of 1991** upholds and strengthens the Civil Rights Act of 1964. Under the 1964 law, an employee has the right to make a claim for discrimination against his or her employer. The EEOC then investigates the claim and makes a decision. If discrimination is found to have occurred, depending on the charge, the employee could receive back pay, be reinstated, or awarded a promotion. The Civil Rights Act of 1991 takes possible actions by the employee farther, by allowing for jury trials and increased monetary awards for employees. Employees may now receive **compensatory damages** for discriminatory actions against them. Compensatory damages cover the actual financial loss of the employee and could cover repayment for lost time off work or payment for medical bills. **Punitive damages** may also be awarded to the employee as a way to further punish the employer and prevent the employer's discriminatory behavior from continuing. It is important that the punitive damages are large enough to deter the employer from allowing the discriminatory behavior to continue. The employer may decide to implement sexual harassment training or start a diversity program to correct discriminatory practices in the organization.

Age Discrimination in Employment Act of 1967

The **Age Discrimination in Employment Act (ADEA)** prohibits discrimination on the basis of age against individuals age 40 and older. Interestingly, the ADEA permits employers to favor older workers based on age even when doing so adversely affects a younger worker who is 40 or older (EEOC 2008). In other words, a 47-year-old employee cannot claim that they were discriminated against on the basis of age if a 53-year-old employee was favored in a hiring or promotion situation. Because benefit costs increase with age, companies were reducing or even eliminating benefits, resulting in a disincentive to hire older workers. An amendment to the ADEA stopped this practice, and now organizations must offer equal benefits to employees of all ages. Enforcement of the ADEA is provided by the EEOC.

The ADEA also affects retirement issues. Mandatory retirement was required at age 65, but the ADEA raised the age to 70; and an amendment to the ADEA in 1986 removed a mandatory retirement age altogether as long as long as a person is able to do the job. Because of certain job requirements, some professions such as police officers and firefighters are allowed to mandate retirement by a certain age. This is an important issue for HIM managers to understand, because if job performance suffers in an older worker, a manager must be careful to separate the job performance from the age so as to avoid a claim of discrimination. Older workers are sometimes offered early retirement incentives. In these instances, employees are usually asked to sign a waiver that prohibits them from filing a claim under the ADEA. The ADEA offers protection to employees by publishing minimum requirements that state such waivers must:

- Be in writing and be understandable
- Specifically refer to ADEA rights or claims
- Not waive rights or claims that may arise in the future

- Be in exchange for valuable consideration in addition to anything of value to which the individual already is entitled
- Advise the individual in writing to consult an attorney before signing the waiver
- Provide the individual at least 21 days to consider the agreement and at least seven days to revoke the agreement after signing it (EEOC 2008)

Similar to the antidiscrimination laws already covered, employees age 40 and older are also protected against retaliation should they make a claim of discrimination.

Family and Medical Leave Act of 1993

The **Family and Medical Leave Act (FMLA)** allows employees to take unpaid time off work for specific family and medical reasons that include the following:

- The birth of a son or daughter or placement of a son or daughter with the employee for adoption or foster care
- To care for a spouse, son, daughter, or parent who has a serious health condition
- For a serious health condition that makes the employee unable to perform the essential functions of his or her job
- For any qualifying exigency arising out of the fact that a spouse, son, daughter, or parent is a military member on covered active duty or call to covered active duty status. (DOL 2012)

An employee is eligible for this benefit if they have worked for their employer for at least 12 months and have worked at least 1,250 hours during the previous 12 months. An employee may take up to 12 weeks of unpaid leave during a 12-month period. Under some circumstances, such as for a planned medical treatment, an employee may take the leave on an intermittent basis rather than in consecutive weeks. This may have the effect of extending the 12-week period. Some organizations choose to offer paid leave, but this is not mandatory. More frequently, the organizations require employees to use their accrued sick, vacation, or other paid time as part of the leave. An employee must continue to receive healthcare coverage, but does not have to continue to accrue paid time off while on leave.

Another provision of the FMLA is that upon return to work, "an employee must be restored to his or her original job or to an equivalent job with equivalent pay, benefits, and other terms and conditions of employment" (DOL 2012). In other words, an HIM supervisor taking an FMLA leave to have a baby cannot be placed in a document imaging position upon her return. In most cases she will return to work as a supervisor, as few other HIM department jobs match the terms and conditions of a supervisory position. For an HIM manager, this means that any position held by an employee taking an FMLA leave must simultaneously be covered and kept open for up to 12 weeks. A manager may have to hire and train a temporary person, use overtime, or leave the position vacant for the duration of the leave. The Wage and Hour Division of the United States Department of Labor oversees the FMLA, but some states have enacted their own family and medical leave laws. In the case where a state has its own law, the more stringent of the two laws takes precedence. An HIM manager should work with the human resources department so the correct laws are followed.

Fair Labor Standards Act

The **Fair Labor Standards Act (FLSA)** is more commonly known as the wage and hour law. The FLSA is a federal law, and is the basis for many state wage and hour laws. When the FLSA conflicts with a state law, the more stringent law applies and is administered by the Wage and Hour Division of the United States Department of Labor. The intent of the FLSA is to determine minimum wage and overtime pay rules as well as definition of a work week. While wage and hours worked are monitored closely by HR and payroll departments, it is important that HIM managers have a familiarity with the legal requirements.

The FLSA defines those categories of employees that are exempt and nonexempt from overtime pay. For example, some executive, administrative, and professional positions, including some nursing positions, are exempt from or do not receive overtime pay. Nonexempt employees do receive overtime pay. Overtime pay is currently defined as time and one-half the regular rate of pay for all hours worked over 40 hours in a workweek (FLSA 2011). This means that a nonexempt employee earning 20 dollars per hour would be paid 30 dollars per hour in an overtime situation.

Overtime pay also becomes an issue for a manager when working with flexible scheduling. A manager must be aware of overtime regulations when using compressed workweeks, flextime, or job sharing. A **compressed workweek** is a work schedule that permits a full-time job to be completed in less than the standard five days of eight-hour shifts. A common example of a compressed workweek is 4/40 or working four 10-hour days, which equals 40 hours per week. **Flextime** is a work schedule that gives employees some choice in the pattern of their work hours, usually around a core of midday hours. Generally, there are specific hours that must be worked during the day, and as long as these hours are covered, the start and end times are flexible. For example, an HIM department might experience 80 percent of their walk-up customers between the hours of 9:00 a.m. and 2:00 p.m. An HIM department receptionist might choose to work 7:00 a.m. to 3:30 p.m. three days a week and 8:00 a.m. to 4:30 p.m. two days a week, allowing her to be present during the core hours of 9:00 a.m. to 2:00 p.m. and accommodate her children's after-school practice schedules. **Job sharing** is a work schedule in which two or more individuals share the tasks of one full-time or one full-time-equivalent position. One EHR implementation specialist may work 7:00 a.m. to 11:00 a.m. each day and the second EHR implementation specialist works 1:00 p.m. to 5:00 p.m. later in the same day. They do the same job, share the same desk, and are available to increase their hours to cover for extended illnesses or vacations. All of these flexible scheduling options have the potential for employees to work more than eight hours in a day or more than 40 hours in a week. Therefore, managers must be aware of overtime rules and regulations.

Health Insurance Portability and Accountability Act of 1996

The **Health Insurance Portability and Accountability Act (HIPAA)** impacts the healthcare workplace in different ways. HIPAA is federal legislation enacted to provide continuity of health coverage, control fraud and abuse in healthcare, reduce healthcare costs, and guarantee the security and privacy of health information. HIPAA limits exclusion from health coverage for pre-existing medical conditions, prohibits discrimination against employees and dependents based on health status, guarantees availability of health insurance to small employers, and guarantees renewability of insurance to all employees regardless of the size of the organization.

Most HIM professionals are familiar with HIPAA from the privacy and security perspective. The HIM department is usually the department within an organization charged with the responsibility of safeguarding and releasing patient information. However, an HIM manager must also be aware of the aspects of HIPAA as it pertains to employee actions in the HIM department. Title II of HIPAA, Preventing Health Care Fraud and Abuse, Administrative Simplification, and Medical Liability Reform, details the **Privacy Rule**. The Privacy Rule requires that a patient's **protected health information (PHI)** be made available only to the providers that have a proven need for access. PHI is individually identifiable health information and contains a piece of information such as patient name, address, phone number, or Social Security number that allows the patient to be identified. The most familiar understanding of PHI is that it applies to patient records, but PHI also applies to employee health records. Employee health records might consist of documentation of medical conditions, medical claims receipts, or employment physicals. Unauthorized release of PHI by an organization can result in legal action and fines. Consequently, an organization must provide HIPAA awareness training to all employees and implement policies and procedures that prevent privacy breaches. Disciplinary action taken in the case of a privacy breach must be clear and disseminated to all employees. An HIM manager works to ensure that both orientation training is taking place and that annual HIPAA update training is done within a healthcare organization. Policies and procedures must be in place and updated annually, and appropriate disciplinary action must be carried out for privacy violations.

HIPAA Title II also covers the **Security Rule**. The Security Rule is similar to the Privacy Rule in that it applies to PHI, but the Security Rule is different in that it applies to PHI only in an electronic form. The Security Rule maintains that employees who need access to **electronic PHI (ePHI)** must be granted access, but employees who do not need access must be prevented from accessing the PHI. In an electronic environment, a manager must decide the level of ePHI authorization for each position in the department. Does a coder need the same level of access as a scanning clerk? Does a data analyst need the same access as a supervisor? The answers will depend on the individual job descriptions, which should address the need for access to ePHI. Security awareness training must be done, and policies and procedures unique to electronic access must be developed. Policies and procedures for changing passwords, computer virus detection, and log-in attempts are examples of what must be covered.

HIPAA also addresses the issues of employee health insurance portability and accountability by allowing employees to move from one job to another without losing insurance coverage or being penalized for pre-existing medical conditions. The intent of the law is that health insurance coverage continues without a waiting period when an individual leaves one employer for another. In addition, an employer cannot deny coverage of a pre-existing medical condition to a new employee who was covered by health insurance at their previous employer. In most cases, such benefits are managed by the HR department in conjunction with the insurance carrier. Enforcement of HIPAA is covered by the **Office for Civil Rights (OCR)**, an agency of the Department of Health and Human Services.

Consolidated Omnibus Budget Reconciliation Act

The **Consolidated Omnibus Budget Reconciliation Act (COBRA)** affects employment practice because it offers continuing health insurance coverage for qualifying employees that have lost healthcare coverage. If an organization offers a group health insurance plan and an employee leaves the organization, the employee is given the opportunity by the organization to continue health insurance coverage. The employee must assume payment for the insurance premium, but does so at the organization's group rate. Generally, the cost of the group plan rate is much less than if the employee tried to secure health insurance coverage on the open market.

There are considerations when dealing with COBRA. An employee must qualify for this benefit, it is not automatically applied. An employee qualifies for COBRA benefits due to any of the following events: voluntary or involuntary job loss (for other than gross misconduct), reduction in the hours worked, transition between jobs, death, divorce, or the employee becomes entitled to Medicare coverage (COBRA 1986). There is also a time limit on how long an employee can receive COBRA benefits. In most cases, an employee may receive COBRA benefits for up to 18 months from the time they qualify, but special qualifying events such as eligibility for Medicare coverage may extend benefits to 36 months. An employer may elect to continue coverage for longer than the law requires. In most cases, the human resources department is responsible for notifying employees of their rights under COBRA. However, an HIM manager should be aware of COBRA rules, and how they are applied at an organization. Due to the specific nature of COBRA, many organizations do not want managers to discuss COBRA benefits directly with employees in case wrong information is communicated. If employees have questions, a manager should refer the employee to the HR department or, at the very least, have an HR representative present during the discussion. Similar to the Fair Labor Standards Act and the Family and Medical Leave Act, COBRA is overseen by the Department of Labor.

Check Your **Understanding**

1. Discuss why it is important for an HIM manager to have an understanding of employment laws.
2. Explain the role of the EEOC in regards to employment laws.
3. What are some reasonable accommodations that might be made in the workplace for disabled workers?
4. Explain the difference between HIPAA and COBRA when providing continuing health insurance coverage for employees.
5. Explain the two different types of sexual harassment.
6. How does the Civil Rights Act of 1991 strengthen the provisions of the Civil Rights Act of 1964?

Applying Equal Employment Opportunity Principles to Health Information Management

Once an HIM manager has an understanding of employment laws, the next step is to use the knowledge to develop sound management practices and implement in day-to-day duties. The laws have a great impact on the interviewing, personnel policies, counseling, and progressive discipline. Interviewing and personnel policies were introduced in chapter 2 and are discussed in more detail in chapter 7, but these topics are discussed from a legal standpoint in this chapter.

Personnel Polices

All employment laws and their corresponding guidelines should be detailed in an organization's policy and procedure manual. A **policy** is a governing principle that describes how a department or an organization is supposed to handle a specific situation or execute a specific process. In the case of employment law, there should be a policy covering the law itself and additional policies to cover aspects of the law that will need to be handled appropriately. For example, there should be a policy in place that addresses discrimination in the workplace and also a policy specific to sexual harassment as an aspect of sex discrimination. A **procedure** details the steps taken to implement a policy. A policy addressing sexual harassment should further detail the procedures, or steps, an employee would take in order to report an incident of sexual harassment, the steps that should be taken by the person responsible for investigating a claim of sexual harassment, and procedures detailing the corrective action that must be taken once a claim has been investigated.

Policy and procedure manuals are usually developed by the HR department in conjunction with attorneys specializing in employment law. The manuals should be made available to all employees, at every level in the organization. Hard copy manuals should be placed in each department or work station where they are easily accessible by all employees. Many organizations publish their policy and procedure manual in a secure location on the organization's website or intranet.

Interviewing

As noted previously, there are laws that prohibit discrimination on the basis of race, color, religion, gender, national origin, and disability. It is therefore illegal for an employer to try and determine the presence (or absence) of any of these in the pre-interview or interview phases of employment. In most cases, this applies to the interview process. There are certain topics that are off limits during an interview unless they are a **bona fide occupational qualification (BFOQ)**. A BFOQ is a job requirement that in most jobs would be illegal to discuss, but in specific jobs is a necessity. The most common examples of BFOQs are a men's room attendant or a female swimsuit model. In both cases, the gender of the person directly relates to the ability of the person to do the job, so screening out women for a men's room attendant or men for a female swimsuit model is not illegal. Certain HIM jobs would appear to have BFOQs. A completely deaf person may not be able to be a transcriptionist, although a blind person could do the job. Likewise, a completely blind person may not be able to be a data quality specialist, but a deaf person could do the job. Listed are areas that should be avoided in a job interview. A sample of inappropriate questions is offered in table 5.1 (on the next page), but is by no means a complete list.

A manager cannot ask inappropriate questions of an applicant, and a manager cannot use inappropriate information gathered in an interview to make a hiring decision. Sometimes an applicant may offer the information, unsolicited, in an interview. An applicant may be nervous or excited and volunteer that they are a single parent, or a cancer survivor, from a certain country, or practice a specific religion. Despite the fact that the information is now known, a manager cannot use the information when deciding which applicant to hire. The list of inappropriate questions can be very long, and it can be intimidating to a new manager who might be worried about asking the wrong type of question and opening up their employer for a discrimination lawsuit. It is good practice to work with a representative from the HR department to develop a list of questions that are approved for use in an interview. The manager then uses this list for each applicant, asking the same questions of everyone. This standardization supports antidiscrimination behavior since all candidates are treated equally. In addition, a manager is not tempted to ask a potentially discriminatory question when there is an approved list of questions from which to choose.

Social media is a constant in today's work environment. Many organizations use social media to post job advertisements and recruit candidates. However, "the improper use of information obtained from social media sites may be discriminatory since most individuals' race, gender, general age, and possibly ethnicity can be discerned from information on these sites" (EEOC 2014). If an organization decides to use social media for background checks, it is advisable to have a third party who has no part in the hiring decision capture only the appropriate information and present it for review. Only public information should be gathered, and an applicant should not be asked for passwords or user names to their social media sites. In fact, it is illegal in some states to request password information from applicants, so a manager must go beyond EEOC guidelines and know state laws as well. Again, consulting with the HR department should help an HIM manager to make the right decision as to whether or not to use social media as part of the interview process.

Table 5.1. Sample inappropriate questions for job interviews

Topic	Inappropriate Question
Age	How old are you? What is your birthdate? When did you graduate from high school? College? When do you plan on retiring?
Religion	Do you regularly attend church? Which one? Do your parents, spouse, or other family members attend church? Do you observe any religious holidays?
National origin	Are you a naturalized or native-born citizen of the United States? Are your parents or spouse naturalized or native-born citizens of the United States? Where were you born? You have an interesting name, where is it from? What kind of accent is that? Where did you learn to speak English? Do you belong to any special clubs, organizations, or groups? You may not ask if an applicant is a citizen of the United States, but you may ask if they have the legal right to work in the United States. You cannot ask about their country of origin.
Marital status	Are you married? Divorced? Separated? Widowed? What is your spouse's name? I see the diamond on your finger, are you engaged? Will you be getting married soon? Do you plan to have children? Does your spouse's job require you to move a lot? Will your spouse be able to help with child care issues? Will your spouse be upset if you are required to work overtime or weekends or holidays? Whom should we notify in case of an emergency?
Children	Do you have children? How many? What are their names? How old are they? Do you have reliable child care?
Height or weight	How tall are you? How much do you weigh?
Worker's compensation	Have you ever had a job-related injury? Have you ever filed a workers' compensation claim? Have you ever received payment for a workers' compensation claim? Has any member of your family ever had a work-related injury? Filed a workers' compensation claim? Received payment for a workers' compensation claim?
Arrest record	Have you ever been arrested? This is different from asking if a person has ever been convicted of a crime, which is allowed.
Military	In what branch of the military did you serve? What type of discharge did you receive? What were the circumstances surrounding your discharge?
Disability	Do you have any current medical conditions? Have you ever been treated for cancer, epilepsy, AIDS, diabetes, high blood pressure, drug or alcohol abuse, mental illness? Does any member of your family have a current medical condition, or been treated for cancer, epilepsy, AIDS, diabetes, high blood pressure, drug or alcohol abuse, mental illness? Are you or any member of you family disabled? It is allowed to ask an applicant if they are able to perform specific functions of a job with or without accommodation. In fact, it is allowed to request that an applicant demonstrate their ability to perform a job function, as long as all applicants are asked to do the same.

Counseling

For some new (or even seasoned) managers, employee counseling sessions are looked at in the same way as interviews: managers are nervous they will say something wrong or against the law. Despite these negative concerns, counseling is one management task that all managers have in common. Counseling is done for many reasons:

- Heading off potential behavior issues
- Addressing declining performance
- Giving career advice
- Training
- Praising and encouraging
- Coaching or mentoring

Regardless of the reason for the counseling, common techniques exist to keep the HIM manager focused on the intent of the counseling session. All counseling should be done in private and, if at all possible, an appointment should be made so that both the manager and employee know to expect a discussion. It is very stressful to an employee for a manager to approach with a request to "step into my office." It is very frustrating to a manager to have an employee appear at the office door five minutes before leaving for a meeting and saying "I have something I need to talk to you about." It is better practice to arrange a time to talk and to give the employee a brief idea of what will transpire. For example, "Let's meet at 3:00 this afternoon to go over the training schedule I created for you," or "I have to leave for a meeting now, can we talk at 10:30?"

Any counseling session should stick to the topic at hand. If there is a behavior problem, be specific about what happened and clearly state how the behavior needs to change. If the meeting is to address declining performance, probe for an underlying cause such as inadequate training or a personal problem that might be distracting the employee from his or her work. Be careful not to get involved in personal problems. Any personal problems should be referred to an appropriate professional or an employee assistance program. Managers are in place to see that the work of the organization gets accomplished, not to solve personal problems for employees. Stick to the facts of the matter. It is fine to for a manager to admit that they will need to research a question that they do not know the answer to, but it is important to respond promptly to the employee with the answer. Behavior and performance issues should be dealt with immediately so they do not get out of hand. Sometimes managers are reluctant to discuss negative issues with employees, but if it is done as soon as a problem arises it is much easier to put it in perspective, handle it, and move on, rather than let the problem continue until it becomes more serious and needs stronger intervention. Finally, regardless of the reason for the counseling, a brief anecdotal note should be written and placed in the employee's department file. This helps the manager to track problems and be reminded of previous conversations.

Progressive Discipline

In some cases, counseling is done as part of disciplinary action. Discipline is a necessary, if difficult, part of an HIM manager's position. Even when expectations have been made clear, some employees fall short and need to be reminded of their responsibilities to their position and to the organization. The need to discipline an employee for an infraction is not something most managers enjoy, but putting it off only makes the situation worse, as violations can continue to build. In addition, when poor behavior is allowed to continue, it negatively affects the morale of the employees who witness the behavior and see that no action is taken. Most organizations use some form of **progressive discipline** to correct unwanted behavior, meaning that the first few infractions are treated with less severity than later infractions. The discipline methods progress in severity as the same offenses recur or offenses become more severe in nature. Despite the negative connotation associated with discipline, the intent of the process is to help the employee correct the behavior and improve. Progressive discipline steps differ among organizations, but common steps are displayed in figure 5.1 and detailed as follows.

A verbal warning is the first step. As soon as possible after the infraction, the manager should schedule a time to privately discuss the behavior with the employee. At this time, it should be made clear what the expected behavior was, what the incorrect behavior was, and what the consequences of the incorrect behavior are, as well as consequences of continued incorrect behavior. The employee should be given an opportunity to explain his or her behavior and also verbalize understanding of the possible consequences. A **corrective action plan** can be developed with both the manager and employee offering suggestions for improvement. A corrective action plan is a written plan of action to be taken in response to identified issues. For example, after discussion with the employee, a manager determines that the majority of an employee's repeated absences are due to having to care for sick children.

Figure 5.1. Typical progressive disciplinary process steps

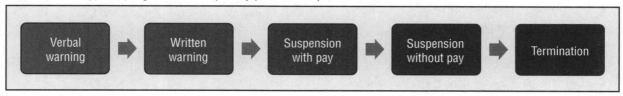

The manager and employee work together to develop a written corrective action plan that results in the employee asking her spouse to begin to take time off from work to help with sick children. The employee and her spouse will work to trade off absences so that their children are cared for when they are sick. Another option might be for the employee to investigate the possibility of using a daycare provider that specifically cares for sick children. The details of the verbal warning should be documented in writing, signed and dated by both the employee and the supervisor, and placed in the employee's department file. Sometimes an employee will refuse to sign a warning document. An employee's signature does not necessarily mean they agree with the verbal warning, but indicates that they were present at the meeting. If the employee still refuses to sign the document, the supervisor should write "employee refused to sign" in the signature space. Generally, the verbal warning is not forwarded to the HR department, but some organizations may request that this be done.

If the corrective action is not successful and the behavior continues a written warning is the next step. The same procedure is followed as for a verbal warning, but this time the written document is forwarded to the HR department. Some organizations also provide the employee with his or her own copy of the written warning. At this time employees are also warned that repeated behavior will lead to further disciplinary action, up to and including termination.

After the written warning, progressive steps are suspension (with or without pay) and, finally, termination. For each of these steps, employee meetings should follow the basic procedures as the verbal and written warning sessions. Once behavior has escalated to the point of suspension from work, it is advisable to have a representative from the HR department or another manager present when discussing this with the employee. If a representative from HR is not available, an HIM manager should review the suspension and termination procedures carefully with someone from HR prior to scheduling the meeting with the employee.

In all cases, discipline should be handled fairly and honestly, but it is possible that the progressive discipline process will not be followed in exactly the same way for each infraction. For example, an employee may have trouble with tardiness, but after a verbal warning adheres to the time and attendance policy for a year, at which time they lapse and are repeatedly tardy again. Since the employee received a verbal warning a year ago, the next step would be a written warning; however, the supervisor may decide to repeat the verbal warning step instead. Another example may be a more serious infraction, such as employee insubordination, in which case the verbal warning may be skipped and a written warning becomes the first step. An organization's policy and procedure manual should list possible infractions and their resulting disciplinary action. In addition, the previously discussed laws must be taken into consideration so that a manager does not appear to be acting in a discriminatory manner.

Termination for Cause and Due Process

Termination (or dismissal) for cause is generally the last step in the progressive discipline process. This occurs when an employee has been taken through the progressive process, but behavior has not changed enough to warrant continued employment. Termination at this point should not be a surprise to the employee, as the documentation should have been clear that termination was the final step.

Termination for cause can also be used for immediate dismissal. In this case, the progressive discipline steps are not implemented. An HIM manager who believes that they have an immediate termination for cause situation should contact the HR department for guidance. In most cases, an employee will be suspended (with or without pay) so that the situation may be investigated. This also allows all parties to gain some distance from the situation; it provides a cooling off period. Reasons for immediate termination for cause vary from one institution to another. Some examples are:

- Abuse of a patient, resident, or another employee
- Falsification of health records
- Falsification of employee records
- Theft
- HIPAA violation of patient privacy
- Use of illegal drugs or alcohol while on the job
- Carrying a weapon while on the job

In all cases, a thorough investigation must be carried out with documentation occurring along the way so there is no question as to the appropriateness of a termination. The HR department must be involved so there is a third party making sure all procedures are correctly followed and no discrimination occurred. However, in most organizations, an employee has the right to **due process** in a termination decision or any progressive discipline measure. Due process means that the employee has the right to make sure their disciplinary action was carried out in accordance with the organization's policies and procedures. Employees should be able to file a grievance or ask for an investigation without the threat of retaliation. As with the other policies and procedures, this process should be covered in the organization's policy and procedure manual. There are many different grievance processes, but the general steps are listed in figure 5.2 and include the following.

- A grievance is generally brought by the employee to the attention of their supervisor. Here, the intent is to resolve the problem informally. However, sometimes the problem involves the supervisor, so an unbiased resolution might not be possible as the employee would feel that they will not get a fair hearing. In such cases, the next-level supervisor becomes the first step in the process.

- If the first or subsequent steps fail, the grievance is then taken up the line to a department head or even to the vice president level. At each step the documentation is reviewed and facts are gathered to support the decision to either uphold or overturn the disciplinary action. Again, the intent is that resolution of the problem can occur at this level.

- The next step is to involve the HR department. Generally, there are individuals or a committee appointed to hear the grievance and make a final recommendation. These individuals are outside the affected department and provide a neutral third party review.

- In extreme cases, an employee has the right to go outside the organization and file a complaint with the EEOC or the appropriate state division of human rights. The EEOC has the power to investigate claims under their jurisdiction (ADA, Civil Rights Act) and even to call for a jury trial if necessary.

Any grievance should be handled fairly and objectively. In addition, a prompt decision at each level lets an employee know that their grievance was considered and acted on in a reasonable time frame. Neglecting a grievance or taking

Figure 5.2. Employee grievance process steps

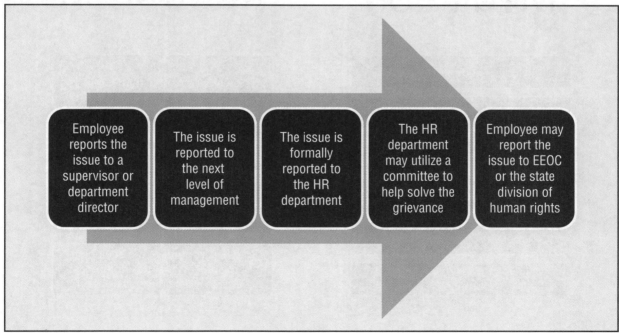

Employee reports the issue to a supervisor or department director

The issue is reported to the next level of management

The issue is formally reported to the HR department

The HR department may utilize a committee to help solve the grievance

Employee may report the issue to EEOC or the state division of human rights too long to answer leads to the creation of hard feelings, if they are not already present. There are alternatives to the grievance process. An organization may offer or an employee may request that mediation or arbitration be used as a means to settle disciplinary action.

Mediation

The EEOC also offers the option of **mediation** as an alternative to the traditional investigative or litigation process (McDermott et al. 2000). Mediation involves both sides of the claim sitting down with a neutral third party and reaching an agreement. The mediator does not decide the issue, but rather helps both sides come to a solution together. Benefits to mediation include the following.

- Mediation is available at no cost to either party
- Each party has an equal say in the process and the settlement terms and there is no determination of guilt or innocence
- All parties sign a confidentiality agreement
- If mediation occurs early enough in the process, many are completed in one meeting, saving time and money
- The intent is to avoid a more expensive investigation or even a litigation
- Mediation uses a problem-solving approach that allows for reduced workplace disruptions, and this can lead to positive feelings after the issue is resolved as each side has had a fair chance to present their side and work to arrive at a joint solution (EEOC 2015b)

Figure 5.3. Comparison of mediation and arbitration

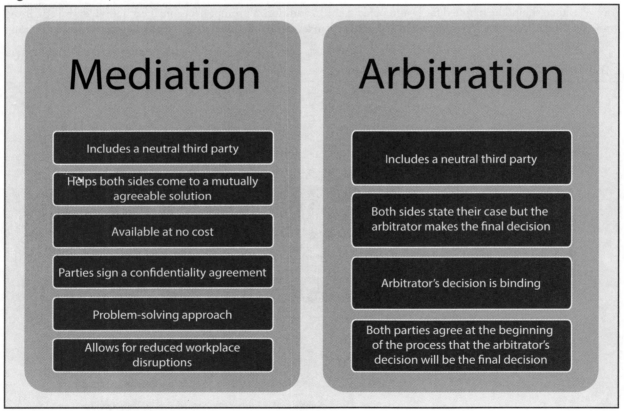

© AHIMA

Arbitration

A second type of alternative dispute resolution is **arbitration**. Arbitration, like mediation, involves a neutral third party. However, in the case of arbitration, each party presents their side, and the arbitrator makes the decision. The arbitration decision is binding, meaning that prior to the start of the arbitration both parties agree that the arbitrator's decision will be final and both agree to abide by the decision in this matter. Figure 5.3 provides a comparative chart describing the traits of both mediation and arbitration.

Check Your **Understanding**

1. Discuss the importance of policy and procedure manuals in applying healthcare laws.
2. Write three inappropriate interview questions and explain why they are inappropriate.
3. Explain the steps in the progressive discipline process.
4. What are some examples of infractions that would result in immediate termination?
5. Explain the difference between arbitration and mediation.

Case Study

Objectives

- Assess employment laws that impact healthcare particularly as they relate to the management of HIM employees
- Develop an educational set of slides on employment laws that impact the management of HIM employees
- Develop a needs assessment and post-education survey to deploy in order to assess the efficacy of the educational session regarding employment laws in healthcare

Instructions

Review the following scenario and create the appropriate deliverables.

Scenario

The HIM department of Memorial Hospital recently hired two new managers, a second shift supervisor and a day shift coding manager. During the hiring process, the HIM director realized that all HIM management staff needed a refresher course on the legal requirements that a manager must be familiar with in regards to employee hiring, training, discipline, and retention. The HIM director and the human resource consultant met and discussed the training needs of managerial employees in light of employment laws and their impact on the healthcare workforce. The HIM management team meets monthly to discuss pertinent topics and next month the HIM director is going to provide training on employment laws and how they impact the management of HIM employees.

Assumptions

- HIM management staff has not received previous training at this facility on the legal aspects of healthcare management.
- HIM management staff are always advised to consult with their human resource consultant if there are any legal issues involving HIM employees.

- The needs assessment results will suggest that HIM management staff require training on all employment laws covered within this chapter.
- The needs assessment and post-education survey will be created, but they will not actually be deployed. If the process were actually performed within an HIM department, the needs assessment would be performed, the training program would be created, and then a post-education survey would be performed to assess learning. There would be data to aggregate to assess pre- and post- learning.

Deliverables

1. Develop a needs assessment reflecting questions regarding the knowledge level of HIM staff in terms of employment laws and how they impact the management of HIM employees. The needs assessment must include one question regarding each of the laws covered within this chapter. The needs assessment should contain at least eight questions and responses to the questions should include a five-point response scale: 5 = Strongly Agree, 4 = Agree, 3 = Neutral, 2 = Disagree or 1 = Strongly Disagree. You may create other responses but make sure that you use a five-point scale.

2. Develop a set of slides to present at a training program that incorporate education on all of the employment laws within this chapter and how they impact the management of HIM employees. The slide set should include:
   - Title slide
   - Learning objectives for the program
   - Six to eight content slides that include the particular law as well as examples of how the law impacts management of HIM employees
   - Summary slide
   - Reference slide to support your research or to provide sites for further research that may be required to fully complete this educational session
   - Each slide should contain notes pages on how the information on the slide will be presented to the audience; the information does not have to be in complete sentences, but must clearly convey the intent of the slide without repeating the slide content.

3. Develop a post-education survey that addresses the topics covered within the educational program to be given to HIM management staff one month after the presentation. Use the same five-point scale that was incorporated within the needs assessment. The post-education survey should include at least eight questions.

Review Questions

1. Jennifer applied for a promotion within her department. During her interview for the new job, John, the department head, told Jennifer that if she agrees to have sex with him the promotion would be hers. For Jennifer, this may constitute an example of what type of sexual harassment?

   a. Hostile work environment
   b. Illegal discrimination
   c. Quid pro quo
   d. Statistical discrimination

2. Maryann resigned her position as transcription supervisor at Memorial Hospital in order to start her own transcription company. She does not have extra money to purchase health insurance, so elects to receive health benefits from Memorial's group health plan for the next six months. Maryann's request is covered under the:

   a. Americans with Disabilities Act
   b. Civil Rights Act of 1964

c. Consolidated Omnibus Budget Reconciliation Act
d. Fair Labor Standards Act

3. Patty is a hearing-impaired coder at Memorial Hospital. In order to comply with the ADA, Memorial Hospital agrees to hire an interpreter for all in-service education and monthly department meetings so Patty can fully understand the proceedings. This is an example of:

   a. Bona fide occupational qualification
   b. Reasonable accommodation
   c. Quid pro quo
   d. Undue hardship

4. The law prohibiting sexual harassment in the workplace is the:

   a. Civil Rights Act of 1964
   b. Consolidated Omnibus Budget Reconciliation Act
   c. Fair Labor Standards Act
   d. Health Insurance Portability and Accountability Act

5. Privacy awareness and training must be provided to all employees in order to prevent privacy breaches. This requirement is covered under which of the following laws?

   a. Civil Rights Act of 1991
   b. Consolidated Omnibus Budget Reconciliation Act
   c. Fair Labor Standards Act
   d. Health Insurance Portability and Accountability Act

6. Heather and her husband recently adopted a little girl. Heather has been saving her paid time off so she may take 10 weeks off to spend with her new daughter. She is confident that her coding position will be available to her upon her return. The ability to return to her job is covered under which of the following employment laws?

   a. Civil Rights Act of 1991
   b. Fair Labor Standards Act
   c. Family and Medical Leave Act
   d. Health Insurance Portability and Accountability Act

7. Good Shepherd Hospital, a Catholic-run hospital, requires the chief executive officer (CEO) be Catholic so that ultimate decision-making responsibility conforms to religious beliefs. Therefore, it is lawful for CEO candidates to be asked what religion they practice during an interview. This is an example of a(n):

   a. Bona fide occupational qualification
   b. Undue hardship
   c. Quid pro quo
   d. Reasonable accommodation

8. Sandra has repeated absences from work and was put into progressive disciplinary action. Today her supervisor met with Sandra, explained the consequences of future absences, and had her sign a form stating she understood the process. The form will be forwarded to Sandra's personnel file in human resources. This is an example of what step in the progressive disciplinary process?

   a. Oral warning
   b. Written warning
   c. Suspension with pay
   d. Termination

9. John filed a discrimination suit against Memorial Hospital. He agreed to sit down with a representative from Memorial Hospital and a neutral third party to reach an agreement. Both sides agreed to accept the decision of the third party as the final word. This is an example of:

   (a) Arbitration
   b. Litigation
   c. Mediation
   d. Termination

10. Which of the following is the first step in an employee grievance procedure?

    a. Immediately file a complaint with the Equal Employment Opportunity Commission
    b. Involve the HR department in resolving the grievance
    (c.) Meet with a direct supervisor to try and resolve the issue
    d. Meet with a vice-president to try and resolve the issue

References

Americans with Disabilities Act of 1990. Public Law 101-336.

Consolidated Omnibus Budget Reconciliation Act. 1986. Public Law 99-272.

Department of Labor. 2012. Fact Sheet #28: The Family and Medical Leave Act. http://www.dol.gov/whd/regs/compliance/whdfs28.pdf.

Equal Employment Opportunity Commission. 2015a. The ADA: Your Responsibilities as an Employer. http://www.eeoc.gov/eeoc/publications/ada17.cfm.

Equal Employment Opportunity Commission. 2015b. Facts about Mediation. http://www.eeoc.gov/eeoc/mediation/facts.

Equal Employment Opportunity Commission. 2014. Social Media is Part of Today's Workplace but Its Use May Raise Employment Discrimination Concerns. http://www.eeoc.gov/eeoc/newsroom/release/3-12-14.cfm.

Equal Employment Opportunity Commission. 2008. Facts about Age Discrimination. http://eeoc.gov/facts/age.html.

Equal Employment Opportunity Commission. 1990. Enforcement Guidance: Policy Guidance on Current Issues of Sexual Harassment. http://www.eeoc.gov/eeoc/publications/upload/currentissues.pdf.

Fair Labor Standards Act of 1938. 2011. Public Law 75-718.

McDermott, E.P., R. Obar, A. Jose, and M. Bowers. 2000. An Evaluation of the Equal Employment Opportunity Commission Mediation Program. http://www.eeoc.gov/eeoc/mediation/report/index.html.

Title VII of the Civil Rights Act of 1964. Public Law 88-352.

6

Job Descriptions and Roles in Health Information Management

Learning Objectives

- Explain job analysis
- Identify typical job description formats
- Differentiate between health information management (HIM) job analyses, job descriptions, and job specifications
- Formulate job descriptions based on evolving HIM roles
- Develop job descriptions that support employee performance and oversight

Key Terms

Ability	Job context	Observation	Secondary data sources for job analysis
Competency model	Job crafting	Occupational Information Network (O*NET)	Sector changes
Demand-control model of job strain	Job description		Skills
Diary or log method	Job diagnostic survey (JDS)	Personal Interviews	Structured questionnaires
Fleishman job analysis survey	Job redesign	Position	Task analysis
Grade level assignment	Job responsibility	Position analysis questionnaire (PAQ)	Technical conference method
Job	Job role		Work design questionnaire (WDQ)
Job analysis	Job specifications	Primary data sources for job analysis	
Job content questionnaire (JCQ)	Job summary	Reporting relationships	Workflow
	Job title		
	Knowledge		
	Needs assessment		

Job roles and responsibilities are changing at a fast pace in health information management (HIM) departments. In addition, HIM professionals are assuming job roles in nontraditional workplaces that require job descriptions reflective of the skills needed specifically for these workplaces. HIM managers and other management personnel need to keep pace, creating new job descriptions and updating current job descriptions to attract and retain HIM employees who have skills and abilities that directly match these job descriptions. This chapter outlines the basic components of job analysis and job design, which include reviewing techniques for assessing job needs, reviewing job analysis methods, and designing jobs that will attract highly-skilled individuals. The second portion of this chapter specifically outlines the typical components of job descriptions and job specifications. The final section of this chapter discusses job crafting and job redesign as methods for improving HIM employee job satisfaction and retaining motivated HIM professionals. The case study provides an opportunity for an HIM professional to assess a job role, create a new job title for an emerging role, and analyze two different methods of job analysis that will be applied when creating a new job description for the emerging role.

Job Analysis and Job Design

As job roles change within healthcare organizations, it is important to ensure that job descriptions are kept current and relevant with the tasks actually performed by the employees. Standardized methodologies can be employed to analyze and design jobs appropriately. It is imperative that all healthcare managers work with the human resources (HR) department to ensure job analysis is performed according to the requirements of the organization. The legal requirements associated with job analysis and the use of job descriptions in the hiring process were discussed in chapter 5. Effective job analysis and design can ensure that healthcare organizations maximize workforce job skills, therefore improving employee job satisfaction. Appropriate job analysis and design results in job descriptions that provide the healthcare organization with a competitive edge when recruiting individuals to fill jobs and provide a solid foundation for monitoring employee job performance. The following sections outline and identify the steps for completing a job analysis project.

Job Analysis Terminology

It is important to clarify several terms within the job analysis process. A **job** "consists of a group of activities and duties that entail units of work that are similar and related" (Fried and Fottler 2008). Examples of typical jobs in HIM are coder, transcriptionist, revenue cycle coordinator, electronic health record (EHR) implementation specialist, and release of information clerk. One job description may be created for each of these jobs or there may be several different job descriptions based on the job requirements or job specifications. For example, coding may be delineated in three different job descriptions: coder level 1, coder level 2, and coder level 3. A **job description** is a detailed list of a job's duties, reporting relationships, working conditions, and responsibilities. Depending on the size of the healthcare organization, each of the jobs mentioned may have one or more employees who complete the tasks and each employee occupies a position within the HIM department. A **position** or **job role** consists of different tasks or jobs that are completed by one employee. A health information manager may be required to perform a job and task analysis for particular jobs within the HIM department when a needs assessment notes a gap in performance. A **task analysis** is a procedure for determining the specific duties and skills required of a job. The term *job analysis* is defined and detailed in the following section.

Job Analysis Method

Job analysis is a structured approach used to identify the unique job tasks performed within each job. Tasks are then organized and aligned appropriately to create a job description that most clearly represents the job being performed. A job and task analysis provides value to an organization whenever there is a substantial change in an organization necessitating new or revised job descriptions for both managerial and nonmanagerial positions (Sleezer et al. 2014). The changes experienced by HIM positions require a job analysis for each of the work processes that are impacted by the change. The end goal of the job analysis process is creation of new or updated job descriptions and job specifications that demonstrate the actual job functions performed within the HIM department. For example,

HIM integrates technology throughout most departmental functions. Technology changes the **workflow**, or any work process that must be handled by one or more employee, of the health record within HIM departments so it is important to assess how these changes impact the completion of job tasks for each job function.

The importance of job analysis cannot be ignored as HIM departments strive to align HIM positions to the mission and vision of healthcare organizations. Job analysis can provide support for departmental and pay structure. Current and relevant job analysis can provide a competitive edge for an HIM department, assist in appropriate candidate selection, and identify gaps in training needs. Job analysis stemming from changes in workflow can result in the design of new jobs or the redesign of existing jobs.

The target of job analysis is not appraising job performance, but rather the information that is obtained regarding the job itself. Questions should be addressed in terms of what knowledge, skills, and abilities are needed for employees who may perform the job or who are already performing the job. A standardized process should be developed in healthcare organizations for performing a job analysis and the HR department may already have a methodology that is used for this process (methodologies are discussed later in the chapter).

A thorough job analysis process is not usually undertaken for all jobs in a particular department at the same time because it is a very labor and time intensive process. The steps in conducting a job analysis are to:

- Perform a job needs assessment
- Obtain approval from administration and the HR department to conduct a job analysis
- Create a team or group to evaluate the job tasks
- Identify the sources of data and the specific job data to be collected; and outline methods of collecting data
- Collect and aggregate data
- Create updated job description content (Fried and Fottler 2008)

Figure 6.1 reflects the steps in performing a job analysis. The steps for conducting a job analysis are discussed in detail and tools are provided to assist HIM professionals in performing a job analysis project systematically. It is important to remember that most of the time the health information manager will perform a job analysis alongside the HR department, which employs individuals who are specifically trained to perform job analyses. In addition, before embarking on the job analysis process, the health information manager should obtain approval from upper management as well as the HR department. In smaller healthcare organizations or nontraditional healthcare settings, an HR consultant may not be available to assist with the job analysis process so the information contained in this chapter is helpful to an HIM professional embarking on the job analysis process alone.

Needs Assessment

A **needs assessment** is a procedure performed by collecting and analyzing data to determine what is required, lacking, or desired by an employee, group, or organization. The needs assessment is a process for determining how to close a learning or performance gap as it relates to jobs performed in a particular department. Needs assessment is a process that relies on data collection and analysis to assess the actual job tasks being performed within a department or entire healthcare organization (Sleezer et al. 2014). In this chapter, needs assessment is discussed in terms of defining the discrepancy of needs between the current job roles in HIM versus the ideal or expected performance of job roles in the futuristic HIM department. To narrow the scope more specifically, job and task analysis and competency-based needs assessment is discussed in relation to the development of emerging job descriptions to meet the performance expectations of a technology-based HIM department.

Figure 6.1. Steps of the job analysis process

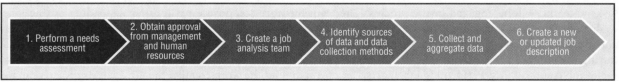

© AHIMA

Job and task analysis needs assessment focuses on the information about the scope, responsibilities, and tasks of a particular job role. Competency-based needs assessment focuses on determining the competencies needed to complete specific HIM job functions. The 2017 Health Information Technology (HIT) or Health Information Administration (HIA) Competencies developed by the American Health Information Management Association (AHIMA) Council on Excellence in Education in appendix A provides an excellent framework for incorporating specific competencies into job functions within HIM departments.

A health information manager or director should regularly assess the jobs and tasks required of the department and assess additional needs based on the gaps between the tasks performed to additional job tasks that need to be completed. The needs assessment may identify current job roles containing tasks that are no longer applicable to the healthcare organization. The needs assessment will then lead to development of job and tasks analyses that will result in new or updated job descriptions.

Obtaining Approval to Perform a Job Analysis

Periodically, the HR department will perform job analyses on positions that have been identified as difficult to fill because of competition in the workforce for the job skills required. Other items that trigger the need for job analysis are sector changes, organizational changes, and employees' perceptions of the jobs being performed in the healthcare organization. **Sector changes** in healthcare are events triggered by "new technologies, new or revised regulations, and new or revised accreditation or certification standards" (Layman 2011). Examples of sector changes that directly impact HIM are the adoption of health information technologies as a result of the American Recovery and Reinvestment Act and the provisions outlined in the Health Information Technology for Economic and Clinical Health (HITECH) Act of 2009 portion of the act. Regulations that impact HIM jobs are changes in prospective payments systems, governmental auditing programs, and implementation of new classification systems.

Organizational-level changes that impact the need for health information job analyses are organization-wide initiatives such as implementation of electronic health record (EHR) systems, mergers or acquisitions of other health systems, or incorporation of new service lines that directly affect the type of health information data required to provide the services. All of these organizational-level changes require assessment of the tasks performed within the department and aligning appropriate tasks to the actual jobs performed. Often, new tasks assumed by the HIM department are layered upon current job tasks without any true analysis of the jobs performed. This may require the health information manager to perform a job analysis about the employees' perceptions associated with the job performed. If job tasks are inappropriately aligned to actual job titles and job descriptions, employees' perception of job value and job performance may decline (Layman 2011).

It is important for health information managers to identify the factors precipitating the need for a job analysis in order to seek approval to begin the process and to ensure the correct individuals are involved in the job analysis process (Wilson 2012). The request for approval to have a formal job analysis performed in the HIM department will occur after a needs assessment has been performed. The HIM manager will need to submit a formal request in writing to the human resources department outlining the results of the needs assessment and the gaps that are occurring within job tasks. The formal request should include the identified gaps in job tasks and how these job tasks impact other jobs within the department. The human resources department may also request approval from the HIM department's executive level administrator prior to starting a full job analysis.

Job Analysis Process Team

The next step in preparing for the job analysis process is to select a team that will assist with the evaluation of the jobs. This team can be comprised of the HIM management, HR consultants, subject matter experts, and individual employees. The team members should be vested in the process and knowledgeable regarding the job tasks to be evaluated. It is important to include average to high job performers who can give appropriate feedback on job tasks and who will be engaged in the process. The team member composition will differ depending on the jobs evaluated. The team should meet on a regular basis with specific agendas, assign homework for all team members, and employ consensus-building techniques at all meetings. The team will provide input based on the data collected during the analysis process about the major job responsibilities and help categorize the job tasks that match each major job responsibility. Performing job analysis as a team divides the work equally; the job analysis process can be very time consuming.

Evaluation of Primary and Secondary Data Sources and Tools for Job Analysis

The job analysis team will evaluate the sources of data and methods of data collection for the job analysis. **Primary data sources for job analysis** are employees or managers who currently perform or oversee the job being evaluated. **Secondary data sources for job analysis** are information obtained from subject matter experts, human resource consultants, job data banks, or competency models. It is important to extrapolate data from the primary and secondary data sources in a manner that will assist the job analysis team by quantifying the information to create a meaningful job description (Fried and Fottler 2008).

Primary data can be collected from employees and managers using several different methods and a combination of tools can be utilized to aggregate job task information. The methods are listed as follows:

- **Personal Interviews** may be carried out by the HIM manager or HR consultant with employees who complete the job tasks being analyzed. These interviews should contain a list of structured questions that are asked of all the selected individuals. The HIM management team should evaluate ahead of time whether or not all individuals who complete the tasks will be interviewed or if a select group of individuals should be chosen. Personal interviews are very time consuming and the person performing the interviews should be skilled in soliciting information from employees so as to gather pertinent information for the job analysis process.

- **Observation** is a method in which the HIM manager or HR consultant observes the employee or employees who are completing the job tasks. Standardized comment sheets are used to capture key elements of observation. A variety of employees may be observed completing the same job tasks to evaluate commonality between job processes.

- The **diary or log method** is a job analysis tool that requires employees to complete a daily diary or log of all job tasks completed within a set period of time. All employees who complete the job tasks being analyzed will turn in the diary or log for that specified time period and the HIM manager or HR consultant will aggregate the information from all the diaries or logs. Guidance must be provided to those completing the diary or log so that similar data is captured by each employee performing the job task.

- **Structured questionnaires** or checklists may be distributed to all employees completing the job tasks being evaluated. Structured questionnaires or checklists allow for a standardized method of collecting data on job tasks and questions related to job tasks can only be answered in one specific manner (Fried and Fottler 2008). The manager familiar with the job or jobs being analyzed should create structured questionnaires or checklists based on job content. There are also some standardized questionnaires or tools that can be used (outlined later in this chapter).

A variety of standardized HR tools can be employed for primary data collection to create a comprehensive assessment of job tasks performed. Some of these tools require extensive training to ensure the data is collected in a systematic manner so the aggregated results of the data provide the necessary information to analyze the job appropriately. The HR department can assist the HIM manager to select a tool that is appropriate for the job being analyzed. The following are standardized tools used most often to provide meaningful data for job analysis.

The Work Design Questionnaire

Frederick P. Morgeson, instructor at Michigan State University, and Stephen E. Humphrey, instructor at Florida State University, created the **work design questionnaire (WDQ)** in 2006 as part of a study to improve work design research. The WDQ surveyed a variety of workers in different settings with a questionnaire in order to assess specific characteristics related to job tasks. The outcome of the study was that the WDQ results showed good promise to assist practitioners in the design and redesign of jobs in the organization. Although this questionnaire is not specific to healthcare, it may be used with some modifications to collect data on job task characteristics (Morgeson and Humphrey 2006).

The Job Diagnostic Survey

Introduced in 1975 by J. Richard Hackman and Greg Oldham, the **job diagnostic survey (JDS)** was developed to evaluate existing jobs to determine if jobs could be redesigned to improve employee motivation and productivity and to study the effects of job changes on employees. The JDS is a questionnaire composed of core job dimensions, critical psychological states, and personal work outcomes. The items assessed in the core job dimensions are skill variety, task identity, task significance, job autonomy, and feedback from the job, management, and peers. The critical psychological factors assessed are employees' perception of the experienced meaningfulness of work, experienced responsibility of work outcomes, and knowledge of work results. Personal and work outcomes are evaluated in terms of general job satisfaction, internal work motivation, and specific satisfactions such as job security, pay, peer, and supervisor relations (Hackman and Oldham 1975).

The JDS has a few limitations that should be taken into consideration when selecting a job analysis tool. The JDS should not be utilized for diagnosing individual jobs but rather a workgroup of individuals to allow for anonymity in survey completion. This survey tool provides useful information about job tasks and is one of the most frequently cited instruments for assessing workers' perception of job characteristics (Taber and Taylor 1990).

The Job Content Questionnaire

The **job content questionnaire (JCQ)** is a self-administered questionnaire, composed of questions that measure four main dimensions of the workplace environment.

- Decision latitude. This refers to the amount of decision making required in the job.
- Psychological demands of the job. These demands are categorized as emotional requirements, mental effort, and relationship problems with peers or management in the job setting. This dimension also measures the perceived psychological stress associated with a job.
- Physical workload. Assesses the amount of physical effort that is required to complete the job.
- Job insecurity. Assesses the factors associated with job security such as job tasks that might be more appropriate for another job or require another skill, degree, or certification level.

The most difficult component of the JCQ was creating appropriate questions that assessed jobs in terms of psychological demands. This is an internationally accepted tool that has been translated into a dozen languages and can be nationally standardized for a variety of detailed occupations in several countries. The **demand-control model of job strain scale** originated from the use of the JCQ and this scale is calculated from score results of the questions related to decision latitude and psychological demands of the job. The demand-control model relates that job strain (stress) is evidenced by the interaction between job demand and job control. For example, a job with high demand and low control would result in high strain while a job with low demand and high control would result in low strain (Karasek et al. 1998).

The JCQ examined the effects of job redesign at a large teaching hospital in Ontario, Canada and was highly effective in measuring and correlating results among the job decision latitude, job psychological demands, physical workload of a job, and job security scale measures. This questionnaire is not available in the public domain but it and component training models can be purchased by organizations. JCQ is a tool most likely promoted for a broad-scale research study, rather than a typical job analysis process within one or two departments (Sale and Kerr 2002). The JCQ is a reliable tool that can assist healthcare organizations understand the psychosocial elements of work that are negatively impacted by poor or inadequate work design.

The Position Analysis Questionnaire

The **position analysis questionnaire (PAQ)** is a structured job analysis instrument created in 1972 by researchers Ernest J. McCormick, Paul R. Jeanneret, and Robert C. Mecham from Purdue University. This tool is used to measure job characteristics and relate them to human characteristics within the following five categories:

- Information input
- Mental processing
- Work output
- Relationships with others
- Job context

PAQ has been used for assessing hundreds of jobs across multiple fields of work and the data collected from these assessments is maintained in a database at Purdue University. The PAQ is a valuable nonbiased tool for translating job analysis data into job evaluation information for a wide variety of jobs (Jeanneret 1980). This questionnaire in its original format or a more up-to-date format can be purchased from Purdue University. The human resources department within a healthcare organization may elect to incorporate this tool as part of the data collection process when performing a job analysis.

This section has only touched on a small selection of standardized, researched tools that may be used during a job analysis process. The HR departments within healthcare organizations may have an entire set of job analysis tools or questionnaires for conducting a job analysis. An HIM manager should work with the HR department to ensure that the tools collecting job task data conform to the standards in that particular healthcare organization.

Secondary Data Collection

In addition to primary data, secondary data collection may be necessary for gathering information regarding emerging job roles or technological changes impacting job roles. The tools that typically collect secondary data during the job analysis process are as follows.

- The **technical conference method** is used for soliciting information about job tasks from a group of supervisors or managers who have knowledge about the job but do not actually perform the job. Individuals from other HIM departments outside of the healthcare organization may be interviewed regarding similar job tasks performed within their HIM departments. This method may be helpful creating a job analysis for a role that is not currently performed in an HIM department, but if the need for this job role was identified in a needs assessment. The technical conference method can be time consuming and expensive so limiting the number of outside individuals involved in the conference may be appropriate (Fried and Fottler 2008).

- The **competency model** is a method of evaluating competencies for particular job tasks and applying them within the job framework. Competencies are measurable knowledge, skills, abilities, and behaviors that are critical to assessing job performance (Washington State Human Resources 2012). The Health Information Technology (HIT) or Health Information Administration (HIA) competencies developed by the AHIMA Council on Excellence in Education (appendix A) are the type of competencies that may be helpful as a secondary data source for performing a job analysis. These competencies can be inserted with a job analysis tool and employees' performance can be objectively evaluated as to whether or not the knowledge, skills, abilities, and behaviors for the competencies are being met. Some healthcare organizations develop their own set of core competencies that are inserted into all job descriptions.

- The **Occupational Information Network (O*NET)** was developed and introduced by the US Department of Labor in 1995. This network is a standardized, comprehensive online system for performing worker and job-oriented job analysis in the development of job descriptions. O*NET provides a tool that describes jobs from a variety of different perspectives and uses cross-job descriptors that provide a common language to describe and compare jobs (O*NET 2015).

- Standardized questionnaires and checklists may also collect secondary data from outside sources during the job analysis process.

It is important to note that the tools listed are standardized HR tools and the HR department can assist the manager and job analysis team in deploying the correct data collection tools for the particular job(s) being analyzed. An HIM manager should be familiar with the concept that there are standardized job analysis data collection tools available. An HIM manager should work with the HR department to select the appropriate data collection tools for the particular jobs being analyzed within the manager's realm.

Data Aggregation

The data collected from the primary or secondary data collection tools requires aggregation using a method that allows the team to evaluate job tasks relevant to each job responsibility. A **job responsibility** is a function that falls under the main job-holder's work-related tasks. Figure 6.2 (on the following page) is an example of a job responsibility or task tool template that can be used to insert data obtained from questionnaires, checklists, interviews, or observations. Each job responsibility or function should be listed and beneath each function is a description of each job's tasks. The specific skills and abilities needed to complete each job function should be noted as well as the competencies associated with the particular job. The goal of aggregating all the tasks associated with each job function is not to create a job procedure, which is discussed later, but rather to create a comprehensive list of tasks that relate to each job function.

Figure 6.2. Job responsibility task tool template

This tool identifies each major job responsibility and the tasks associated with this responsibility during the job analysis process.

Job title (current):

Job responsibility:	
Job tasks:	
Skills or abilities:	
Job competencies:	

© AHIMA

After all tasks are entered into the tool, essential and nonessential job tasks should be grouped together. Then, each major job responsibility associated with the job being analyzed along with the essential tasks for that particular job should be outlined in the tool. Next, the skills and abilities associated with each task should be added. Finally, apply competencies or domains from HIT or HIA program competencies (appendix A) or individual healthcare organization competencies to each job task. Tasks and competencies should be linked together by HIM managers in order to demonstrate the job task relationship to each competency.

All tasks should be documented on the job responsibility task tool in the same manner and a general format for writing task items will need to include what task is being performed and to whom is the task being performed in order to produce a given job outcome—including the what, why, and how of the job outcome. An example of an HIM task for a release of information clerk would be: Scan incoming release of information authorizations paper documents (the task) into the release of information request system (to whom or what the task is being performed) for processing by the release of information coordinators (the task outcome). Some additional tips for writing tasks are:

- Remove unnecessary words in the tasks to make it as clear and concise as possible.
- Do not combine two tasks with the word "and;" break apart multiple tasks into two or more separate items.
- Do not be overly specific with each task; for example, "Create a spreadsheet to total the numbers of charts copied by each ROI clerk and divide by the total number of hours worked." Better wording is "Use spreadsheets to track ROI clerk productivity."
- Do not use vague terms outlining job tasks. Replace subjective adjectives or adverbs (good, excellent) with more descriptive terms (verify, create, identify) with all tasks.
- Do not use acronyms or abbreviations for job tasks. Make sure that you spell out all terms whenever possible (University of California, San Diego 2015).

After all job tasks for each major job responsibility area are collected, the tasks should be ranked or prioritized into how frequently the task is performed and how important the task is to the entire completion process. See figure 6.3 for an example of a task frequency rating scale and figure 6.4 for an example of a task importance rating scale. The job responsibilities that fall into the three to five categories (important, very important, and extremely important) should be identified as the major job responsibilities for the current job title and listed on the job responsibility task tool ranked in order of frequency performed (US Office of Personnel Management 2015).

After a job responsibility or task tool has been completed for each job responsibility, the next step requires aggregation of all similar tasks performed by a position. If the job analysis process evaluated a variety of tasks performed by several individuals, the end result of the process may be several new job descriptions or several current job descriptions rolled into one job description.

Figure 6.3. Task frequency rating scale example

Indicate how often you perform the task as part of your job using the following scale:

Task Frequency Scale

0 = Not performed

1 = Every few months to yearly

2 = Every few weeks to monthly

3 = Every few days to weekly

4 = Every few hours to daily

5 = Many times each hour to hourly

Source: US Office of Personnel Management 2015.

Figure 6.4. Task importance rating scale example

Indicate how important the task is to successfully performing the job using the following scale:

Task Importance Rating Scale

0 = Not performed

1 = Not important

2 = Somewhat important

3 = Important

4 = Very important

5 = Extremely important

Source: US Office of Personnel Management 2015.

The basic premise behind collecting job analysis data is to determine the job requirements and delineate appropriate position classification and **grade level assignments**. Grade level assignments set forth the criteria between or among the various levels of jobs within an organization that represent the pay level of the position. It is important in the job analysis process that the level of tasks performed for each job are assigned to the correct grade level so that pay is equitable throughout an organization (US Office of Personnel Management 2009). Some additional features of the job analysis process are identify training needs and other personnel actions such as promotions and performance evaluations (US Office of Personnel Management 2015).

Check Your **Understanding**

1. Discuss the role of a needs assessment in the job analysis process.
2. Explain the six steps in the job analysis process.
3. What are potential triggers that would require a manager to obtain approval to complete a job analysis?
4. Differentiate between primary and secondary data sources for a job analysis.
5. Discuss the four primary data collection methods used in a job analysis.

Job Descriptions

The final step in the job analysis or job design or redesign process is to create meaningful job descriptions that will match the jobs that were analyzed during the job analysis process. A job description is an official document developed within a healthcare organization for job recruitment; it creates a repository for job tasks and provides the basis for evaluating annual job performance. A job description states the purpose of a specific job along with the duties or tasks for completion of the job, job standards, job context, job specifications, and reporting relationships (Law 2009). Job descriptions for all positions within a healthcare organization are created using a standardized job description template. The statements given in the job responsibilities section of the job description template should be written clearly and simply stated with a verb at the beginning of each responsibility. For example, a scanning job responsibility would be to scan records from outside sources with a 98 percent accuracy rate.

The verbs employed in each of the job responsibilities should mirror the level of competency required in order to complete the job task. An association of the level of competency or learning can be reflected by using Bloom's taxonomy—which identifies the different levels of learning—to create the verb. Figure 6.5 provides a list of verbs along with the level of learning required for the particular verb. Job tasks are often required to be performed at different levels throughout a healthcare organization. For example, a coder and coding manager job description will include the job responsibility of assigning appropriate diagnosis and procedural codes for all patient discharges using appropriate clinical classification systems such as ICD-10 and CPT. However, the verbs used in the job responsibility

Figure 6.5. Bloom's Taxonomy job task verbs and levels of learning

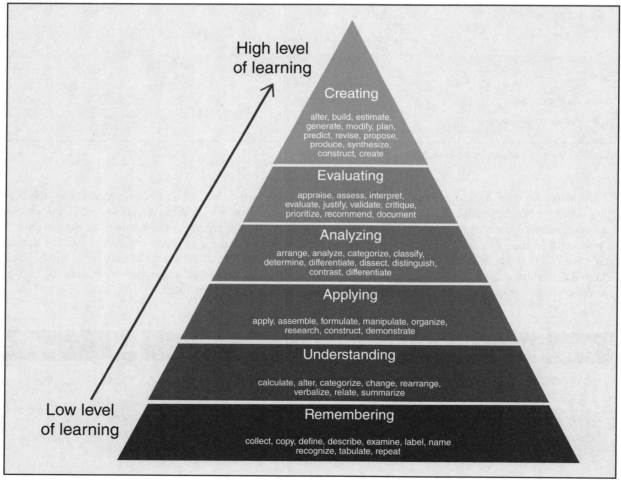

will differ between the coder and the coding manager. The coder will be responsible for *applying* and *analyzing* the code assignments whereas the coding manager will be responsible for *evaluating* the overall appropriateness of coding. As noted in figure 6.5, the coding manager has a higher level of responsibility according to the Bloom's taxonomy versus the coder's level of responsibility.

The AHIMA Body of Knowledge (BoK) is the primary knowledge base for HIM practitioners and is located on the AHIMA website (AHIMA n.d.). The AHIMA BoK is an excellent resource to consult when creating job descriptions as it contains job descriptions for a variety of job titles utilized by health information practitioners. These job descriptions provide key action words that can assist health information managers in the creation of the job tasks related to the specific job description being developed. The US Department of Labor developed a website that can assist with writing descriptions for many positions including the positions of health records and health information technicians (CareerOneStop 2015).

The components of a typical job description are title, to whom the employee reports, job responsibilities or duties, position goals, relationships, job specifications or qualifications, job context, and position summary, scope, and purpose. Most healthcare organizations will have standardized job description formats required for all new or updated job descriptions. The guidance provided outlines how to complete each section of the job description.

Job Title

The title of a job description is very important in today's competitive workforce market as it provides the foundation for attracting qualified candidates for open positions as well as providing a descriptive categorization of jobs in an organization. The **job title** should be comprehensive in that it clearly describes the level of skills and knowledge required for the role such as supervisor, coordinator, manager, director, analyst, or technician. In healthcare, it is very important that job titles reflect where individuals fit within the organization. Job titles could change when a job analysis is performed. For example, implementation of new technologies in healthcare could require new job titles to be developed to accurately depict the tasks performed (Smith 2012).

Health information managers need to ignite their inner creativity for developing job titles. Researching titles employed by other HIM departments in the region or within a similar healthcare organization can be very useful. For example, if the HIM department at Mercy Hospital is recruiting for similar positions as other HIM departments within the same region, a creative job title could be a great asset for attracting qualified individuals to the position over other job titles. It is important to realize that if an out-of-the box thinker is required for a position, do not use an inside-the-box title (Linker 2014). Figure 6.6 (on the next page) provides a list of job titles that are emerging as potential job roles for HIM professionals. This is not an all-inclusive list but it does provide some good ideas for updating or creating new HIM job titles.

The following are some tips when assessing if job titles can or should be changed:

- If several employees in an organization share the same title and one individual requests a title change, an assessment should be performed on the entire subset of individuals to decide whether or not a formal job analysis is required. For example, the position title "data quality specialist" may be assigned throughout the healthcare organization to individuals who perform data quality tasks on patient records or healthcare statistics. If one department requests a job title change, this department should work in conjunction with the HR department to perform an analysis of any positions throughout the organization also using this title.

- If an individual in a healthcare organization is performing tasks that do not match the individual's job title, the title needs to be updated in order to reflect appropriate job performance. For example, the title "chart management clerk" does not reflect the scope of skills required for an "electronic record management clerk."

- Job titles are usually associated with standardized job categories that are connected with pay scales, so managers should always work in conjunction with the HR department when initiating title changes.

- It is important to remember that job titles for individuals reflect a career progression and individuals often look for future positions based on advancing skills within the organization or outside of the organization. By adding the word leader or coordinator in a title, it usually reflects some type of managerial or supervisor role. Also, adding levels such as coder I or coder II reflect a career progression in a similar role. HIM professionals may be looking for positions in a healthcare organization where there is room for career progression and evidence of different levels of job roles for both supervisory and non-supervisory positions. A comprehensive, well-constructed job title is an excellent way to recruit individuals who are looking for mobility within a healthcare organization.

Figure 6.6. HIM emerging job titles

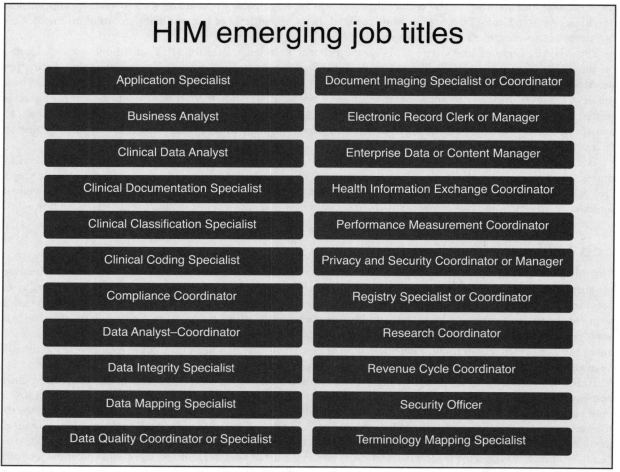

HIM emerging job titles

Application Specialist	Document Imaging Specialist or Coordinator
Business Analyst	Electronic Record Clerk or Manager
Clinical Data Analyst	Enterprise Data or Content Manager
Clinical Documentation Specialist	Health Information Exchange Coordinator
Clinical Classification Specialist	Performance Measurement Coordinator
Clinical Coding Specialist	Privacy and Security Coordinator or Manager
Compliance Coordinator	Registry Specialist or Coordinator
Data Analyst–Coordinator	Research Coordinator
Data Integrity Specialist	Revenue Cycle Coordinator
Data Mapping Specialist	Security Officer
Data Quality Coordinator or Specialist	Terminology Mapping Specialist

© AHIMA

Reporting Relationships

Reporting relationships are an important component of job descriptions because they define the working hierarchy—who manages whom. For example, an HIM manager reporting relationship would indicate that the position reports to the director of HIM and that all department technical and clerical employees report to the HIM manager. When health information managers recruit for open positions, it is important that this section of the job description is accurately completed as qualified individuals may be looking for positions that appear to have some job progression or provide guidance of the span of control the individual will have in the job.

Job Summary

A **job summary** (or job purpose or scope) describes the key tasks and responsibilities of a job. The basic content of the job summary outlines how the job fits within the department and provides an overview of the job requirements. This job summary is usually what is used for posting any job openings in regards to the position.

Job Tasks or Duties

There are different levels of job tasks or duties that should be included in the job description, classified as broad, intermediate, and specific. The broad level tasks are the major function areas of the position such as coding, transcription, and release of information. The intermediate task level is what activity is performed when carrying out the function of the job. The intermediate task level also includes the skills associated with carrying out the activity. Specific level tasks are the actual steps required to complete the activity within the functional area of the job description. The job responsibility task tool in figure 6.2 allows a health information manager to build job descriptions that accurately reflect the tasks completed by specific job positions.

The largest content area in job descriptions are the tasks that should have been identified during the job analysis process. Each major task or responsibility will be described with an appropriate level verb and these major job tasks or responsibilities will be the basis for creating measurable job standards or goals for the performance appraisal process.

Job Specifications (req.)

The **job specifications** or requirements section of the job description outlines the knowledge and specific skills required for a position. Job specifications are qualifications that individuals must possess in order to perform the duties and responsibilities contained within a particular job description. The knowledge, skills, abilities, and other characteristics (KSAOs) necessary to be present upon employment, educational qualifications, and working conditions are all outlined in the job specifications section of a job description. KSAOs provide a basis for recruiting qualified individuals for positions as well as providing a career ladder for those already employed in the organization. When KSAOs are identified in all job descriptions, individuals internal and external to the organization can assess their current skill level against any job description within the organization. Employees who have been in a current job for a period of time may actually acquire KSAOs that are applicable to a higher level job within the organization and thereby create an ability to move up in the organization.

Knowledge is the formal organized body of factual information that must be present in order to be considered for the position. An example of knowledge is: an individual can apply HIPAA guidelines when evaluating privacy breaches. **Skills** refer to the abilities related to the verbal, manual, and mental processing of data and information for a particular job. An example of a skill is: an individual can utilize a spreadsheet application when analyzing statistical data. **Ability** refers to the capacity to effectively engage in activities outlined by the job description. An example of an ability is: the individual performs coding of diagnoses employing appropriate classification systems. *Other characteristics* are items that do not fall into the previous three categories but are necessary in the job environment such as working well in teams or listening to and following directions. Other characteristics are often the people skills required to function within a work setting. The KSAOs for all positions are usually described with the minimum necessary qualifications required to be hired for a particular position. KSAOs are often employed as a screening mechanism by the HR department to sort through job applicants (Community for Human Resource Management 2015).

Job Context

Job context, the situations or conditions where the employee performs the job, should also be included in the job description. This includes working conditions such as the requirement to sit or stand for long periods of time and weight-lifting requirements. This section of the job description should also include the risks involved with the position such as those associated with long-term computer use like eye strain or carpal tunnel syndrome (Management Study Guide 2013b). Job context may be rolled into the job specification section of a job description. This is the section that should include the potential for the individual to perform job tasks remotely either on a full or part-time basis.

The HIM team of an organization should follow some best practices to ensure job descriptions and job titles are relevant to the overall healthcare schema. Best practices are outlined as follows:

- Assess job titles on a regular basis (at least annually) by comparing HIM job titles at healthcare organizations within the region and with other HIM peers to ensure that the HIM department keeps pace with the industry.
- Tune in to employee grumblings that HIM job titles might not actually reflect the job tasks performed based on the implementation of new technologies and new processes.
- Evaluate turnover rates in the HIM department particularly in regards to job titles and job descriptions.

Check Your **Understanding**

1. Define the components of a job description.
2. Discuss at least three different uses for job descriptions in the HIM department.
3. Differentiate among the levels of job tasks in a job description.
4. List items included in the job specifications section of a job description.

Job Crafting

Job crafting impacts job roles within organizations and is the unsupervised or spontaneous changes to jobs that may or may not be congruent to the goals of the organization. Job crafting is redefinition of a job by an individual to incorporate his or her own motives, strengths, and passions (Wrzesniewski et al. 2010). Job crafting is the "action that employees take to shape, mold, and redefine their jobs" (Wrzesniewski and Dutton 2001). In situations where it would be appropriate to initiate a job analysis but only one employee is affected, a formal job analysis may not be realistic to perform for one individual so employing a job crafting exercise with the affected individual may be the best solution.

The precipitating factor for job crafting is that it should come from the affected individual and not driven by management; it is a proactive behavior exhibited by an employee. Job crafting happens at an individual level whereas job redesign is a process in which management decides to change something with an employee's job (Tims and Bakker 2010). Job crafters tend to be initiators, independent decision makers, intrinsically motivated, and perceive work as a part of their well-being (Tims and Bakker 2010). Research indicates that "employees (at all levels and all kinds of occupations) who try job crafting often end up more engaged and satisfied with their work lives, achieve higher levels of performance in organizations, and report greater personal resilience" (Wrzesniewski et al. 2010).

The dimensions that should be assessed by an individual during a job crafting exercise are tasks, relationships, and perceptions. Tasks can be reevaluated and new or different processes can be engineered to complete the tasks as long as the result remains congruent with departmental or organizational goals. Relationships can be revamped and mentorship or succession planning can be considered within the employee's job role. Creation of a new image regarding the employee's job role in the department or organization can impact the actual perceptions of how the employee's role is viewed by others. By evaluating and changing job tasks, relationships, and perceptions, an employee embraces role innovation, creates a voice for his or her position, develops ideals, and demonstrates personal initiative. All of these tasks require the individual to actively participate in and, if implemented appropriately, he or she can greatly improve job performance (Tims and Bakker 2010).

The Three Dimensions of Job Crafting

It is important to analyze each of the dimensions (tasks, relationships, and perceptions) of job crafting comprehensively in order to understand how this process can be utilized to redefine job roles.

Tasks

Job crafting by assessing job tasks allows an individual to develop his or her job by incorporating a variety of tasks along with providing the identity and significance of these tasks. The individual will add, emphasize, or redesign tasks (Berg et al. 2013). For example, a health information coding manager's duties may be to provide education to coders but the frequency and depth of training for coders needs to be reevaluated. The coding manager can provide more frequent coder educational sessions to highlight the ability to train others as an important attribute for his or her job. In another example, a coding manager redistributes tasks to individuals within his or her workgroups, allowing the coding manager time to focus on higher-level job tasks that bring value to his or her job.

Relationships

The second aspect of job crafting is reevaluating and creating meaningful job relationships that enhance an individual's well-being. The three functions of job relationships that need to be evaluated are building, reframing, and adapting relationships (Berg et al. 2013). For example, the HIM coding manager may realize in order to craft his or her job so that it is more meaningful, he or she will have to build relationships with others in the healthcare organization that value the HIM skills inherent to the coding manager. The HIM coding manager may reach out to the manager in the decision support department who typically runs reports for other healthcare managers and he or she can share information regarding clinical classification code sets. Sharing this information with another department will allow the HIM coding manager to demonstrate coding skills knowledge as well as build a new relationship between two departments. Helping other departments understand the clinical coded data they are using to make business decisions adds value to the organization and credence to the HIM profession.

The HIM coding manager can also reframe existing relationships by changing the nature of the relationship for a different purpose (Berg et al. 2013). Networking with other HIM individuals who have similar job roles may provide the HIM coding manager with ideas for additional job tasks that will broaden the position's scope and create more meaning for the coding manager role. When adapting relationships one adjusts a relationship to cultivate meaningfulness by providing others with valuable help and support (Lyons 2008). For example, an HIM coding manager has an HIM management team within his or her department but the relationships between managers have been adversarial rather than supportive. The HIM coding manager may adapt the daily interactions with his or her peers to be more caring and supportive of other managers within the department.

Perceptions

Linking perceptions of job tasks to other skills and interests can make the job more meaningful. For example, the HIM coding manager may have inordinate persuasive and collaborative skills and these skills can be linked to daily management tasks by motivating employees to perform at their best (Berg et al. 2013). An individual can cultivate meaningfulness in his or her position by thinking of the job as a whole rather than as a set of tasks. For example, if an HIM coding manager perceives the tasks that he or she performs as an important piece of the entire revenue management cycle within the healthcare organization, he or she has an expanded perception of his or her job. Focusing on the more pleasing aspects of a job rather than the tasks an individual does not like can provide a more positive perception of the entire job. In this example, the HIM coding manager should focus on the positive aspect of teaching coders new skills and improving revenue flow within the organization rather than on the less pleasant aspects of management such as disciplining employees, backlog management, and such.

Alignment

Although job crafting is employee driven, the role of management in the process cannot be overlooked. Feedback and communication between the employee and manager are essential to ensure that the employee's job role is still in alignment with departmental or organizational goals (Tims and Bakkar 2010). Positive results demonstrate reinforcement for employees who executed the changes effectively. If the job changes are not aligned with or are contrary to the workgroup objectives, the job crafting is considered a problem and must be addressed by management (Lyons 2008).

Job crafting may be an ideal way to embrace some of the fast-paced changes occurring in HIM departments, allowing motivated individuals to engage in more meaningful work. Job crafting may eventually lead to creation of new job descriptions and create additional pathways for growth inside an HIM department.

Check Your **Understanding**

1. Explain the concept of job crafting.
2. Discuss both the positive and negative aspects of job crafting.
3. Explain the three dimensions of job crafting and give an example of each.

Job Redesign

The change in workforce dynamics and increased use of technology in HIM departments has altered the alignment of job tasks for many roles ranging from HIM clerks to those managing frontline employees. **Job redesign** is the process of realigning the needs of the organization with the skills and interests of the employee and then designing the jobs to meet those needs. For example, in order to introduce new tools or technology or provide better customer service, new positions may be created. Job redesign uses a range of techniques that attempt to increase the variety of tasks employees perform in order to improve motivation and satisfaction at work (Heery and Noon 2008). Three general concepts emerge from job redesign: job enlargement, job enrichment, and job rotation (refer to chapter 3 for definitions and examples of these job redesign categories).

Job redesign allows HIM managers to evaluate employees' job tasks and define each employee's responsibilities without performing a full-blown job analysis. It is important for a healthcare organization to use a model of job redesign that is flexible, given the changes that are occurring. There are five premises associated with a flexible job redesign model:

- Job redesigns are flexible and adjustable for the short term and some employees are proactive in the process to ensure jobs keep pace with change.

- An employee's job performance and perception are important factors in facilitating job redesign initiatives.

- Job knowledge by both the manager and employee is a key factor in understanding the impact of job redesign.

- Job changes have an impact on an employee's self-efficacy and provides a prediction for an employee's behavior in terms of job performance.

- Job redesign processes are dynamic and circular, not just linear, and should be performed whenever changes in job tasks emerge (Clegg and Spencer 2007).

Job redesign can increase employee job satisfaction and motivation by including employees in the design process. The following activities should be performed by the HIM manager in conjunction with the employee when performing a job redesign.

- Revise the job content by collecting and analyzing job-related information to identify inconsistency between the actual job description and tasks performed by the employee.

- Analyze the job-related tasks and categorize them into similar job-task groupings

- Compare documented job description tasks against the new job-task groupings

- Alter the job tasks based on the actual technology or processes employed, as long as the tasks remain congruent to the job's outcomes.

- Realign job tasks and responsibilities in order to increase employee satisfaction and employee motivation (Management Study Guide 2013a).

Job enlargement allows employees to continue performing their current job tasks employing the same skill sets but expanding tasks to include more of the same type of tasks. Job enrichment allows employees to actually broaden their skill set by adding additional tasks that require more or advanced skills. Rotating job tasks with other employees helps strengthen and broaden the workgroup's capacity to understand the bigger picture of the work performed.

Participative job redesign interventions are important to ensure the well-being of the employees involved in the process. The job characteristics that can positively impact employee job satisfaction and overall job performance are job control, skill utilization, participation, and feedback (Holman et al. 2010). The advantages associated with job redesign are:

- Enhancing the quality of work life for individual employees

- Increasing organizational productivity as employees complete job tasks congruent with job skills

- Increasing on-the-job productivity

- Creating the right fit for a job with the right person

- Enhancing the sense of employee belongingness (Management Study Guide 2013a)

Figure 6.7. Differentiating between job redesign and job crafting

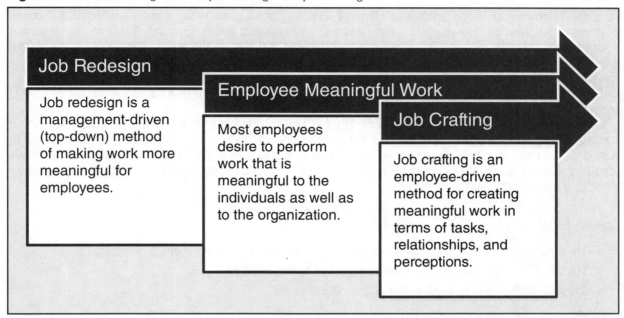

© AHIMA

Although the premise behind job crafting and job redesign look very similar, it is important to remember job crafting is initiated by employees and job redesign is initiated by management. Figure 6.7 illustrates how job redesign and job crafting are related but different. The end result in either activity is increased employee performance and job satisfaction.

Check Your **Understanding**

1. Explain how job redesign differs from job analysis.
2. Explain how job redesign differs from job crafting.
3. Discuss the three components of job redesign.

Case Study

Objectives

- Evaluate job tasks performed by two distinct coding positions applying two methods of job analysis
- Research current literature for an appropriate job title for a new, combined coding position or job description

Instructions

Review the following case study and answer the questions posed within the scenario by writing a two page paper that contains a comprehensive new job title, identifies two job analysis tools, and explains how the tools will assist in development of a new job description for the new job title.

Scenario

Consider the position of coding specialist at University Hospital, which currently is comprised of two distinct coding positions or job descriptions—inpatient coding specialist and outpatient coding specialist. As the coding supervisor, you have been asked to conduct a job analysis that will be used to determine the need to create one coding position with a new job title. In other words, the two current coding positions will be combined into one position and the job role will have a completely new name.

Research a job title reflective of today's coding market. All coders will perform inpatient, outpatient, and emergency room coding.

Select two methods of job analysis to collect primary and secondary data on this proposed new position. For each method, explain why the method was selected and describe how the methods will be applied to analyze the coding positions. The purpose of this assignment is not to create an entirely new job description but rather outline the new job title and the methods used to perform an analysis on the job tasks performed in a combined position. Please provide references to support your response.

Assumptions

- The duties for each job description will be combined into a single job description
- The title will reflect the job role and position within the HIM department
- Job analysis tools will be assessed for appropriateness

Deliverable

A two-page paper containing the following:

- New (combined) job title and a two paragraphs describing why this title was selected
- Selection of two job analysis tools and an explanation of how these tools will be used to collect information to assess the combination of the job tasks
- Four references as additional research may be required to complete this paper

Review Questions

1. Before the actual job analysis process begins, an HIM manager must complete the following:
   a. Collect primary data to support the job analysis
   b. Execute a workflow analysis
   c. Perform a needs assessment
   d. Write a job description

2. As the assistant director of the HIM department, Judy is responsible for creating a job description for the new application specialist position. As part of the data collection phase, Judy researches the AHIMA Body of Knowledge to locate similar job descriptions already on file. The Body of Knowledge is what source of data?
   a. Primary
   b. Secondary
   c. Tertiary
   d. The Body of Knowledge should not be a source of data

3. Jane is responsible for developing the positions needed for scanning inactive records in anticipation of EHR implementation. Since she has no scanning experience, Jane called the supervisors of the scanning function

at three different facilities to pick their brains in regards to scanning jobs. This method of data collection for job analysis is the:

a. Competency model technique
b. Diary method
c. Observation method
d. Technical conference method

4. Which of the following would be an example of a job specification?

a. Assigns ICD-10-CM or PCS codes to all inpatient records
b. Performs chart analysis in accordance with department procedures
c. Able to type 90 words per minute with 98 percent accuracy
d. Supervises second and third shift HIM department staff

5. Elizabeth has been a privacy officer at University Hospital for four years. She likes her job, but feels she could be doing more challenging work. Elizabeth approaches her boss, the corporate director of HIM, with a proposal to begin traveling to hospital-affiliated physician practices to perform privacy audits and educational workshops for the office staff. This is an example of:

a. Job analysis
b. Job crafting
c. Job interviewing
d. Job redesign

6. Which of the following would be an example of a job task?

a. Holds an HIM credential of such as RHIA, RHIT, CCS, or CCS-P
b. Excellent written and oral communication skills
c. Required to sit for extended periods of time
d. Releases patient records to third parties in accordance with department procedures

7. Which of the following is not a component of job redesign?

a. Job analysis
b. Job enlargement
c. Job enrichment
d. Job rotation

8. Kevin is responsible for updating all job descriptions in the HIM department. In order to gather information about the data analyst position, he spends time interviewing and observing Sophie, who has held this job for three years. Kevin is using what source for data collection?

a. Primary
b. Secondary
c. Tertiary
d. Definitive

9. Which of the following is not a function of the job redesign process?

a. Creates the right person for the job fit
b. Enhances the quality of work life for the employee
c. Realigns the needs of the organization
d. Involves employee-driven changes to the job role

10. What is the final goal of the job analysis process?

    a. Aid in department strategic planning
    b. Create a new or updated job description
    c. Increase employee job satisfaction
    d. Increase employee job productivity

References

American Health Information Management Association. n.d. Body of Knowledge. http://library.ahima.org/xpedio/groups/public/documents/web_assets/bok_home.hcsp.

Berg, J.M., J.E. Dutton, and A. Wrzesniewski. 2013. *Job Crafting and Meaningful Work.* Washington, DC: American Psychological Association. 81–104.

CareerOneStop.org. 2015. Medical Records and Health Information Technicians. http://www.myskillsmyfuture.org/TargetOccupationMatch.aspx?onetcode=29207100&keyword=Health%20Information%20Technician&detailonetcode=29207100&highestmatch=Medical%20Records%20and%20Health%20Information%20Technicians&zipcode=0&radius=0&workPref=0&showWorkPref=0&indgroup=0&indsize=0&TargetRequest=T

Clegg, C. and C. Spencer. 2007. A circular and dynamic model of process of job design. *Journal of Occupational and Organizational Psychology* 80(2):321–339.

Community for Human Resource Management. 2015. What does KSAO stand for? http://www.chrmglobal.com/Qanda/55/1/What-does-KSAO-stand-for-.html.

Fried, B.J. and M.D. Fottler. 2008. *Human Resources in Healthcare: Managing for Success.* Chicago: Health Administration Press.

Hackman, J.R., and G.R. Oldham. 1975. Development of the job diagnostic survey. *Journal of Applied Psychology* 60(2):159–170.

Heery, E. and M. Noon. 2008. *A Dictionary of Human Resource Management.* Oxford: Oxford University Press.

Holman, D., C. Axtell, C. Sprigg, P. Totterdell, and T. Wall. 2010. The mediating role of job characteristics in job redesign interventions: A serendipitous quasi-experiment. *Journal of Organizational Behavior* 31(1):84–105.

Jeanneret, P.R. 1980. Equitable job evaluation and classification with the position analysis questionnaire. *Compensation Review* 12(1):32.

Karasek, R., C. Brisson, N. Kawakami, I. Houtman, P. Bongers, and B. Amick. 1998. The job content questionnaire (JCQ). *Journal of Occupational Health Psychology* 3(4):322–355.

Law, J., ed. 2009. *A Dictionary of Business and Management,* 5th ed. Oxford: Oxford University Press.

Layman, E. 2011. Job Redesign for Expanded HIM Functions. AHIMA Convention Proceedings.

Linker, J. 2014. The 21 Most Creative Job Titles. Forbes.com. http://www.forbes.com/sites/joshlinkner/2014/12/04/the-21-most-creative-job-titles/.

Lyons, P. 2008. The crafting of jobs and individual differences. *Journal of Business Psychology* 23(1/2):25–36.

Management Study Guide. 2013a. Job Redesign—Meaning, Process and Its Advantages. http://www.managementstudyguide.com/job-redesign.htm

Management Study Guide. 2013b. What to Collect During Job Analysis? http://www.managementstudyguide.com/what-to-collect-during-job-analysis.htm.

Morgeson, F.P. and S.E. Humphrey. 2006. The work design questionnaire (WDQ): Developing and validating a comprehensive measure for assessing job design and the nature of work. *Journal of Applied Psychology* 91(6): 1321–1339.

O*Net Online. 2015. US Department of Labor/Employment and Training Administration. http://www.onetcenter.org/overview.html.

Sale, J. and M.S. Kerr. 2002. The psychometric properties of Karasek's demand and control scales within a single sector: Data from a large teaching hospital. *International Archives of Occupational and Environmental Health* 75(3):145–152.

Sleezer, C.M., D.F. Ruff-Eft, and K. Gupta. 2014. *A Practical Needs Assessment,* 3rd ed. San Francisco: Wiley.

Smith, A. 2012. It's All in the Name: How to Ask for a Better Job Title. http://www.forbes.com/sites/dailymuse/2012/07/31/its-all-in-the-name-how-to-ask-for-a-better-job-title/.

Taber, T.D., and E. Taylor. 1990. A review and evaluation of the psychometric properties of the job diagnostic survey. *Personnel Psychology* 43(3):467–500.

Tims, M. and A.B. Bakker. 2010. Job crafting: Towards a new model of individual job redesign. *SAJIP: South African Journal of Industrial Psychology* 36(2):12–20.

United States Office of Personnel Management. 2015. Assessment and Selection: Job Analysis. http://www.opm.gov/policy-data-oversight/assessment-and-selection/job-analysis/.

United States Office of Personnel Management. 2009. Introduction to Position Classification Standards. Determining Grade Level. https://www.opm.gov/policy-data-oversight/classification-qualifications/classifying-general-schedule-positions/positionclassificationintro.pdf.

University of California, San Diego. 2015. Staff Human Resources: Writing Tasks Statements for Job Descriptions. https://academicaffairs.ucsd.edu/staffhr/classification/task-statements.html.

Washington State Human Resources. 2012. Competencies. http://www.hr.wa.gov/WorkforceDataAndPlanning/WorkforcePlanning/Competencies/Pages/default.aspx.

Wilson, K.L. 2012. Job Analysis. Chapter 52 in *Encyclopedia of Human Resource Management,* Volume 1. Edited by Rothwell, W.J. and R.K. Prescott. San Francisco: Pfeiffer.

Wrzesniewski, A., J.M. Berg, and J.E. Dutton. 2010. Managing yourself: Turn the job you have into the job you want. *Harvard Business Review* 88(6): 114–117.

Wrzesniewski, A. and J.E. Dutton. 2001. Crafting a job: Revisioning employees as active crafters of their work. *Academy of Management Review* 26(2):179–201.

Recruitment, Selection, and Retention in Health Information Management

Learning Objectives

- Evaluate the role of human resources in the recruitment of health information management (HIM) professionals
- Compare recruitment methods used for HIM job positions
- Discuss employee selection in relation to job hiring
- Evaluate retention strategies in terms of effectiveness in retaining employees
- Discuss compensation practices in relation to recruitment and retention

Key Terms

360-degree interview	Headhunters	Market pricing	Selection
Bonus	Incentive program	Negligent hiring	Semi-structured interview
Compensable factors	Internal candidates	Networking	Structured interview
Cost-of-living adjustments (COLA)	Involuntary turnover	Offer of employment	Turnover
Dysfunctional turnover	Job autonomy	Outsource	Unstructured interview
External candidates	Job evaluation	Pay grade	Validity
Factor comparison	Job grading	Point method	Voluntary turnover
Functional turnover	Job ranking	Recruitment	
	Job retention	Reliability	

ecruitment, selection, and retention are basic functions of any health information management (HIM) manager's responsibilities. As the electronic health record (EHR) becomes the standard in healthcare organizations, HIM positions continue to change and develop. The need for file clerks disappears, but the need for scanning clerks increases. Voice recognition applications mean that transcriptionists do less typing and more editing. Coding personnel develop new skills as they work with physicians and other healthcare providers to improve clinical documentation in the record so that *International Classification of Diseases, Tenth Revision, Clinical Modification (ICD-10-CM);* and *International Classification of Diseases, Tenth Revision, Procedure Coding System (ICD-10-PCS)* can be implemented and used to its fullest potential. Chapter 3 discussed the fact that population statistics indicate the younger workforce is declining. The competition for younger workers will be strong. An organization must hire and retain qualified individuals as part of any strategic plan. This chapter examines the recruiting tools available to managers, details the selection process of new employees, and discusses the impact of turnover and retention on the workforce.

Job Recruitment

Recruitment is the process of finding, soliciting, and attracting employees. For most HIM managers, the process of finding a new employee begins when one of two things has happened: a current employee has vacated a position and a replacement must be found, or a new or additional position has been approved and now must be filled (addressed in chapter 6). For a current position, the job description is reviewed and updated as necessary. If it is a newly created position, it is likely that the job description was recently written as part of the position approval process. If not, a new job description will have to be created. The job description contains the qualifications necessary for the position such as required credentials, experience, and level of education. These elements are important to include in any recruiting tool so potential applicants or recruiters know up front what a position needs. It is a waste of time for a grossly unqualified person to apply for any job. On the other hand, a potential applicant with the necessary credentials and required level of experience may decide to take a chance on the position.

Early in the recruiting process, the HIM manager partners with a representative from the human resources (HR) department to create a plan for filling the open position with a goal of finding a qualified pool of applicants and then selecting the individual who presents as the best fit for both the position and the organization (see figure 7.1). The HR department should be instrumental in providing a history of the position in regards to how long it has taken to fill previous positions and, if possible, provide a list of applicants that are still available from the last time the position was filled. It should be noted, however, that in a small organization there may not be an HR department, so the HIM manager may be on their own when it comes to recruiting. If there is a representative from the HR department, it is a good idea to take the time to educate them about HIM in general, and the open position in particular. Sometimes HR personnel are not as familiar with HIM as they are with other areas in the organization such as nursing or rehabilitation services. Invite them to the department to see firsthand what tasks the new employee will be performing.

Early in the recruiting process, it is necessary to determine the competitive nature of the position. Will the position be easy to fill? Is there a shortage of qualified applicants for the position, making it potentially difficult to fill in a timely manner? What is the prevailing wage for the position? This information is especially important if the position is new to the organization. Generally, an organization will prefer that someone from the HR department conduct a survey of local or even regional competitors to collect this information. Salary data and other job specifications such as experience and education will be gathered. Comparisons will be made to the same or similar jobs at other organizations so that a fair wage and benefit package may be put together for the position. An HR representative usually gathers this information so that survey practices throughout the organization are uniform. An HR representative has the background and experience to collect data on different types of positions, and they know what questions to ask to efficiently gather the right information.

Figure 7.1. Recruitment plan workflow

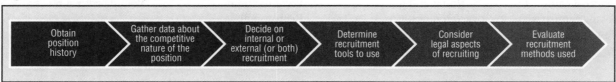

A decision must be made as to whether a position should be internally or externally recruited, or a combination of both. **Internal candidates** are individuals already employed by the organization. An internal candidate may be promoted from within the HIM department or promoted or transferred from another department in the organization. There are advantages to recruiting from within an organization:

- The candidate is already known and has proven themselves to the organization
- Candidates have an understanding of the culture and procedures of the organization
- Acts as a motivating factor for current employees' performance
- Improves morale and a sense of loyalty for current employees
- Is generally a quicker process than recruiting externally

There are also disadvantages to recruiting from within an organization:

- Contributes to a culture of sameness
- May promote discriminatory hiring practices over time
- May lead to hard feelings and lowered morale if an employee is not chosen for the position
- Some managers may recommend poor performers for transfer to other departments

External candidates are individuals from outside of the organization. External candidates come from educational institutions such as high schools, community colleges and universities, other competing organizations, or vendors. There are advantages to recruiting from outside an organization:

- Candidates contribute new ideas to an organization
- New graduates are trained in the most up-to-date methods
- Candidate may introduce a specific skill or knowledge set not present in the organization
- Usually offers a larger pool of candidates
- Candidates do not have predetermined opinions of the organization and can start fresh

There are also disadvantages to recruiting from outside an organization:

- Can be a demoralizing factor to current employees
- Time is lost while a candidate adjusts to the new organization
- It is unknown as to whether the candidate will fit the culture of an organization despite having the necessary technical skills

Most organizations have a "promote from within" policy to encourage employees to stay with the organization. Qualified employees are promoted to new positions and outside candidates are recruited into the lower level positions, allowing for both internal and external recruiting.

The next step in the recruitment plan determines which recruitment tools to use. Again, the HIM manager should work with the HR representative to decide the appropriate tools to use for each position. The plan continues with a consideration of the legal aspects of recruiting and finishes with an evaluation of the recruitment methods used.

Recruitment Tools

There are many different types of recruitment tools. Some methods are more appropriate than others for different positions in the HIM department. Also, recruiting tools come at a price and an HIM manager must be mindful of any approved recruiting budget set for a specific position. For example, it does not make sense to hire a search firm to recruit for an entry-level position such as release-of-information clerk, but using a search firm may make sense for a corporate-level HIM director that will oversee four different facilities. Recruitment tools include the following:

- Advertisement: Newspapers, business journals, and industry publications (such as the *Journal of AHIMA*) can be found both locally or nationally. Web-based ads are placed on industry or professional websites. Television and radio ads may also be effective. An ad should be designed by a professional and include the basic requirements of the position. Ads can be expensive so there may be a time limit placed on how long the ad can run in a specific medium. Ads may be used to recruit locally if there is a known supply of potential candidates in the region. For example, in a large metropolitan area there may be many healthcare facilities, so placing an ad in a local newspaper for a privacy officer might make sense. On the other hand, a rural long-term acute-care hospital also needing a privacy officer may decide not to advertise locally as the population is generally known. It may be better for them to place ads in professional journals or newspapers in neighboring cities.

- **Networking:** Networking—cultivating a mutually-beneficial, active circle of acquaintances and associates—gets the word out about a job through personal contacts. Networking occurs in person through contacts made at conferences or professional events. Job openings are discussed among friends, relatives, neighbors, and other acquaintances to get the word passed from one person to another. Managers may contact their peers at other organizations or previous instructors at educational institutions with information regarding job openings. Networking may also be done via social media sites. Networking is free and works for almost any type of open position. The benefit is that a manager can target a certain population—at a state HIM association meeting, for example—and spread the word about a specific job opening to a select audience for no cost.

- Internet: The Internet offers access to job search websites. Job openings can also be posted on job boards on social media sites. According to one survey, 92 percent of employers indicate reaching qualified candidates through social media is a worthwhile recruiting strategy (*i*CIMS 2014). Job search websites allow candidates to post their resumes for review. The Internet offers the ability to reach a large amount of potential candidates without the high cost of direct advertising. However, the large amount of information available also increases the time to review and discard any undesirable applications.

- Job fairs: Job fairs bring a number of employers together in one physical location in an effort to reach many potential candidates. Job fairs are held on college campuses, at business conventions, and by community civic organizations. Interested candidates can meet face-to-face with employers who have job openings and discuss employment opportunities. Employers have the opportunity to meet a number of potential applicants at one time and collect resumes or contact information for the future should a need arise. Job fairs are usually staffed by HR department personnel, but an HIM manager may be asked to participate if the job fair is expected to appeal to HIM professionals. The downside to this method is that there are often multiple types of health professionals in attendance, all looking for jobs, and an HIM manager may have to talk to individuals who are neither qualified nor interested in the HIM positions available. Timing is also an issue. Job fairs are usually scheduled in advance and there may not be any open positions at the time of the job fair. When there are open positions, candidates from a job fair may have found employment elsewhere.

- Search firms: Search firms employ professionals, or **headhunters**, to seek out job openings and match specific individuals to specific jobs. Headhunters represent both job seekers and organizations looking to fill positions. Search firms may represent an organization recruiting for a highly specialized position, an upper management position, or may even perform a confidential search for a job that is not publicly available. Due to the high cost, headhunters are usually not the first method chosen to recruit for a job. It is not uncommon for a search firm to charge up to one-half the annual salary of the position they have been contracted to fill.

- School affiliations or professional practice experiences: Colleges, universities, and even high schools can be a source of potential job candidates. An HIM manager should connect with local or regional HIM programs to post job openings and recruit graduates. New graduates have up-to-date knowledge and an enthusiasm for the profession that can offset a lack of experience. Often an HIM manager is asked to speak to graduating seniors on topics such as interviewing techniques, real-world work experiences, or the future of the HIM profession. An HIM manager should use this opportunity to represent their employer in a positive manner, or personally network with seniors who may be looking for post-graduate employment. An HIM manager who opens her department to professional practice experience (PPE) students from an HIM program gets a firsthand look at how students conduct themselves in a work setting. When a job opens up the manager has a list of available people who might be interested in applying.

- Outsourcing: Organizations also **outsource** certain positions, designating certain positions or functions to be filled on a permanent basis by contracted employees. These individuals are employed by a third-party company that specializes in the required function. Common examples of outsourced functions in the HIM department are transcription, coding, release of information, and management staff. Outsourcing is an option when there is a serious lack of qualified applicants for a position. Having an outside company take over the function fills the position quickly and can be cheaper than paying a full salary with benefits. Outsourcing may be appropriate for a task that is performed on an occasional basis, such as preparation of a cancer program's annual report. Outsourcing is also an option when an organization restructures and decides to focus on core initiatives, leaving other functions like HIM department management to an outside company. Any organization considering outsourcing HIM functions should perform due diligence to verify business practices, ensure conformance to contract terms, and mitigate potential risks of Health Insurance Portability and Accountability Act of 1996 (HIPAA) violations (Sett et al. 2014).

- Temporary agencies: One alternative to filling open positions is to work with a temporary agency. A temporary agency hires its own employees in a variety of areas such as clerical, healthcare, industrial, and engineering, and then contracts with organizations to provide coverage on an as-needed basis. Temporary employees can fill positions that are empty due to family and medical leave absences. If a position is expected to be difficult to fill, a temporary employee may be hired until recruiting efforts secure a permanent employee. Temporary agencies are used for short-term replacement of open positions, whereas outsourcing is used for long-term or even permanent replacement of open positions. Temporary or outsourced employees may be hired as permanent employees if their skill set matches the opening, but before offering employment to a temporary or outsourced employee it is important to review the contract with the agency or company to determine if there are any stipulations that prohibit this practice.

- Employee referral: Current employees of the organization can be an excellent source of recruiting if they can recommend potential applicants. The employee has knowledge of both the organization and the candidate, and can offer insight to both parties. Often there is a monetary reward if the candidate is hired. Part of the money is paid to the referring employee upon hire and the remainder of the money is paid after the new hire completes a specific term of employment.

In some cases, these traditional recruitment methods do not result in any candidates for a position. It may be a specific issue such as the advertisement is poorly written or poorly placed, but often the demand for a position exceeds the supply of qualified candidates. Such is the case with HIM coding professionals, as the demand for coders in the United States is expected to grow. The United States Bureau of Labor Statistics classifies coders as health information technicians and the employment of these professionals is projected to grow 22 percent through 2022, much faster than the average for all occupations (BLS 2015). The shortage results in unique recruiting and staffing models implemented throughout the industry. One such program is to "grow your own" coders (Endicott 2014). Hospitals are developing their own in-house training programs and offering them to internal eligible candidates. The successful programs range in time from 8 to 12 weeks, to 8 months. Most programs require candidates to hold a current coding or HIM credential in order to participate, but it is possible to create a program that is open to all employees, regardless of whether or not they hold a coding credential (Endicott 2014). Typical courses include medical terminology, anatomy and physiology, and both ICD-10-CM/PCS and Current Procedural Terminology (CPT) instruction. Candidates complete the courses and are slowly introduced to real-world coding so their speed and accuracy can be closely monitored. The intent is to hire the graduates of these grow-your-own programs for permanent coding positions.

Another method used to recruit and keep coders and other positions such as clinical documentation improvement specialist, business analyst, and data analyst is a post-graduate apprenticeship program developed by the American Health Information Management Association (AHIMA) Foundation. The AHIMA Foundation's mission is to "improve lives by supporting leadership in health information governance and informatics through research, education, and life-long learning" (AHIMA Foundation 2015a). The AHIMA Foundation accomplishes this mission with advancement programs such as the apprenticeship program. The program accepts applications for apprenticeships from candidates who are new graduates of HIM programs and who possess the required HIM credential. The specifics of the apprenticeship program are:

- An apprenticeship is a paid position that bridges education and employment in an organization.
- Apprentices start at an entry level pay scale of an occupation that increases as certain checkpoints are reached. They learn while both the apprentice and organization earn, financially and professionally.

- Apprentices may be temporary or permanent employees and are usually full-time positions.
- Apprentice qualifications vary according to role. For example, a coder apprentice must hold a Clinical Coding Associate (CCA), Registered Health Information Technician (RHIT), or Registered Health Information Administrator (RHIA) credential while a data analyst apprentice must hold a minimum of an RHIA credential.
- An apprenticeship program lasts from one to two years, with the goal of permanent placement in the position. The apprentice candidate gains real-world working experience that can be of substantial work to any company (AHIMA Foundation 2015b).

Legal Aspects of Recruitment

Regardless of the source of the candidates and tools used to recruit them, an HIM manager must be mindful of the legal aspects of the recruiting process. Chapter 5 covered the antidiscrimination laws and Equal Employment Opportunity Commission (EEOC) guidelines that must be followed when interviewing individuals for open positions. The same information applies to the recruiting process. It is illegal to discriminate against potential candidates on the basis of age, race, color, religion, national origin, sex, or disability on application forms or when screening candidates. Application forms and position advertisements generally include the statement that the organization is an equal opportunity employer. When using social media for recruiting, an HIM manager must be careful not to allow pictures of candidates available to prejudice their decisions to move a candidate forward in the hiring process. When placing advertisements, a variety of publications should be used to ensure that the position is known to a diverse population. For example, if a position is to be advertised in trade magazines, seeking out additional organizations with diverse memberships should be done to ensure wide distribution of the position. The HR department should provide direction for an HIM manager who is unsure of the legalities of recruiting.

Evaluation of Recruitment Methods

Once recruiting has ended and a position is filled, it is important to evaluate the effectiveness of the recruiting methods so an organization can begin to gather data on which methods produce the best applicants and ultimately the best employees. Some measures of effectiveness include:

- Evaluating each recruitment tool to determine how many qualified applicants were cultivated, hired, and how long they worked at the organization
- Measure direct costs for advertising, search firms, travel to job fairs, and employee referral bonuses
- Measure indirect costs such as lost productivity due to open positions and training new employees
- Measure the time from job requisition to interview, offer, acceptance, and start date
- Evaluate the diversity of the applicant pool

Most organizations have an HR information system (HRIS) that provides extensive history and data on each position. An HIM manager does not need to keep their own data if the organization's HRIS can provide the necessary information.

Check Your **Understanding**

1. Explain the importance of the job description in the recruitment process.
2. Discuss the advantages and disadvantages to hiring from within and outside the organization.
3. Explain the various recruiting methods available to HIM managers.
4. What legal considerations must be in place when recruiting for HIM professionals?
5. Discuss the importance of measuring recruiting methods.

Job Selection

If properly executed, the recruitment process should yield a number of applications and resumes from qualified candidates. Candidates who do not meet the basic job requirements are eliminated from the group and the HR department offers only qualified candidates to the HIM manager for consideration. The next step is **selection** or the process of choosing the right person for the job. The manager has many selection tools from which to choose to rate candidates in order to determine the best applicant. There are different types of interviewing techniques as well. As with recruitment, the HIM manager should work closely with the HR department to determine which applicants to interview and include in the final selection.

Selection Tools

Once qualified candidates for a position are identified, it is necessary to decide which ones are suitable to advance to an interview and an eventual offer of employment. It may be that an HIM manager received the names of 10 candidates from the HR department who fit the requirements for a posted position, but in most cases time constraints will not allow for all 10 candidates to be interviewed. The manager must therefore decide among the candidates who will be eliminated from consideration. It may be that only three qualified candidate names are put forward by the HR department, but a manager must still eventually decide which candidate will be chosen for the position. There are numerous tools that can be used to rate candidates; the choice depends on the job. In general, the more complex the job, the more complex and time consuming the selection tool. For example, an HIM manager hiring a new supervisor may use a variety of selection tools, but may use only one or two tools when hiring a scanning clerk.

- Employee application form or resume: An application form is a standard form developed by the organization to collect basic information from candidates such as name, contact information, education and work history, credential or license numbers, references, and volunteer experience. A resume serves the same purpose but is created and submitted by the applicant. Application forms and resumes are used in some combination for almost all open positions. Some organizations ask each candidate to complete an application form regardless of whether or not they have a resume. Some organizations will accept a candidate's resume in lieu of an application. Information collected must comply with EEOC guidelines in regards to discrimination. To prevent inaccurate or falsified information, applications should have a statement for the candidate to sign that attests to the truth of the information. Applications and resumes should be reviewed as an initial check to make sure the candidate meets the minimum qualifications for the job. If the minimum qualifications are not met, a candidate should not be moved forward for further consideration, but it might be possible to consider the candidate for a different position. Applications of qualified candidates not chosen for the position are often saved for a period of time in case the position comes open again.

- Ability tests: Ability tests measure the ability of the candidate to perform certain functions of a job. HIM examples would be coding tests for coders and typing tests for transcriptionists. Such tests are appropriate if they pertain directly to the job functions and measure what they are intended to measure. For example, if a coding test is going to be used to test coding ability, all candidates must be given the same test under the same circumstances. One candidate cannot take the test in a quiet room with access to an encoder and another candidate take the test in an open office environment using code books. Also, if the position is for an outpatient coder, there should be both ICD-10-CM/PCS and CPT coding on the test.

- Simulations: Simulations are similar to ability tests in that they demonstrate a candidate's job-related skills. A simulation is more hands-on and real-time; for example, a candidate for a data analyst position may be asked to extract data and format a report from a database application.

- Reference checks: Reference checks include both telephone calls to and letters of reference from previous employers, professors, or other individuals who might be able to attest to the candidate's work habits. They are a good way to verify the employment and education history provided on applications and resumes. Some organizations go beyond traditional reference checks and delve into the background of candidates by performing credit checks and checking driving and criminal records. It is unlikely that a candidate would provide a reference from anyone who would not give a positive recommendation, which is why some managers are hesitant to check references and view them as a waste of time. In addition, previous employers may be reluctant to provide any negative information about a candidate, because if they do they run the risk of being sued for defamation should the candidate find out what was said. Despite the disadvantages to checking references, there are reasons to do so. An organization may run the risk of being charged with **negligent hiring**. A charge of negligent hiring can be made against an organization if a current employee in some way harms a patient or another employee, or commits a serious offense and the organization should have known about the employee's tendencies had a thorough background check been done prior to hiring. For example, while driving a hospital vehicle, the driver is in an accident with serious injuries to patient passengers. If the driver has a poor driving record, a claim could be made that the driver should not have been hired for that position. Because of the sensitive nature of reference checks, most organizations require them to be handled by the HR department. Information given to potential employers is usually restricted to what is available in the employee's personnel file. Information gathered relates only to the position for which the applicant is being considered. The question that most prospective employers want answered by a previous employer is: Would you rehire this person?

- Assessment centers: Traditionally, assessment centers are used for managerial and executive positions, but some organizations choose to use them for a variety of jobs, including very specialized or high-turnover positions. Testing is done by professionals and applicants are given a series of individual and group exercises that are then scored and shared with the employer. Paper-and-pencil tests such as personality, psychological, and aptitude tests are given, and oral and written communication skills are measured. An individual applicant may be asked to perform an *in-basket* exercise. In this case, a pile of memos or list of emails is presented, and the applicant must handle each item in some way within a given time period. Team behavior may be measured with leaderless discussion groups. These involve applicants being placed together to solve a common work situation such as recommended disciplinary action for an employee with a behavior problem; this exercise demonstrates team behavior. Role-playing activities are also used to test team behaviors. Applicants assume managerial and subordinate roles and respond to scenarios such as employee disciplinary action, budget requests, and employee appraisals.

Each of the selection tools should be measured for both reliability and validity. **Reliability** is a measure of consistency of data items based on their reproducibility and an estimation of their error of measurement. In other words, the chosen tool should produce the same results regardless of who administers the tool or how it is administered. Consider whether reference checks are a reliable tool. Information gathered through a reference check could certainly vary depending on who was asking for the information. If a letter of reference is provided, there is no consistency from writer to writer and no common questions asked, so the information provided cannot be considered reliable. **Validity** is the extent to which an instrument measures what it purports to measure. If a coding test is created using examples of coding scenarios at the facility, the test will measure what it is supposed to measure. However, a coding test with one- or two-word phrases may not be as valid an instrument. In other words, the coding test must show that those who score well on the test will be good coders after they are hired. Data should be kept that illustrates that connection between scores and coder performance so that the validity can be proven if questioned.

Interviewing Techniques

The job interview is a popular selection tool used by organizations. At some point, almost everyone in the working world has been interviewed for a position. Interviews are done one-to-one or with another person present. Interviews may be done by a group (panel), either with all group members present or with each group member individually. A **360-degree interview** involves three different interviews, with the supervisor of the position, peers of the position, and subordinates of the position. Interviews are done in person, over the telephone, or through video conferencing software. The location of the interview depends on the cost relative to the position. For example, if there are five or more candidates for an open department head position, it might be too expensive to set up an in-person interview for each applicant. In this case a telephone interview may be appropriate as a first-interview screening for the position. The telephone interview process would result in two or three top candidates who would then be brought on site for the personal interview.

Interviews are generally categorized as structured, unstructured, or semi-structured. A **structured interview**, also called a directive interview, focuses on the job to be filled, using the job description as the starting point. The job description is reviewed in detail, giving the applicant a clear idea of the job requirements and expectations. The interview has a predesigned format that is followed with each applicant; questions are developed prior to the interview and usually asked of each applicant in the same order. This structure makes it easier for the HIM manager to compare candidates, as each person is presented with the same information and asked the same questions.

Structured interviews have a higher degree of reliability than other interview types due to the fact that the questions are replicated. Structured interviews have a lower degree of validity, however, due to the fact that their inflexible nature does not allow for detailed probing about the candidate or areas not covered by the questions. The following types of questions may be asked during a structured interview:

- Situational: Situational questions are intended to show how the candidate would react in hypothetical situations. They begin with "How would you..." or "What would you do if...." For example, a candidate interviewing for an evening supervisory position might be presented with a scenario of two or three night shift employees calling in sick at the last minute and asked how they would handle such a situation.

- Behavioral: These questions are experienced-based and the intent is that the best predictor of future behavior is how a person acted in a similar situation in their past. Behavioral questions are "Tell me about a time..." or "How did you...." For example, a candidate interviewing for an HIM audit technician position might be asked to describe a time when they disagreed with their supervisor and to explain the outcome of the encounter.

- Job knowledge: Job knowledge questions are intended to determine if the applicant knows how to do the job. For example, a person interviewing for a privacy officer position might be asked about their experience with HIPAA regulations and privacy breaches. A potential data analyst might be questioned about their knowledge of spreadsheet and database applications.

- Work requirement: While an interviewer must be careful not to ask any illegal questions, it is perfectly allowable to ask if a potential employee is available to work weekends or holidays if that is a job requirement. If travel is a part of the job, an applicant might be questioned on their availability for overnight travel. The questions must be framed so as not to be discriminatory, and all applicants must be asked the same question.

An **unstructured interview**, also called a nondirective interview, is the opposite of a structured interview. In general, no questions are planned in advance, although certain topics may be targeted. An interviewer may begin with one question, and then ask follow-up questions based on the interviewee's answer. The questions are not necessarily job-related, and the interview may resemble a conversation rather than a question and answer period. The random nature of an unstructured interview makes it better suited for identifying unsuitable candidates rather than suitable candidates. This type of interview is less reliable because it cannot be replicated among candidates and is difficult to do well. An interviewer must be able to ask open-ended questions and adjust to the interviewee's responses while still trying to gather useful information on how the candidate would fit the job.

A **semi-structured interview** is a combination of the structured and unstructured interviews. Generally, the interviewer will have a few predetermined questions to start the interview, but then will respond to the interviewee's answers with more probing follow-up questions. For example, the interviewer asks a behavioral question and based on the answer might follow up with a request for a second example, or ask for further insight or details about the first answer. While less reliable than a structured interview because all the questions are not the same, the semi-structured interview has a higher validity rating because the probing follow up questions can shed light on characteristics and behaviors not elicited during a structured interview.

Once the type of interview is determined and questions are written, it is time for the HIM manager to prepare for the interview itself. The following suggestions will help make the interview go smoothly and be less stressful for both the HIM manager and the candidate.

- Prepare. Read over the job description a few times and review the questions that will be asked. Even an unstructured interview will have a few questions or topics that must be covered. Become familiar with the candidate's resume or application form so that gaps in employment or other areas of concern or interest are highlighted for discussion.

- Arrange for privacy and no interruptions. If the interviewer does not have an office, try to borrow an office or arrange to use a conference room or an isolated area of a location such as a cafeteria or library.

- Set a time for the interview to be over. This helps to keep the interview on track.

- Put the candidate at ease by being welcoming. Offer a glass of water, ask general questions intended to relax the interviewee such as "Did you have trouble locating the office?" and, "How did you find out about the job?"

- Listen carefully and take notes if necessary. The candidate should do most of the talking. A good rule of thumb is for the interviewer to talk only about 30 percent of the time.

- Maintain a professional yet friendly tone. Do not let the conversation get too personal.

- Make sure the candidate has a thorough understanding of the job responsibilities and expectations. It is a good idea to share the job description if they have not already seen it.

- Ensure the candidate has an opportunity to ask any questions they may have about the job or the organization.

- Explain the rest of the selection process such as how much longer interviews will last, when a decision is expected to be made, and how they will be notified of the outcome of the search.

Candidate Selection

Once the results of the selection tools are compiled and all interviews are complete, the HIM manager must make a decision about which candidate to hire. Consideration should be given to the experience of the applicants, the attitude and personality demonstrated during the interview, and any other results that are pertinent—drug testing, ability test results, promotion status. A manager may decide to use a rating system, assigning point values to each selection tool used and then rank the candidates. Using the job description as a guide, an HIM manager should be careful to match the person to the job, not the job to the person. One option that remains is that if an ideal candidate is not found, reopen the recruitment and selection process. It may be necessary to review the job posting to make sure the qualifications were clear, to expand the search area, or to even consider an apprenticeship or grow-your-own program to locate the best candidates.

When the decision has been made on which candidate to hire, an **offer of employment** is presented to the candidate. The offer of employment is a formal job offer usually in a letter or a telephone call followed by a letter. The offer of employment should include, at a minimum, the position title, salary, and start date. Most organizations prefer to have an offer of employment come from an HR representative rather than from the department manager. Having the HR department make the offer provides consistency and prohibits a department manager from giving out erroneous information if the candidate asks about salary or benefits. Once the candidate has accepted the offer, all other candidates should be notified that the position has been filled. Again, this should be done by the HR department and not the HIM manager. No reason needs to be given to unsuccessful candidates, and an HIM manager who is contacted for a reason should refer the person to the HR department.

Check Your **Understanding**

1. Discuss the advantages and disadvantages to using reference checks as a selection tool.
2. Why is it important to consider the reliability and validity ratings of a selection tool?
3. Which selection tools are rated the highest in regards to reliability and validity?
4. Explain the difference between structured, unstructured, and semi-structured interviews.
5. What are the best practices for conducting an interview?

Job Retention

If recruitment and selection are attracting and choosing the right people for the right jobs in an organization, **job retention** is keeping those people from seeking employment elsewhere. The cost of recruiting, selecting, and training employees is high, and represents an investment the organization makes in its workforce. If an organization builds on the work done during recruitment and selection, they will retain their employees. If the right employee is hired, the chances are better that the employee will remain with the organization. It is important to understand the difference between turnover and retention. Retention means keeping the right people employed; **turnover** means people are leaving the organization.

Turnover

No manager likes to lose good employees, and a good manager pays attention to the turnover in their department. There are many different factors that influence an employee's decision to leave an organization. Some factors such as transfer of a spouse, retirement, life choices (such as returning to school or deciding to stay home with children), and medical problems are out of the control of the HIM manager. Other factors such as job-related stress, lack of recognition, and low morale are concerns that need to be addressed. One survey found that the top five reasons employees reported voluntarily leaving an organization are better growth and earning potential, more time and flexibility, increased financial compensation, enriched culture and work environment, and improved benefits (DeScherer and Myers 2007). When employees choose to leave an organization it is called **voluntary turnover**. When an employee is fired, laid off, or otherwise terminated by the organization it is called **involuntary turnover**.

There are two other types of turnover: functional and dysfunctional. **Functional turnover** occurs when poor performing or disruptive employees leave the organization. Functional turnover also occurs when an organization downsizes out of financial necessity. This action allows for the organization to make a commitment to refocusing efforts on their long-term fiscal health. Generally there are organizational benefits with functional turnover. Morale and productivity improve when sub-par performers leave and are replaced by new, motivated employees. Even layoffs and restructuring benefit the organization in the long run, allowing the organization to improve its financial position. **Dysfunctional turnover** occurs when valued or highly skilled employees leave the organization or a number of employees leave a critical work area. For example, if half the coders left a hospital months before the October 1, 2015 implementation of ICD-10-CM/PCS, it would have a devastating effect on productivity, morale, and reimbursement. Dysfunctional turnover can hurt the organization from both a quality and financial standpoint. Recruiting and selection costs are much higher for difficult-to-fill positions. If multiple positions are vacated in a short period of time, quality and productivity suffer. If the positions are in critical areas, patient care could suffer too. Considering the various categories of turnover, the type that managers must be most concerned with is voluntary, dysfunctional turnover. Some voluntary turnover is unavoidable as in the cases of retirement or a spouse transferred out of town, but for voluntary turnover that can be avoided, such as leaving a high-stress position, an HIM manager must look at how the turnover affects the organization. The cost of employee turnover is high, as displayed in table 7.1.

Retention Strategies

Organizations invest considerable time and money into bringing a new employee on board and an HIM manager needs to pay attention to retention as well as turnover. Retention strategies are designed to keep employees interested and satisfied enough in their workplace that they want to remain with the organization. A review of motivational theories from chapter 3 shows that employees have levels of needs (Maslow's hierarchy of needs) as well as satisfiers and dissatisfiers (Herzberg's two-factor theory) that impact how they feel about their jobs. Retention strategies across organizations are numerous and varied, but can be summarized into the following best practices.

Select the Right Employee

The recruitment and selection processes are key to finding the employee who will want to remain with the organization. Taking the time to craft the right job posting using an updated job description to use recruitment methods that are proven to work for your organization, interviewing thoroughly to find the right fit for the

Table 7.1. The costs of employee turnover

Direct costs	Indirect costs
• Payouts of accrued vacation and sick time and severance pay • Unemployment insurance and COBRA administration costs • Time lost while recruiting and interviewing for the open position(s)	• Lost productivity of departed employee(s) • Lost productivity of co-workers and supervisors who must cover open positions • Decrease in patient or customer satisfaction due to low staffing levels • The effects of knowledge lost due to employee departure

organization, and applying appropriate selection tools can pay off in the end with a motivated new hire. Relying on professional practice experiences, apprenticeships, or grow-your-own programs to identify new employees can also result in increased retention, as these employees are looking for specific employment in the position for which they have been recruited. On the other hand, rushing through the interview process, not checking resume information, and hiring someone who is "close enough" rather than the right fit can lead to a dissatisfied new hire who soon leaves the organization either by choice or by termination. A continued pattern of poor hires leads to increased turnover and increased recruitment costs.

New Employee Orientation

Orientation is covered in more detail in chapter 9, but some items are mentioned here as part of a retention strategy. Orientation is the organization's opportunity to sell itself to a new employee. This is not the time to bore new hires with lecture after lecture on the organization's policies and procedures. Creative methods of welcoming new employees with breakfast, balloons, and an introduction by the chief executive officer (CEO) help set a positive atmosphere. Many organizations pair new employees with a seasoned employee or buddy to show them how to get around and get along in their new workplace.

Monitor Turnover

The HR department should monitor turnover on an organizationwide basis, and HIM managers should monitor turnover in their departments. Trends may identify key areas in the department that experience higher turnover, or specific managers or supervisors that experience higher turnover among their direct reports. Both are opportunities to examine if improvements can be made to processes or workflows that result in decreased employee turnover. For example, mandatory overtime in the coding area may take its toll over time and cause coders to look for less demanding jobs elsewhere. Implementing a team approach to overtime allows for employees to contribute ideas and work together to find a solution. The amount of overtime may not be reduced, but employees now feel as though they have some control over the situation and feel more satisfied and willing to remain at the organization. A supervisor with high turnover among direct reports may be connected to a mentor who will help build communication skills and create a less stressful environment for employees.

Exit interviews and surveys completed by employees as they leave the organization can provide additional information about areas that might need improvement. Interviews are done face-to-face, and surveys are given to employees to complete on their own and return to the HR department. It is important that exiting employees believe that the interviews and surveys will be kept confidential so they feel they may be honest in their responses. This is more difficult than it would seem, as exiting employees may be concerned that their comments might be reflected in a poor reference or be shared with their supervisor. For this reason, surveys provide more anonymity than interviews, and exit interviews or surveys should be administered by a neutral third party such as an HR representative or a firm contracted for this purpose.

Periodic employee satisfaction surveys are another way to gather information about why employees may be thinking about leaving the organization. Satisfaction surveys can be organizationwide or department-specific. Either way, managers must be prepared to show good faith and act on information received in this manner. If you ask for employee opinions, it is not good practice to ignore them.

Communication

A common saying in the workplace is, "employees do not quit their jobs, they quit their bosses." Improved communications can go a long way to mitigating this statement. Managers must listen to ideas and concerns presented to them by their employees and then act in good faith to resolve or address them. Taking the time to listen and respond is imperative—during the interview process, a manager must do more listening then talking; understanding employee motivation depends on communicating with employees; and job design and analysis require both written and oral communication skills. Job crafting (chapter 6) is a collaboration, but depends on the employee bringing the idea to the manager. Performance appraisals (chapter 8) require trust and honest communication about goals and productivity. Open communication allows for positive relationships to develop, encouraging subordinates to trust in and want to work with their bosses; as a result, the employees are more likely to stay committed to the organization.

Working Conditions

Working conditions include the environment in which an employee works such as noise levels, lighting, compensation, stress, overtime, benefits, and safety. Employees care about their physical working conditions just as they care about the psychological or mental aspects of their working conditions. Methods for improving physical working conditions include flexible scheduling such as compressed workweeks, job sharing or flextime (chapter 5), working remotely from home, safety measures provided in the workplace, and on-site childcare.

One strategy for influencing the psychological aspects of working conditions is providing a sense of **job autonomy**, or individual control, to a position. For example, one aspect of a release of information (ROI) job is to monitor and respond to requests for copies of health records. As requests are logged into the ROI system, the turnaround time for requests is calculated. The intent is to keep the turnaround time for requests as short as possible. In some HIM departments, the ROI manager scrutinizes this report daily, reporting the turnaround time to the ROI staff, and shifting schedules or using overtime to improve the numbers on the report. ROI staff has little, if any, autonomy in this example. The ROI manager controls the distribution of and the reaction to the turnaround time report; he or she makes all the decisions and communicates the solutions. In other HIM departments, ROI staff works together as a self-directed team (chapter 3) to manage the turnaround time. The staff monitors the report and shifts their schedules as necessary to maintain a target turnaround time. The ROI manager only becomes involved when certain thresholds are reached, allowing the ROI staff a degree of autonomy over this particular job task.

Other retention strategies include providing adequate training for job competency, equal treatment across the department on disciplinary matters, opportunities for career development, award and recognition programs, and the presence of performance appraisals and fair job performance standards. These latter two strategies link to the goal-setting theory of motivation detailed in chapter 3.

Competitive Compensation Practices

Financial compensation may not be the only reason that employees leave an organization, but it is certainly one of the reasons (DeScherer and Myers 2007). Compensation practices are discussed in more detail later in this chapter, but there are retention strategies that impact employee compensation worth mentioning here. Retention strategies with a financial component include tuition assistance or reimbursement programs, free parking, forgivable loans, retirement plans, and benefit plans. Flexible benefit plans, or cafeteria plans, allow employees to choose those benefits that appeal to them the most. For example, an employee with young children may choose a dental plan that offers orthodontia services while an older employee may opt to increase contributions to the retirement program.

Other Retention Strategies

Not all retention strategies will appeal to all employees. The ability to work remotely may not be an attraction to an employee who enjoys the social aspect of the workplace. An employee with no children does not need on-site childcare as a benefit. It is the responsibility of the organization to continually monitor through data collection and employee feedback, which strategies are working, when they are working, and why they are working, and then make the necessary changes based on that feedback. An HIM manager can implement retention strategies on a smaller scale. A manager may not be able to impact the benefits package, but may begin a reward or recognition program or implement flexible scheduling to a practical extent within an HIM department. Communication issues are within the control of the individual manager. An HIM manager can be sure to keep communication lines open and set realistic performance goals in collaboration with employees. Performance appraisals and necessary disciplinary action should be carried promptly and fairly with no discrimination involved. An HIM manager can also monitor turnover within their department and investigate when data indicates there may be a problem area or supervisor. Even though setting compensation is outside the scope of a manager's position, a manager must understand and support the overall compensation practices implemented by the organization.

Compensation Practices

Compensation is all direct and indirect pay earned by employees. This includes wages, mandatory benefits such as unemployment insurance and workers' compensation, and benefits such as medical insurance, life insurance, child care, elder care, retirement plans, and longevity pay. How an organization compensates its workforce is generally established by senior management with the assistance of the HR department. It would be very unusual for an HIM manager to be part of the decision-making process in determining what compensation methods to use, but an HIM manager would be involved in influencing the compensation methods at the department level. A manager may be involved in explaining overtime or incentive pay to a new hire, fielding questions about annual wage increases or benefit changes from other employees, and overseeing an operating budget in which more than half of the expenses fall under wage and salary administration. Compensation issues such as wage and salary and benefits administration affect everyone in an organization. Not only do managers influence the compensation of their employees, they are subject to the same compensation influence from their superiors.

Employees generally have two concerns about what they are paid. The first is that they are paid what they feel they are worth to the organization in general, and their department specifically. The second concern is that employees expect to be paid correspondingly to what other employees in the same or similar positions receive. They may adjust the amount for longevity but, overall, they expect the pay to be the same. The equity theory of motivation (chapter 3) reminds us that employees pay attention to the balance of their inputs in relation to their outputs, compared to both the organization and other workers. This theory is illustrated using compensation. In this case, an employee views their inputs to be the work they perform, and their outputs to be the pay they receive for that work. First, when comparing their pay to that of the work they do, employees expect to see equity or balance. They want to be paid a fair wage (output) by the organization according to how much effort, time, and skills (input) they provide. Second, when comparing their pay to that of others doing the same work, they expect to see equity too. An employee who views his inputs as equal to that of others will expect the same outputs as others doing the same tasks (chapter 3). For example, a director of HIM at a large urban teaching hospital will expect to earn more than an HIM director at a small rural hospital. However, the HIM director at a large urban teaching hospital does not expect to earn as much as the vice president of nursing services at the same hospital. If an employee perceives this relationship to be out of balance, the manager will be the first person asked to address the issue. Therefore, a manager must have an understanding of compensation administration and the objectives of a compensation plan.

Objectives of a Compensation Plan

An organization has four purposes when creating a compensation plan. First, any compensation plan should link to an organization's strategic plan, their mission and vision statements, and support their corporate culture. There must be a belief that compensation is part of the culture of an organization and matches the values set forth by the mission and vision statements. Second, the overall compensation should be high enough to recruit quality employees to the organization. Third, compensation practices should be such that they motivate current employees to remain with the organization. Lastly, an organization must be able to pay its staff and remain fiscally solvent. In addition, a compensation plan must be antidiscriminatory, as discussed in chapter 5.

An overall compensation plan is the responsibility of upper administration. The HR department will have input, and some organizations bring in a consulting company to review and revise compensation practices. An organization does not often start from scratch when developing a compensation plan; other factors influence the need to align pay structures. Over time salaries for hard-to-fill positions may have increased faster than the rest of the organization, or efforts to keep people in highly skilled positions may have resulted in pay inequities. Technological advances have impacted jobs as well. As new jobs are created and previous jobs change as a result of EHRs and other forms of technology in healthcare, the compensation rates may not have been properly assigned or adjusted.

Job Evaluation

Internally, the first part of beginning a compensation plan is to perform a job evaluation on each position. A **job evaluation** is the process of applying predefined compensable factors to jobs to determine their relative worth to the organization. A job evaluation begins with an in-depth review of the job description, job specifications, and any job analysis that might have been done (chapter 6). A job is evaluated to determine the necessary skills, education, complexity, responsibility, and working conditions to perform the job effectively. The intent of job evaluation is twofold:

- Jobs that are more complex, require specialized skills, or have adverse working conditions will receive higher pay than less complicated or specialized jobs
- Jobs that are similar across the organization will be grouped together into the same pay grade

Job evaluations are generally performed by the HR department with input from the HIM department. Once the job evaluation is complete, the data collected are analyzed and jobs are assigned to specific pay grades. There are different ways to assign the jobs and each organization will chose the method that works for them. Three of the most common methods are ranking, grading, and factor comparison.

Job Ranking

In **job ranking**, each job is rated according to how valuable it is to the organization. Organizationwide, this process is completed by the HR department with input from other departments as necessary. Because the HR department has access to pay data across the organization, one method is for HR to rank jobs as a whole, with the more valuable (higher paying) jobs at the top of the order and the less valuable (lower paying) jobs ranked at the bottom. A second method is to rank jobs within departments and then the HR department combines the department rankings into an organizational report. In an HIM department, one ranking may result in a department head job ranked at the top, then a data quality specialist, then a scanning clerk. Another ranking may place the department head at the top, but the scanning clerk above the data quality specialist. The job ranking method is fairly easy to do, but highly subjective. Since there is no criteria attached to the ranking, decisions are based on perception of value to the organization and this may be difficult to defend to employees. Feelings of inequity are more common when the job ranking method is used.

Job Grading

Another method of assigning jobs to a pay grade is **job grading**. Job grading, or job classification, requires the establishment of predetermined categories and the various jobs sorted into these categories. Again the HR department is the best choice for creating categories and sorting jobs due to their organizationwide knowledge of jobs. The categories are then assigned to a pay range. Categories may be established according to responsibility such as department head, supervisor, lead position, or nonsupervisory. They may be established according to patient care such as direct patient care, indirect patient care, or no patient contact. Similar to job ranking, jobs are sorted into classifications using the entire job and there is a degree of subjectivity, although not to the level found in job ranking. Difficulties may also arise if jobs seem to fit into multiple categories, or if jobs do not fit easily into any category.

Factor Comparison

The final job evaluation method is **factor comparison**. Factor comparison is more quantitative than job ranking or grading because it breaks down each job into compensable factors and assigns a dollar value. **Compensable factors** are characteristics used to compare the worth of a job (skill, effort, responsibility, or working conditions). Each compensable factor is further broken down into subfactors. An organization may decide that the compensable factor of skill is further divided into education and experience. For example, the HR department, with input from other departments, assigns a dollar value of $3.47 to an associate's degree, $5.25 to a bachelor's degree, and $8.68 to a master's degree. Under responsibility, supervising 5 to 10 employees is assigned $9.45 and supervising more than 20 employees is assigned $13.51. Once each factor and subfactor are assigned dollar values, a job is analyzed to see which compensable factors are part of that position. The dollar values are then added to determine the monetary value of that job. Jobs with similar monetary values are grouped together in a pay range. A variation on the factor comparison method is the point method. The **point method** places weight (points) on each of the compensable factors in a job and the total points associated with a job establish its relative worth. Jobs that fall within a specific range of points are assigned to a pay grade with an associated wage. Because of the quantitative nature of the factor comparison method, it is less subjective than either job ranking or grading. There is a greater sense of fairness associated with factor comparison, and this makes it easier for all employees to support. Both the factor comparison and point methods are extremely time consuming to implement, making them more expensive to use as well.

Wage Determination

Once the job evaluation process is complete, the next step is to determine what wage will be associated with each pay range. To help with this, organizations look to external forces and use a market pricing approach. **Market pricing** is determining the going pay rate for similar jobs in a particular labor market. For example, the compensation rate for an EHR application specialist position would be compared to other similar positions in a labor market to determine what the job would be worth. An organization may choose to conduct its own salary survey to collect this data, and this may be the best choice to compare wages in a local or regional labor market. For hard-to-fill jobs, or jobs that are recruited nationally (for example, chief executive officer), an organization may obtain salary data from surveys conducted by private consulting firms, the Bureau of Labor Statistics, or professional organizations. AHIMA conducts periodic salary surveys and breaks down responses based on work setting, job level, and credential. Care must be taken to obtain salary surveys from reliable sources, and also to make sure similar jobs are being compared to one another. The job tasks assigned to an HIM technician in one organization may not be comparable to job tasks for an HIM technician in a different organization.

Once salary information is gathered, an organization must decide how they want to position themselves relative to external competition. Most organizations place themselves in the middle of the market, or what is referred to as the second quartile. A quartile represents one quarter of the market position: the first quartile is 0 to 25 percent, the second quartile is 25 to 50 percent, the third quartile is 50 to 75 percent, and the fourth quartile is 75 to 100 percent. A second-quartile approach means that an organization belongs to the quartile where 50 percent of organizations pay below-market wages and 50 percent pay above-market wages. A first quartile strategy positions an organization so they belong to the 25 percent of organizations that pay below-market wages while 75 percent of organizations pay market or above-market wages. An organization would chose the first-quartile strategy if they do not have the financial resources to pay market or above-market wages, or if there is an abundance of workers in the market place. Organizations that pay below-market wages will experience higher turnover rates as employees leave for better-paying jobs. Some organizations choose to place themselves in the third quartile. This means they belong to the 25 percent of organizations that pay above-market wages while 75 percent of organizations pay market or below-market wages. Organizations that pay above market wages can be more selective in who they hire and generally experience higher retention. However, these organizations also expect higher productivity from their employees to justify the higher pay rates.

A combination of job evaluation and market pricing allows for jobs to be placed into **pay grades**. Each pay grade has a minimum, midpoint, and maximum range that allows an employee to progress through the pay grade, receiving pay increases for longevity or improving skills. For example, a new department director may be hired at the minimum amount of pay within the pay grade. Upon successfully earning her master's degree, she may be given an increase to just above midpoint in the pay grade. Pay-for-performance (chapter 8) increases also move an employee along the pay scale. Longevity increases are in the form of **cost-of-living adjustments (COLA)**. COLAs are generally pay increases tied to a change in the consumer price index (CPI) published by the US Department of Labor, which measures purchasing power between time periods (usually one year). These increases are not linked to performance or acquisition of new skills, but are in place to keep wage and salary administration in line with inflation in the United States. Each year the minimum and maximum pay rates are adjusted within the pay grades, and employees receive an adjustment to keep their wage in line with the rest of the pay grade.

Each employee receives a base pay rate, but the employee's amount of pay may increase through incentive or bonus programs. **Incentive programs** are intended to motivate employees through increased productivity, while a **bonus** is a reward given related to the performance of an entire organization or individual (Fottler et al. 1998). Incentive programs in HIM are most often found in transcription and coding. Individual transcriptionists are paid a base rate and then earn a per character or per line incentive amount once they reach a standard character or line count. The procedure is similar in coding, where coders are paid a per chart amount once they reach a standard production amount. The incentive pay is then added to their hourly base rate. Bonuses are generally awarded based on the meeting of performance goals of an entire organization. The performance goals are stated in advance, and bonuses are awarded either to the entire organization or to those individuals deemed to have had the most effect on reaching the goals. This might be an upper management team, an individual, or a combination of both. Team compensation can be tricky to administer as the team is made up of individuals, each having contributed their own part. There are sometimes problems with inequity if some team members have not done their fair share, or are not perceived by the group or team members as having done their fair share. Regardless of how teams are compensated, successful plans start with clearly defined and agreed upon goals so that there are performance outcomes based on common performance standards.

Benefits

The final component of a compensation plan is employee benefits. Offering benefits to employees is a significant investment for any organization. Research shows that the cost of benefits can be anywhere from 20 to 40 percent of wages and salaries. That means if an HIM supervisor makes $40,000 per year and the organization's benefit package is 30 percent, the supervisor is realizing an extra $12,000 in benefits for a total compensation package of $52,000 per year. Benefits are also considered part of a recruitment and retention program. Creating and administering a benefits plan is the responsibility of the HR department, but managers still must understand the basics of the benefits package. Employees may approach first-line managers with questions about benefits before contacting the HR department or visiting the organization's intranet site. As with direct compensation, a manager should refer most questions to the HR department, so as not to give out wrong information; but in some cases, an HIM manager may be in a position to help with certain benefits administration. For example, a tuition reimbursement program may require that a course be related to the employee's job. It may fall to the supervisor to determine to what extent a course meets this requirement.

Some benefits are mandated by law to be covered: Social Security, unemployment, family and medical leaves, and workers' compensation benefits fall into this category. Other benefits, considered voluntary, include the following:

- Health, dental, and vision insurance, and prescription drug coverage
- Disability insurance
- Life insurance equal to a portion of or full salary
- Wellness programs such as providing a fitness club membership
- Employee assistance programs for behavioral and mental health wellness
- Retirement plans
- Tuition reimbursement
- On-site child care or adult day care

This list is by no means exhaustive. The cost of providing benefits changes each year and organizations evaluate their benefits package to determine if a specific benefit is cost effective.

Check Your **Understanding**

1. Explain the difference between voluntary and involuntary turnover and give an example of each.
2. Explain the difference between functional and dysfunctional turnover and give an example of each.
3. How does monitoring turnover affect employee retention?
4. Why is it important for an HIM manager to understand the compensation practices of a healthcare organization?
5. Why would an organization decide to set their pay ranges over or under the average market price in a geographic region?

Case Study

Objectives

- Develop a job posting for an HIM coding position
- Collaborate with the HR department to decide the recruitment methods most appropriate for recruiting for HIM coding positions
- Develop specific HIM coding job-related questions to be asked during the interview process

Instructions

Review the scenario provided and the Clinical Coding Job Description in figure 7.2 to develop a job posting and appropriate interview questions. Provide a written report to the HIM director that contains all the deliverables outlined.

Scenario

A large healthcare organization is expanding HIM centralized coding services based on the recent acquisitions of a rural hospital, long-term acute-care hospital, skilled nursing facility, and a behavioral health facility. All the coding functions for these newly acquired facilities will be centralized within the HIM department. Based on a work volume study it is estimated the HIM department will need four additional full-time equivalent (FTE) clinical coding specialists to perform the additional coding from the acquisition of these new facilities. Laura, the HIM coding manager, is responsible for working with the HR department consultant to develop a recruiting plan for these four open positions. Laura will need to provide a written recruitment plan to the HIM director of the organization.

Assumptions

- The job description for the clinical coding specialist has recently been updated by Laura and is provided following this case study in figure 7.2.
- Interviews for both internal and external candidates will be performed as structured interviews.
- Follow the standard HR department recruitment process: All jobs are posted internally for two weeks and qualified candidates will be referred to the coding manager for interviewing. If qualified individuals are not hired internally, the job posting will then be advertised externally using the recruitment methods identified in the recruitment plan.
- A different advertisement may be necessary for the internal and external job postings.

Deliverables

Develop a clinical coding specialist recruitment plan in collaboration with the HR consultant. The plan needs to include the following items.

1. Three recruitment methods outlined in this chapter with an explanation as to why each of these methods was chosen.
2. A job posting based on the clinical coding specialist job description in figure 7.2 that advertises for these positions. If necessary, a different one may be done for the internal and external job postings.
3. Two interview questions for each of the four categories of questions: situational, behavioral, job knowledge, and work requirement for a total of eight questions. The questions must be specifically focused toward clinical coding specialist job tasks.
4. Create a clinical coding specialist recruitment plan report (in a memo) that includes the previous items.

Figure 7.2. Clinical coding specialist sample position description

---

Clinical Coding Specialist Sample Position Description

Initial Date: 01/01/2016

Review Date: **Department:**   Health Information Management

Job Title: Clinical Coding Specialist   **Reporting Relationship:**   Reports to HIM Coding Manager, Health Information Management; no direct reports

Pay Grade: Non-Exempt, Grade IV

Job Purpose: The purpose of this position is to apply the appropriate diagnostic and procedural codes to individual patient health information for data retrieval, analysis, and claims processing.

Job Responsibilities and Tasks

1. Clinical Classification Coding
   - Assigns ICD-10-CM/PCS, HCPCS, and CPT codes accurately utilizing the 3M encoder.
   - Assigns Present-on-Admission (POA) indicators appropriately.
   - Groups all coded data to MS-DRGs, APR-DRGs, and APCS utilizing the 3M encoder.
   - Keeps abreast of coding guidelines and reimbursement reporting requirements.
   - Distinguishes appropriate coding as outlined by facility's coding guidelines.
   - Abides by the Standards of Ethical Coding as set forth by AHIMA and adheres to official coding guidelines.
   - Queries physicians when code assignments are not straightforward or documentation in the record is inadequate, ambiguous, or unclear for coding purposes by utilizing the appropriate facility querying process.
   - Analyzes health record documents to ensure that the information is timely, complete, and accurate according to facility standards.
2. Abstracting
   - Performs abstracting from the EHR as appropriate.
   - Ensures that data adheres to data standards as outlined within the HIM policies and procedures.
3. Electronic Health Record
   - Utilizes the health record documentation contained in the EHRs as the source of truth for coding.
   - Utilizes dual screens for coding and reviewing EHR documentation efficiently.
   - Identifies issues with copy and paste in patients' EHRs and reports them to the HIM coding manager.

Job Requirements and Specifications

- Proficient in the utilization of the following classification systems: ICD-10-CM/PCS, CPT, and HCPCS.
- Ability to maneuver within EHR systems.
- Proficient in the use of encoders within the coding process, 3M encoder preferred.

HIT Job Competencies

Subdomain I.A. Classification Systems

1. Apply diagnosis or procedure codes according to current guidelines. Level of Learning: Applying
2. Evaluate the accuracy of diagnostic and procedural coding. Level of Learning: Evaluating
3. Apply diagnostic and procedural groupings. Level of Learning: Applying
4. Evaluate the accuracy of diagnostic or procedural groupings. Level of learning: Evaluating

(Continued)

Figure 7.2.   Clinical coding specialist sample position description (*Continued*)

Subdomain 1.B. Health Record Content and Documentation

1. Analyze the document in the health to ensure it supports the diagnosis and reflects the patient's progress, clinical findings, and discharge status. Level of Learning: Analyzing.

2. Verify the documentation in the health record is timely, complete, and accurate. Level of Learning: Analyzing.

Subdomain 1.C. Data Governance

1. Apply policies and procedures to ensure the accuracy of health data. Level of Learning: Applying

Subdomain 1.D. Data Management

1. Collect and maintain health data. Level of Learning: Understand.

Job Qualifications

- Associate degree in health information technology with RHIT credential or bachelor's degree in HIM with an RHIA credential.
- Additional AHIMA coding credential preferred: CCS, CCS-P.
- At least one year previous coding experience within a healthcare organization is required.

Job Context

- Ability to work in an office environment and perform repetitive computer tasks related to coding.
- Potential to work from home after six months of required in-hospital training.

© AHIMA

Review Questions

1. Hiring a known and proven employee with an understanding of the organization and improving morale among current employees are:

   a. Advantages to external recruitment
   b. Disadvantages to external recruitment
   c. Advantages to internal recruitment
   d. Disadvantages to internal recruitment

2. Which of the following types of selection tool has a low reliability rating compared to other tools?

   a. Application forms
   b. Aptitude tests
   c. Reference checks
   d. Resumes

3. Which of the following is true about organizations that pay wages according to a third-quartile strategy?

   a. They care more about patient care than organizations that adopt a first- or second-quartile strategy.
   b. They experience higher turnover in the less skilled positions within their organizations.
   c. They must depend more on their intrinsic reward programs to attract employees.
   d. They usually expect higher productivity from their employees.

4. New ideas, knowledge of the most up-to-date methods, and no preconceived thoughts about organizational politics are:

   a. Advantages to external recruitment
   b. Disadvantages to external recruitment
   c. Advantages to internal recruitment
   d. Disadvantages to internal recruitment

5. Charles is recruiting for a position that requires five to seven days per month of overnight travel. During the interview, he asks each candidate if they would be able to commit to this travel schedule. This is what type of interview question?

   a. Behavior
   b. Job knowledge
   c. Situational
   d. Work requirement

6. When interviewing candidates for a job, Angela likes to get a feel for how their past experiences will shape their future actions. She likes to ask the question, "Tell me about a time when you had to prioritize three or four courses of action, what they were, and how you decided to prioritize each one. Did you choose correctly? How did it work out?" This is what type of interview question?

   a. Behavior
   b. Job knowledge
   c. Situational
   d. Work requirement

7. This type of interview has a high reliability rating due to the fact that the same questions are asked of each candidate and answers can be compared.

   a. Nondirective
   b. Semi-structured
   c. Structured
   d. Unstructured

8. Emily is an experienced cancer registrar who has been with University Hospital for almost 10 years. She is one of two registrars, and has complete responsibility for preparing the annual report. Emily recently submitted her resignation and will be taking a similar job at a hospital where she does not have to pay to park and will be able to work from home two days a week. This is an example of what type of turnover?

   a. Dysfunctional and voluntary
   b. Functional and voluntary
   c. Dysfunctional and involuntary
   d. Functional and involuntary

9. This type of job classifies positions based on predetermined categories such as supervisory level, physical effort, or working conditions. Each job is then assigned to a category with a particular pay range.

   a. Factor comparison
   b. Job grading
   c. Job ranking
   d. Point method

10. Which of the following benefit offerings is not mandated by law?

    a. Social Security
    b. Tuition reimbursement
    c. Unemployment insurance
    d. Workers' compensation

References

AHIMA Foundation. 2015a. The AHIMA Foundation Mission. http://www.ahimafoundation.org/about/mission.aspx.

AHIMA Foundation. 2015b. Registered Apprenticeship Program—Sponsor. http://ahimafoundation.org/prodev/Registered_Apprenticeship.aspx.

Bureau of Labor Statistics, U.S. Department of Labor. 2015. Occupational Outlook Handbook, Medical Records and Health Information Technicians. http://www.bls.gov/ooh/healthcare/medical-records-and-health-information-technicians.htm.

DeScherer, D. and T. Myers. eds. 2007. Employee turnover. *Payroll Manager's Letter* 23(9):6.

Endicott, M. 2014. DIY: Grow your own coders. *Journal of AHIMA* 85(4):60–61.

Fottler, M.D., S.R. Hernandez, and C.L. Joiner. 1998. *Essentials of Human Resources Management in Health Services Organizations*. Albany: Delmar.

iCIMS. 2014 (April 29). Know the Facts and Improve Social Recruiting ROI. http://www.icims.com/hire-expectations-institute/for-employers/infographic-know-the-facts-improve-social-recruiting-roi.

Sett, A., G.T. Hickman, and K. Karban. 2014. Trust but verify: Safeguards in contracting for outsourced coding services. *Journal of AHIMA* 85(6):40–44.

Performance Management in Health Information Management

Learning Objectives

- Interpret healthcare organization policies and procedures in relation to performance outcomes
- Describe the role performance appraisals play in the oversight of health information management (HIM) functions
- Demonstrate use of performance improvement plans in relation to performance appraisals
- Illustrate completion of self-evaluations in the performance appraisal process
- Conduct effective performance appraisal interviews

Key Terms

360 performance appraisal
Benchmarking
Contingent reward
   leadership style
Critical incident method
Essay evaluation method
Forced ranking
Graphic rating scales
Incentive effect

Job complexity
Job experience
Job performance
Job performance
   standards
Management by objectives
   (MBO)
Merit pay
Meritocracy

Noise
Organizational tenure
Pay for performance
Performance appraisals
Performance
   improvement plan
   (PIP)
Performance management
Performance standards

Personalization
Privacy
Probationary
   performance
   review cycle
Situational strength
Sorting effect
Spatial density
Work sampling

Performance management is a set of tools and practices for setting performance goals and designing sustainable job improvement strategies with employees, monitoring employee progress toward job performance goals with feedback, and coaching by managers and measuring individual or group performance (Fried and Fottler 2015). Performance is the act of doing a job (Merriam-Webster 2015). Performance management assesses job performance based on job descriptions and job performance standards set in conjunction with annual performance appraisals.

Job performance is the "work-related activities expected of an employee and how well the activities were executed" during a set time frame (Business Dictionary 2015). **Job performance standards** measure work performance and the stated expectations for acceptable quality and productivity associated within a job or job function. These standards form the basis for annual performance reviews. Performance management is the ongoing process of communication between a manager and an employee that occurs throughout a selected time frame (usually annually). The communication includes whether or not the individual meets established job performance standards and the process includes outlining job expectations, setting job performance objectives, identifying performance goals, and providing regular feedback on actual job performance against expected performance.

Health information management (HIM) professionals are involved in the performance appraisal process within healthcare organizations, both as recipients and providers of evaluations. **Performance appraisals** are an evaluation of an employee's performance during a designated period of time and can also be referred to as performance evaluations or performance reviews. This chapter begins with a discussion in regards to the role that the human resources (HR) department plays in the performance management process and outlines the components of performance management in healthcare organizations.

The second section describes the performance appraisal life cycle and the typical performance management tools utilized in healthcare organizations. The development of performance standards is discussed in detail and rating of performance is provided. The assessment of performance in terms of short- and long-term performance variability is delineated along with describing the contributing factors that can impact performance variability.

The next section of the chapter discusses the actual completion of performance appraisal documents and the HIM manager's role in this process. This section also addresses the different methods that can be adopted in performance appraisals and the advantages and disadvantages of each of these methods. The final section describes the outcomes of a performance appraisal process, which includes self-appraisal and pay for performance.

Human Resources and Performance Management

The HR department within healthcare organizations typically utilizes a standardized performance management plan to handle employee performance on a regular basis. The HR department along with executive management develops the performance management process for the entire healthcare organization. Healthcare organizations are required to monitor employee performance and productivity as many of the accrediting bodies (such as the Joint Commission or the Commission on Accreditation for Rehabilitation facilities) require that employee performance appraisals be provided as evidence to meet accreditation standards in regards to employee performance. Healthcare organizations should create ongoing performance appraisal processes that ensure all personnel are annually meeting the goals and standards outlined within their jobs. In order for performance management systems to be successful in healthcare organizations, performance needs to be linked to employees' daily job tasks and the resulting outcomes resulting of these tasks.

Performance appraisals are an important component of the entire performance management ecosystem within a healthcare organization. These appraisals provide confirmation of an employee's performance by providing standardized documentation that allows for individual performance comparisons from year to year and allows for comparisons between individuals with similar jobs. They provide a common basis for evaluating an employee's promotion readiness by reflecting on competency and job task mastery for particular jobs. Performance appraisals provide standardized documentation on an employee's ability to meet or exceed competency standards throughout the evaluation period. They also open the communication lines between an employee and manager by allowing the employee to provide a self-appraisal and develop individualized goals for the next evaluation time period. Performance appraisals can reflect individual training and development needs particularly if an individual does not accomplish select job tasks efficiently or effectively. They also help the employee develop goals that will allow him or her to achieve success at a higher level or be promoted when training and development needs are identified specific to the goals. In turn, a performance appraisal can reflect the outcomes of training and development programs provided when an employee demonstrates improved completion of particular job tasks that were the focus of the training programs. The employee is provided with a mechanism to provide positive and negative feedback regarding organizational and supervisory items that may impact the employee's ability to do his or her job (Performance Appraisal Methods 2010).

The major components involved in developing a performance management plan are:

- Maintaining updated job descriptions with current major tasks or functions outlined for each job.
- Determining performance standards for each major task or function.
- Evaluating performance based on the process and components outlined by the performance appraisal. Items included in the appraisal process are:
  - Length of the evaluation period (usually annually)
  - Timing of the evaluation cycle
  - Interim contact points for assessing performance, providing ongoing coaching, and feedback
  - Inclusion of annual performance goals (employee and management driven)
  - Standardized evaluation ratings
  - Documentation required to substantiate performance (Performance Appraisal Methods 2010)

Performance Appraisal Life Cycle

The performance management plan is the stepping off point for providing management; it starts with baseline information regarding employees' performance. The plan encompasses a performance appraisal life cycle that begins upon an employee's hire and continues throughout his or her tenure at the organization. Some synonyms for the performance appraisal process are employee annual evaluations, professional development planning, and merit rating. The life cycle of the performance appraisal is depicted in figure 8.1. The cycle includes planning—setting performance goals based on an employee's job description—which sets the stage for the employee's expected performance for the following year. The next phase of the performance appraisal life cycle is a periodic review that requires managers to collect performance data on a regular basis and review progression toward expected goals throughout the year, as established in the planning phase. The performance appraisal annual review between the

Figure 8.1. Performance appraisal life cycle

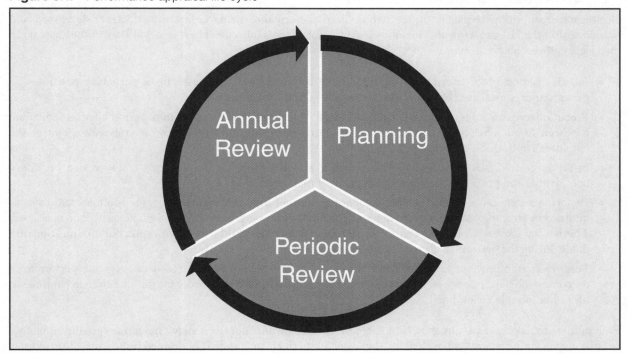

© AHIMA

employee and his or her manager completes the cycle. It starts over with setting performance goals for the following year at the time of the annual performance appraisal review.

Upon hire, an employee may be entered into a probationary performance review cycle. Although there is no law that requires organizations to provide a probationary period upon hire of new employees, it is general practice that this occurs both for the benefit of the employee and the organization. A **probationary performance review cycle** is a set period of time that allows an organization to ascertain whether the new employee will be able to handle the job tasks and challenges associated with the new job. This time period allows employers time to evaluate an employee before making the hire permanent (USLegal 2015). Depending on the skill development required for the job, the employee has a limited amount of time (usually 90 days to 6 months) to develop skills appropriately and if the individual successfully meets the mutually agreed upon goals and expectations for job performance, he or she is then considered a permanent employee. If the new employee does not meet the mutually agreed upon job goals and expectations, the individual is either rendered an extended probationary period or the individual's employment is severed. As discussed in chapter 5, healthcare organizations must follow all legal rules and regulations in regards to hiring and firing individuals. Probationary evaluations set the tone for how new employees perceive the overall performance management system so these evaluations must be completed professionally, efficiently, and effectively. Training and development should be provided to new employees so that job performance standards can be reasonably achieved within the probationary period.

After the new employee successfully completes the probationary period, the individual is then entered into the annual performance appraisal program. The employee's manager should meet with the individual to set up goals and expectations for the next phase of employment. The actual job performance standards should be discussed with the employee and the manager should outline how feedback will occur periodically in regards to job performance outcomes. For example, an HIM manager would share the productivity and quality standards for the release of information types that a release of information (ROI) coordinator will be performing on a regular basis. The HIM manager would share an example of the report that the ROI coordinator will receive on a monthly basis reflecting actual turnaround time and quality and what is expected of the employee when the report is received. A mechanism should be in place so the ROI coordinator can review the actual report results and deliver feedback to the manager in terms of work process decisions. Also, turnaround time productivity calculation should be shared with the ROI coordinator.

Performance Management Tools

Healthcare organizations typically utilize standardized performance management tools that are developed and housed within the HR department. The following are a list of tools (also described in detail later in the chapter) to manage employee job performance.

- Job descriptions: Job descriptions outline all the responsibilities and tasks for a particular position. Job performance is measured based on the tasks outlined in the job description.

- Probationary performance reviews: This evaluation is performed within a set time period after an individual has been hired. This evaluation sets initial performance goals and provides an overall assessment of the employee's initial job performance.

- Multisource feedback (360 forms): The feedback provided in a 360 form allows employees to provide a confidential and possibly anonymous assessment of their peers.

- Performance appraisal forms: The performance appraisal forms contain the job responsibilities and tasks as outlined in an employee's job description and the job standards against which the employee will be measured. This is a standardized form that is used for all individuals in the healthcare organization but modifications are made during the performance appraisal process for each employee.

- Performance improvement plans: These are standardized plans initiated based on negative performance outcomes. Job performance standards that must be met and improved in order for the employee to continue in his or her job role are outlined.

Each of these tools plays a part in appraising job performance throughout the review time frame (usually annually). All managers who have a role in evaluating employee job performance should be trained on the use of these tools upon hire and retrained on the use of them whenever necessary.

Check Your **Understanding**

1. What are the components of a performance management plan?
2. Explain the three phases of the performance appraisal life cycle.
3. Discuss how the performance appraisal life cycle is different for a newly hired employee.

Performance Standards

Performance standards measure work performance and the stated expectations for acceptable quality and productivity associated with a job or job function. Job descriptions are the basis for the development of performance standards as performance is measured against the job tasks outlined in job descriptions. There are four dimensions of performance that should be measured in a performance management system and evaluated on the annual performance appraisal: productivity, quality, timeliness, and fiscal responsibility. It is important for the HIM manager to develop processes for collecting performance data on a regular basis and sharing this information with individual employees on a regular basis.

The sources of performance data for HIM job tasks are typically work sampling and benchmarks. **Work sampling** is a statistical method that reviews a select portion of tasks performed and provides baseline data for further job performance assessment. For example, work sampling is done to calculate the average time for completion of coding an inpatient record, coding an outpatient record, processing a release of information request, transcribing a dictated report, and scanning a defined set of paper records. Work sampling then takes into account the quantity of activities that can be completed within a certain time frame. This aggregation of work sampling provides the framework for a performance standard for the particular activity.

Benchmarking is another source that can be utilized in measuring job performance within the HIM department. **Benchmarking** is a measurement that takes into account the quality aspect of completing a job task from start to finish. Benchmarks can be developed internally within an HIM department or can be solicited externally from professional organizations or other similar healthcare organizations. HIM managers often solicit other HIM departments to compare coding quality, document imaging quality, and release of information turnaround time benchmarks.

Tables 8.1 and 8.2 depict job performance standards for HIM job tasks and HIM management job tasks. These standards are developed and assessed by work sampling or benchmarking over a period of time. The measurements

Table 8.1. Examples of job performance standards for HIM job tasks*

Job task	Quality accuracy	Quantity performance indicator
ROI: Processing request for health information—medical	98 percent accuracy	Average request turnaround time: 4 days Requests per hour: 4
ROI: Processing request for health information— legal or subpoena	100 percent accuracy	Average request turnaround time: 5 days Requests per hour: 2
Coding: Inpatient records	95 percent accuracy	3.2 charts per hour
Coding: Outpatient records	95 percent accuracy	6.0 charts per hour
Transcription	98 percent accuracy	100 lines per minute
Document imaging	97 percent accuracy	Scanning 75 documents per hour
Chart analysis	98 percent accuracy	Inpatient Charts—6 per hour Outpatient Charts—10 per hour

*The tasks are not all inclusive but provide examples of typical HIM performance standards.

Source: BusinessDictionary.com 2015 and Merriam-Webster 2015.

Table 8.2. Examples of job performance standards—HIM management job tasks*

Job tasks	Quantity or quality performance indicator
Completes all employees' performance appraisals	Utilizes approved methods for completing performance appraisals and provides feedback to 100 percent reporting employees
Employs continuous quality improvement methods	Identifies performance gaps and provides opportunities for improving processes through the use of standardized performance methods
	30 percent of manager's time should be spent on quality improvement initiatives
Provides coaching and development to all employees	Identifies employee development and training needs and provides coaching and education as appropriate
	20 percent of manager's time should be spent on coaching and educating
Monitors employee performance on a monthly basis	Provides productivity and quality reports to all reporting employees (100 percent) on a monthly basis
	Provides feedback on both positive and negative performance
	20 percent of manager's time should be spent on assessing employee performance
Attends all department management meetings	100 percent of all meetings

*This is a sample of a manager's tasks and is not meant to be all inclusive.

are based on aggregated data and provide an average job standard against which all employee performance is measured for the particular job tasks. Standard performance measures may need to be recalculated when new processes are integrated into a job or when there is a significant shift in the amount of work to be completed. The HIM manager must periodically reassess these standards to ensure they accurately reflect the average performance for each particular area. These standards are shared with new employees upon hire and are incorporated into the annual performance appraisal.

Another key component of creating job performance standards is that they should be written employing the SMART technique. SMART is an acronym where each letter stands for one component of a job performance standard or objective.

- Specific: Job standards should be written so that they specifically represent the job tasks being performed
- Measurable: Each of the job performance standards should be written so that it can measured in an objective manner
- Attainable: All job performance standards should be written so that they are attainable by the employees performing them
- Realistic: All job performance standards should be written with a realistic expectation that the employee can meet the standard
- Timely: The job performance standard should be written so it is bound by time in some manner (Wayne State University 2015)

This concept can be applied to all job performance standards so they are understood by both the employee and the manager (Wayne State University 2015). An example of a SMART objective for a transcriptionist in an HIM department would be: Types operative reports with 95 percent accuracy on all inpatient encounters within 24 hours of the surgery. If performance standards and goals are written appropriately, assessment of performance can take place in an objective manner.

Assessment of Performance

Job performance has a dynamic component in which employees can experience either short-term or long-term variances in job performance. While employees may experience variances in job performance over the years, their perception may be tainted in that they feel their performance remains stable over time (Barnes and Morgeson 2007). Individual variances in job performance should be assessed separately from overall variances in group performance. It is important to assess individual job performance regularly so variances in productivity or quality of tasks are caught early on (Minbashian and Luppino 2014). An example of a job variance in the HIM department would be when a document imaging specialist's quality decreases for a month or two or when his or her productivity for the year does not match the previous year's overall document imaging productivity.

Early intervention of variances in job performance allows management to intercede quickly and provide additional training, support, or resources as necessary to negate the variances. Short-term fluctuations of job performance are often related to situational cues such as increased job complexity and issues related to resource allocation (Minbashian and Luppino 2014). Personal issues such as illness or loss of a loved one may also cause a variance in job performance. An HIM manager knows when variances are occurring in a workgroup by regularly monitoring employee productivity and quality job performance standards. This routine monitoring allows an HIM manager to address variances in job performance and intervene with the employee early on before overall job performance or group performance is impacted.

There is a direct relationship between job satisfaction and job performance. **Situational strength**, the cues employees experience in their workplace that allow particular job performance behaviors to occur, provides a link between job satisfaction and job performance as well. The climate of an organization can fluctuate from very strong to weak. In strong situations, there are uniform expectations and adequate incentives for job performance. Employees have a common framework and know what is expected of them. In weak situations, there are no uniform expectations and the organization does not offer sufficient incentives for performance. The situation is not construed the same by all employees and there is not a common framework for performance in place (Bowling et al. 2015).

Managers interested in maximizing job performance should recognize that satisfied employees are more likely to be productive employees when they have a common framework for performance. Unconstrained (weak) environments do not offer the same amount of job satisfaction because employees do not feel the work performance parameters are outlined. The management style exhibited by a workgroup leader (discussed in chapter 1) also impacts employees' perception of the situational strength (Bowling et al. 2015).

In evaluating employee performance it is important to understand the impact of different factors that may enhance or hamper employee performance. Job engagement in terms of physical, emotional, and cognitive components influences job performance. Engagement relates closely to predicting job performance in terms of job involvement, job satisfaction, and intrinsic motivation (the employee's inner drive to perform). Managers should focus resources on practices that assess and enhance employee engagement. In terms of job performance, one aspect that can engage employees from the start of employment is developing goals and standards that are congruent with the employee's motivations. If an employee relates to the goals, the individual will more likely perform the tasks adequately or exceeding what is expected (Rich et al. 2010).

The Physical Working Environment

The physical working environment can be a connection between employee behavior and outcomes that impacts job performance overall. The four broad issues that are associated with an employee's work environment are:

- Personal space
- Spatial density or crowding
- Workplace personalization and identity
- Task or workflow interdependence (Ashkanasy et al. 2014)

Traditionally, because of its non-revenue generating status, HIM has not been allocated an optimal work environment or enough square footage to handle all the tasks required. The typical offices of the 1970s were open office areas with no dividers between workspaces; and the workspaces of the 1990s were "cubbies" or work desk cubicles where workspaces were separated by high or low dividers. Work desk cubicles are still the typical set up for most HIM departments. Storage in terms of shelving for paper health records was a necessity for the HIM workspaces in the 1970s, 80s, and 90s. The HIM department of today and the future does not have to worry about space for paper records but space is still required for completion of the electronic work and the use of computers, dual monitors, and keyboards.

Privacy in the Workplace

Personal space in terms of privacy and noise are environmental factors that can affect an employee's job performance. **Privacy** is the quality or state of being hidden from, or undisturbed by, the observation or activities of other persons; or freedom from unauthorized intrusion (Merriam-Webster 2015). An employee needs to feel that there is some control over the amount of privacy that is experienced on a day-to-day basis. It is important that HIM managers have personal office space allowing private employee-manager communications, particularly in regards to sensitive issues.

Noise in the Workplace

Noise in an office environment can aggravate the perception of the loss of privacy and can cause overstimulation for many individuals. Noise is any sound that is undesired or interferes with one's hearing of something or concentration (Merriam-Webster 2015). Critical thinking skills required for HIM jobs can be hindered by too much noise in the office. The use of headsets and personal music devices has improved the noise level in many offices and allows individuals to enjoy their own music without infringing upon the rights of others.

Spatial Density in the Workplace

Spatial density refers to the number of items within a specific area or space and for this discussion it refers to the square footage available to employees in a given work area. The more individuals there are working in a small area can result in the perception of overcrowding. Allowing no personal space for employees can result in overstimulation and provoke conflict and emotional reactions between employees, cultivating a negative work environment, and affect an employee's overall work performance. The positive side of having individuals performing similar jobs within a small area can result in improved communication and cooperation among workgroup members. The type of jobs completed and the interdependence between one another may be directly impacted by spatial density both in a positive or negative manner.

Personalization and Identity in the Workplace

Personalization and identity are important particularly for employees who associate their workplace as not only the place to work but also a home-away-from-home. **Personalization** allows individuals to decorate or mark their workstation with items of interest (within reason) such as favorite quotes, family pictures, and sports team memorabilia. The personalization of a workspace allows employees to feel more at home and to work in a comfortable environment. Personalization of work areas also provides an outward identity for an employee. If an employee decorates his workstation with sports memorabilia from their favorite team, this reflects to others that the employee enjoys sports or is invested in a particular team. Collectively all workstations in an employee workgroup or department may provide an identity for the area as well. A messy workgroup or department may signify to others in the organization that this area is sloppy or that this group cannot get their work done as evidenced by piles of papers, charts, and such.

There is a connotation between the size of offices and the status of the individual who uses the office. For example, the CEO of a large healthcare organization will most likely have a nicely decorated large office with windows; this provides an identity of authority for this individual. Workspace personalization and identity can provide employees with the necessary motivation to perform in the workplace, thereby affecting individual job performance as well as workgroup performance.

Task or Workflow Interdependence in the Workplace

If the necessary resources are not located centrally to all employees completing the job tasks, job performance can be hindered. With the advent of electronic health records, the physical interdependence of job tasks is not nearly as important to completion of HIM jobs as in the past. It still is optimal for those individuals who complete similar tasks within the HIM department to be physically located near one another but if this is not possible electronic tools such as email and instant messaging can eliminate communication gaps between individuals who are not physically next to one another.

Working from Home

It is important for health information managers to be aware of the five items discussed previously as they impact employee job performance. As more and more employees work remotely for HIM departments, it is important to educate employees on the same topics for their home office. Best practice guidelines for at-home (remote) office setup should be developed by the HIM manager. When the employee first sets up the home office, the HIM manager should perform a site visit in-person or virtually to ensure the office is set up appropriately. If an employee lives quite a distance from the healthcare organization, the manager should perform a site visit virtually utilizing some kind of technology, such as video conferencing, that allows the manager to see the work area setup. Distractions in a remote work environment are not as easy to quantify and their bearing on employee performance is not as evident as when the employee works within the HIM department.

Job Experience

Job performance is also impacted by the relationships between job experience, organizational tenure, and age (Sturman 2003). **Job experience** is the accumulation of job knowledge from action and practice and is linked to the tasks and duties associated with a particular job. Job experience leads to the amassing of relevant knowledge, skills, and abilities that should positively impact job performance. The paradigm of job experience has changed over the past several years as long-term HIM professionals acquire different skills with the advent of health information technology such as electronic health records, computer-assisted coding, and speech recognition for transcription. Job experience that was translated easily from job to job is no longer as applicable and HIM professionals need to develop skills and abilities at different stages of their job experience years. HIM managers need to develop different management skills to address the changing HIM workforce such as managing remote workers and a diverse workforce of individuals who have varying levels of HIM technological skills. Job experience was often a relatively stable factor for HIM professionals but now job performance variability is occurring for HIM professionals at all stages of their career.

Organizational tenure is an accumulation of work-related information from job experience and the information gathered is only relevant to the current organization climate or culture. With the multitude of mergers and acquisitions between healthcare organizations, organizational tenure is also a fluctuating factor that influences job performance as long-term employees strive to adjust to changing cultures and climate. Long-term HIM professionals may find it difficult to adjust to centralized HIM functions that often occur with healthcare mergers and acquisitions, this in turn will affect job performance and cause performance variability even among those employees with organizational tenure.

Age is another aspect that can impact job performance negatively; although as addressed in the legal chapter of this text (chapter 5), age cannot be a basis for job discrimination. Chapter 3 discusses the aging workforce; and the reality is that aging impacts how all individuals function in the workplace, ranging from deterioration in motor coordination and strength, memory, reasoning, and cognition to the motivation for developing new job skills. This is clearly evident in the HIM workforce with the number of coders who retired as a result of the adoption of ICD-10-CM/PCS. Some members of the aging workforce just did not have the motivation or perhaps even the cognitive ability to learn the skills that are required for utilizing ICD-10-CM/PCS.

Job Complexity

Another aspect that affects job performance is **job complexity**. Complexity is the quality or condition of being difficult to understand or lacking simplicity (Merriam-Webster 2015). The greater the level of job complexity, the harder is it is for an employee to acquire the skills necessary to perform the job. Also the more complex the job tasks, the more time it takes for employees to adequately perform these tasks. There are two distinct stages of job performance development: the transition stage and the maintenance stage. The transition stage occurs when an employee starts a new position or when tasks and responsibilities are changed. The more complex a job, the longer the employee may remain in the transition stage, which in turn affects individual and overall workgroup performance. The maintenance stage occurs when an employee is sufficiently trained and the individual is using well-learned and developed processes but needs to learn a new technique in an established process, or should receive a refresher course about these processes. When evaluating job performance it is important to take into account the stage at which the employee is actually developing and to make sure that performance goals match the skills and abilities that are in transition (Sturman 2003).

It is important for HIM managers to be cognizant of the impact that the changing HIM work environment has on job experience, organizational tenure, age, and job complexity. Research notes that some of the dynamics in job performance can be attributed to these factors. The HIM role that is highly impacted by job complexity is an HIM coder, who is required to learn multiple new classification systems. The transition to a new classification system not only affects the coders but also the individuals who utilize the data in the healthcare organization and make decisions based on the administrative coded data. Job performance may be variable for all of these individuals as healthcare organizations transition to this new classification system.

Completion of the Performance Appraisal Document

In healthcare organizations, the HR department is responsible for maintaining standardized performance appraisal documents that are utilized by everyone throughout the organization. Training should take place for all new managers on the appropriate completion process of these performance appraisals along with the timelines for completion, periodical collection of data, and ongoing feedback to employees regarding performance. One of the performance objectives for most managers is that all employee performance appraisals are completed in a timely manner according to the healthcare organization's policy. Most healthcare organizations migrated to utilizing some kind of online performance management system that tracks the performance appraisal process for all employees. Managers must follow the standardized processes to ensure that fair and consistent appraisals are performed on a regular basis. Most healthcare organizations utilize systems that impact an employee's pay so it is imperative the manager can provide evidence that supports the increase or denial of increase in pay based on the annual performance appraisal. Pay for performance is described in detail later in this chapter.

Measuring Performance with Qualitative and Quantitative Data

At the completion of the performance appraisal, qualitative and quantitative data will be analyzed for each job task (as appropriate) and employee performance will be aggregated for the year. Periodic reviews of performance should happen throughout the evaluation period so the data aggregation process should not be overwhelming for any manager. Tools should be developed by the HIM manager to collect and maintain periodic review of job performance data as seen in figure 8.3. Each job performance standard that has quantitative or qualitative scores attached will be aggregated and an overall score for job performance standards and goals will be given to the employee.

Performance appraisals will include other items for evaluation and many of these items are standardized by the healthcare organization. One section may delineate specific employee values that match the mission and vision of the organization. These values may be rated as met or not met with no other categorization of the items. Examples of

Figure 8.3. Example of qualitative and quantitative data to evaluate job performance

Performance Standard 1: Performs coding on all assigned inpatient charts within three days of discharge

Category	Points	Performance standards
Exceeds performance	4	96–100%
On target	3	94–95%
Needs improvement	2	91–93%
Does not meet expectations	1	<90%

Performance Standard 2: Assigns appropriate DRGs to inpatient discharges with 98% accuracy

Category	Points	Performance standards
Exceeds performance	4	96–100%
On target	3	94–95%
Needs improvement	2	91–93%
Does not meet expectations	1	<90%

© AHIMA

job performance values that can be assessed for all employees are whether or not the employee is respectful, honest, reliable, and if he or she works as a team player. It is important that the HIM manager understands how these values can be objectively exhibited by employees and how the manager can assess these values during the performance appraisal process.

Evaluating Job-specific Responsibilities

The second section of the performance appraisal document includes the major job responsibilities and the specific performance standards that were developed for each particular job task. The HIM manager will compare standardized performance measures for all employees performing similar tasks. All employees, nonmanagement and management, should be well versed on the performance standards against which they are being evaluated. The job performance standards are set upon hire and initial job performance standards are reviewed during the probationary performance review cycle. During the probationary performance review cycle, job performance standards that evaluate specific employee performance and how frequently communication will occur regarding the employee's actual job performance should be discussed. Managers should also receive communication in regards to the job performance standards for which they will be evaluated throughout the performance plan time frame. The HR department should provide training to managers on all aspects of the job performance appraisal in regards to providing ongoing evaluation of job performance and how to communicate evaluation results to employees.

Individual Goals

The third section of the performance appraisal document includes individual employee goals that are developed in collaboration with the manager. These goals may also include development or training needs for the next performance year. The goals should include specific measurable outcomes and be agreed upon by both the employee and the manager.

Pay for Performance

The term **pay for performance** as related to job performance refers to remuneration for job tasks completed throughout a certain time frame. Pay for performance programs can be a potential driver of performance and can also provide a way to differentiate employment from other healthcare organizations competing for the same job pool of candidates. The major component that makes pay for performance programs successful is the way in which it defines and measures performance. One method of pay for performance that is utilized by most healthcare organizations is referred to as merit pay. Merit pay is used in roughly 90 percent of all US companies including healthcare organizations (Gerhart et al. 2009). **Merit pay** is an increase to base salary (often annually) that is based on performance appraisal ratings by an employee's manager (Gerhart et al. 2009). This concept can also be referred to as **meritocracy**, where employees are evaluated by positions and rewarded based on individual merits and contributions. The final ratings from these evaluations are linked to the employee's pay, thus the term *pay for performance* (Han et al. 2015). There has been very little research on the influence of merit pay on employees' actual performance but what does exist reflects a positive relationship. Performance ratings are usually statistically related to the amount of merit raises (Gerhart et al. 2009). The overall performance rating or score (aggregated within the performance appraisal) for an individual employee will be directly related to the percentage of merit increase that he or she may receive for the next year.

Pay for performance impacts performance in two ways: incentive effect and sorting effect. The **incentive effect** relates to how pay influences the level or intensity of individual motivation toward job performance. The **sorting effect** relates to the effect of pay for performance on the composition of the actual workforce. Individuals who are not able to meet the performance standards required to obtain pay for performance may be weeded out more quickly than in organizations where performance standards are not tied directly to compensation. Different pay systems may attract different job applicants and it may be more difficult to maintain employees within a strictly pay for performance work environment (Gerhart et al. 2009). It is important for healthcare organizations to understand the impact of their pay for performance initiatives on employee performance as well as how it affects managerial performance. Pay for performance initiatives that require an extensive management time commitment as in aggregation of data for assessing an employee's job performance in a pay for performance model may affect actual managerial performance in the long run. Performance appraisal programs should be designed to account for the nature of job performance and build in dynamic performance ratings that take into account variable work performance (Reb and Greguras 2010).

The HR department typically designs and implements pay for performance but individual managers are responsible for the actual delivery of the program to their employees. Managers are the individuals in the organization who evaluate employee job performance and communicate the actual outcomes of the performance appraisal process. An outcome would be how an employee's pay for performance is calculated, so the HR department must provide adequate training to managers about this process. Ensuring all managers are trained on the use of the performance appraisal system upon hire and are updated when any changes occur to the system are key factors to the successful outcome of any pay for performance initiative.

The **contingent reward leadership style** has been found to be an excellent deployment method for ensuring that managers and employees are on board with the outcomes of annual performance appraisal. Chapter 1 discussed aspects of contingency leadership that provides insight into this type of leadership style. Contingent reward leadership is "an active and positive exchange between employees and managers whereby employees are rewarded or recognized for accomplishing agreed-upon performance objectives" (Reb and Greguras 2010). This type of leadership can contribute to employees' belief in performance rewards that are provided by annual merit pay raises as it engages employees directly in the performance appraisal process.

Check Your **Understanding**

1. Differentiate between work sampling and benchmarking as sources of performance data.
2. Explain each step in the SMART method used for setting job performance standards.
3. Discuss the five areas of the work environment and how each area affects job performance.
4. Identify at least five items that are usually found on a performance appraisal form.
5. Define pay-for-performance as it relates to job performance.

Performance Appraisal Process

The performance appraisal process is the third component of an overall performance management system in a healthcare organization (as reflected in the performance appraisal life cycle). Often there are negative connotations associated with actual performance appraisals if they are not managed appropriately. Some of the myths associated with performance appraisals are that it is a painful process and is very emotionally charged. A negative outcome is that the employee did not understand initial expectations in regards to performance. Another common negative outcome is bad timing of when the evaluation is given either for the manager or the employee. The manager should allow ample, appropriate, and uninterrupted time to perform a performance appraisal with an employee. Performance appraisals should not be given at the end of an extremely difficult or stressful day—for either the employee or manager. Many employees feel that performance appraisals are very subjective even when the evaluations contain objective criteria for evaluation. Performance appraisals are often considered unnecessary by many employees if the outcomes of the performance appraisal are not aligned to compensation or promotion. If the department or organization does not provide adequate development or training opportunities for employees to perform their jobs adequately, the performance appraisal process is negated.

Performance management systems should be in place to attempt to avoid these types of negative outcomes. If a standardized performance management system is in place, positive outcomes should be the result of the performance appraisal process. Some of the positive outcomes resulting in a good performance management process are that communication improves between the employees and management because more frequent and regular communication occurs regarding job performance. A standardized performance management process keeps all employees in the loop so they know the process and expectations required to meet job performance standards. Performance appraisals become more relevant to employees and employees connect learning and development to growth in performance (11 Performance Appraisal Methods 2010).

Performance Appraisal Methods

There are a variety of different performance appraisal methods that can be applied and it is the responsibility of the HR department along with senior leadership to develop the methodology most appropriate for that healthcare organization. The healthcare organization may implement several different methods of assessment based on job roles and what is the most appropriate tool for assessing job performance. The six most common methods that are widely adopted and used in health information management departments will be discussed along with the advantages and disadvantages for each methodology.

Critical Incident Method

The **critical incident method** involves maintaining a log or documentation of critical incidences, both positive and negative, throughout each employee's performance cycle. Each incident will be described in detail at the time the incidence occurs. This can be very time-consuming documentation for the manager as each incident needs to be specifically documented and then shared with the employee at the time of occurrence. The manager can also require the employee provide feedback on the incidence, why it occurred, and what can be done to prevent it from happening again or ideas for incorporating new processes that impact positive performance. At the time when the annual performance appraisal is completed, all incidences will be included within the actual performance document and mostly likely will be rated or ranked depending on the quantification process used with the evaluation system.

The advantages for this methodology are that detailed incident documentation can be maintained and shared with the employee on both positive and negative occurrences. There should be no surprises during the evaluation process as incidences were shared with the employee throughout the year.

The disadvantages for this methodology are that detailed documentation is very time consuming and frequently only negative incidences are tracked by managers rather than also including positive incidences. Also it may be difficult to quantify the impact of the incidences on performance in the overall scheme of job performance for the year (11 Performance Appraisal Methods 2010).

Graphic Rating Scales

Graphic rating scales are the most common methodology employed in HIM departments. Checks or monitoring are conducted on an employee's performance throughout the performance cycle. The content of the performance monitoring includes quantity of work, quality of work, dependability, judgment and critical thinking, cooperation, and initiative or motivation. Rating scales are assigned to each key performance indicator and a typical scale might look like that in figure 8.3.

The advantage in regards to this methodology is graphic rating scales take less time to develop than other more subjective evaluation types. Quantitative comparison of job performance can be performed within each segment of the performance cycle or against the previous year's job performance for individual employees. The disadvantage in regards to the use of the graphic rating scale is that scoring can vary between managers or managers can vary how they use the scoring for each individual employee (11 Performance Appraisal Methods 2010). Common rater errors often appear when using graphic rating scales and the most common rater errors are:

- Halo effect—The rater subjectively assesses all performance for an employee as either positive or negative based one specific aspect rather than the performance overall.

- Central tendency—The rater feels that the performance of all employees should be rated as average rather than objectively assessing each employee individually.

- Leniency or strictness—The rater subjectively leans toward being more tolerant or rigorous when evaluating employee performance.

- Bias or similar-to-me—The rater judges the employee's performance on how similar the performance is to the rater's own performance (Dartmouth College 2015).

Essay Evaluation Method

The **essay evaluation method** is mostly applied in combination with another methodology such as the graphic rating scale. This method requires that the manager develop an employee appraisal by qualitatively identifying the strong and weak points of each employee's behavior and documenting each of these items in a written essay. The information the manager may use when assessing the employee's behavior are job knowledge, application of the organization's policies and procedures, working relationships with peers and management, attitude, and organizational abilities. Each of these items will be included in the performance appraisal and the manager will be required to write an essay regarding the strengths and weaknesses exhibited by the employee. The advantage of this methodology is that it requires the manager to perform research on each individual and really get to know the employee's job performance. The disadvantages to this methodology are that the manager may not take time to objectively assess the employee's behavior and the performance appraisal may be very subjective in nature (11 Performance Appraisal Methods 2010).

360 Performance Appraisal

The **360 performance appraisal** is a methodology most often used in conjunction with other more traditional methods such as graphic rating scales and critical incident methods. It measures the manner and capacity of work performance and concentrates on the more subjective areas of work such as teamwork, character, and leadership. The 360 performance appraisal method requires that employees obtain confidential and anonymous assessments from their colleagues. Healthcare organizations develop a standardized process that employees can use when requesting 360 performance appraisals from others within the organization. This process will be outlined in a performance appraisal policy and procedure that is available to all employees of the healthcare organization. "360" implies that the entire picture of an employee's job performance can be assessed with this type of performance methodology. These assessments are not directly shared with the employee but rather forwarded to the employee's manager for incorporation into the performance appraisal process.

The advantages of the 360 performance evaluation are that it provides a more comprehensive and accurate assessment of an individual's performance. Employees tend to feel part of the entire performance appraisal process when they have the ability to provide feedback to both peers and management.

The disadvantages of the 360 performance appraisal method are that it is a time-consuming process and requires training for both administration of the process and for those who are completing the evaluations. An employee may select individuals to perform the 360 evaluations that will only provide positive feedback and avoid those peers and managers who may provide a more negative evaluation of the employee's performance. It is also very difficult for a manager to quantify the results particularly if there is a great variance between the 360 evaluators in terms of the employee's performance.

Forced Ranking

Forced ranking or forced distribution is starting to appear more frequently in healthcare organizations when in the past it was often utilized inside larger corporations such as major energy and car companies. This methodology ranks employees in terms of forced allocations meaning that only 10 to 20 percent of the employees' performance will fall into the higher levels of job performance, 70 to 80 percent will fall into the middle ranges of job performance, and the rest will fall into the lowest levels of job performance (11 Performance Appraisal Methods 2010). The high, middle, or low levels of performance ratings are based on the aggregate performance standard scores calculated within annual performance appraisals. For example, based on the job standard scoring outlined in figure 8.3, a high level of job performance would be an aggregate score of 3.5 to 4, middle range job performance would be an aggregate score of 2.5 to 3.49, and the low range of job performance would be an aggregate score below 2.5. Employee increases for the next year would be based on the forced ranking allocation—high, middle, or low range job performance. In addition, the department or workgroup will only be allowed to have so many employees fall within each range of job performance regardless of how well each individual performs.

The advantage to this methodology is that it forces management to really assess personnel performance and categorize the employees who are the highest performers versus those who are the lowest performers. This method also creates and sustains a high performance culture in which the employees continuously strive to improve performance (11 Performance Appraisal Methods 2010).

The disadvantages to this method are that it can harm morale, discourage collaboration and teamwork, and it can create a more competitive or cutthroat workforce. The forced ranking system results in a heightened focus on individual performance rather than on the importance of teamwork (Lipman 2012). This methodology can be a detriment to employee morale because it forces managers to rank employees on a scale and against one another rather than just on objective performance. This could result in negative work outcomes because the forced ranking requires the manager to rank employees higher than others even when the overall team is performing at a high level of performance (11 Performance Appraisal Methods 2010).

Management by Objectives

Management by objectives (MBO) is another technique used in performance appraisals that addresses the assessment of performance at the management level. MBO is a management approach that defines target objectives for organization work and compares performance against those objectives. MBO is a participative approach to performance and requires goals and objectives to be defined by management-level employees to provide a framework for managing performance outcomes for a given time period. Often management teams within particular departments will have goals and objectives for performance that are interrelated and outlined in each manager's performance appraisal.

The advantage to this method is that collaboration and teamwork within the management group is essential in order to meet the performance objectives. The disadvantage to this method is if one of the team members within the particular management group fails to achieve a component of the goal, all of the team's performance objectives will be impacted and may result in a negative outcome for everyone (Hutchinson 2014).

Self-evaluation of Performance

In the previous section of this chapter, performance appraisal was discussed in terms of the manager's evaluation or colleagues' evaluation of job performance. Another aspect of performance appraisal that is key to a good performance appraisal process is the ability for employees to complete self-evaluations of performance. In order to engage employees during the performance appraisal life cycle, employees should be involved in assessing their own performance on a regular basis. A good performance appraisal allows employees to regularly provide feedback and input on their performance. The feedback should be related to the goals set by the employee and management at the beginning of each annual performance appraisal cycle. It is important that each employee takes the initiative to write an accurate and reflective self-assessment of job performances as this is a way to improve the relationship with his or her manager. As a manager, it is important to document a professionally written self-assessment of your job performance for the year. This process opens and improves communication between the manager and the employee and provides the manager with valuable insight regarding the employee's initiative.

Some tips for writing a self-assessment are:

- Be proud. Do not hesitate to highlight the tasks and projects that provide examples of commendable work.
- Be concise. Clearly articulate insight to performance in terms of both strengths and weaknesses.
- Be honest. Indicate areas that require improvement and be open to training and development to enhance performance.
- Be professional. Provide reflection on why goals were not met and what resources are needed to attain these particular goals (Arline 2015).

Managers should allow employees sufficient time prior to the actual performance appraisal process to provide self-assessments regarding job performance for the particular time frame in review. Standardized forms should be used for collecting self-assessments and the employee's self-assessment should be a component of the formal performance appraisal.

Communicating Performance Appraisal Results

As noted earlier in the chapter, upon hire, all employees should receive an explanation of the purpose of the performance appraisal process and this information should outline the employees' role in the entire process. Standardized policies and procedures regarding performance management and the performance appraisal process should be available online or in hard copy for all employees to view. Upon hire, managers should be trained not only on how to complete the required documents for employees but also on the soft skills required to communicate performance appraisal results. Monitoring and evaluating employee job performance is a key role for HIM managers and HIM managers should be trained on the use of the healthcare organization's performance management plan.

Performance management training should incorporate methods for conducting the performance evaluation. The overall performance appraisal should be a positive experience for both the manager and employee, even if the employee's performance was below the standard for the year. There should never be any surprises in the actual performance appraisal document or during the actual performance appraisal meeting. The manager should select a setting that is quiet and free from interruptions. If the performance appraisals are given inside the manager's office, the office phone and the manager's cell phone should be silenced. This is the time when an employee deserves the manager's undivided attention so no interruptions should be allowed.

It is important to allow enough time in both the employee's and manager's schedule to thoroughly discuss the performance appraisal. As a rule, it is not a good idea to simply hand the employee a copy of the performance appraisal and state, "review this and let me know if you have any concerns." Employees are the greatest asset for any organization and they deserve to receive adequate time and appropriate feedback face-to-face regarding performance. Constructive feedback should be provided in the performance appraisal regarding both negative and positive job performance. During the appraisal process, the following should be done by the manager:

- Provide feedback to the employee on the self-assessment completed prior to the meeting.
- Solicit suggestions on how the manager can assist the employee in reaching his or her performance goals.
- Develop new performance goals for the next performance appraisal cycle.
- Solicit feedback on the manager's performance.
- Wrap-up the performance appraisal by thanking the employee for his or her contributions to the workgroup, department, and the healthcare organization (Buhler 1991).

Not all performance appraisals will be positive in nature particularly if the employee has had a variable year in terms of job performance. Based on periodic reviews throughout the performance appraisal period, an employee should understand what to expect in the outcome of the year's performance appraisal. If he or she has had a variable year, he or she will then understand the appraisal may not result in the optimal pay increase or desired promotion. Often employee performance improvement plans are required if the employee's job performance is suboptimal. If an individual's performance necessitates improvement at any time during the appraisal cycle, an employee improvement plan should be initiated.

Employee Performance Improvement Plans

An employee **performance improvement plan (PIP)** is initiated whenever an individual's job performance is substandard or the employee violates a departmental or healthcare organizational policy. For this chapter, the focus will be on the PIP in terms of employee job performance. The PIP—a strategic roadmap for the employee to utilize to achieve more positive results within his or her job—begins whenever a manager identifies that an employee is performing below the expectations for a particular job standard(s). The focus of improving employee performance can reflect two methods of thought or a combination of both–either by altering an employee's weaknesses or reinforcing performance by focusing on the employee's strengths. Focusing on employees' strengths can result in a positive work climate and can result in motivated employees who perform above and beyond average (Van Woerkhom and Meyers 2015). Developing strength-based performance improvement goals can result in motivated employees who strive to meet performance standards.

As noted previously, job performance should be reviewed on a regular basis so there are no surprises during the annual performance appraisal review. Employees should receive regular communication on how job standards are being met or not being met. An example of this in the HIM department is that coders are expected to maintain a level of coding productivity (quantity) and quality. Coding productivity is monitored on a regular basis, weekly or monthly, and the results of the monitoring should be shared with each coder on a regular basis. Whenever a coder falls below the required standard for coding productivity or quality, the coding manager should identify whether this is a trend or a single event. If substandard performance in either productivity or quality becomes a trend for the coder, the coding manager should initiate a PIP. The department or healthcare organization should have a policy that addresses when a PIP should be initiated because of substandard work performance. The following steps should be followed when initiating an employee PIP:

- *Step 1:* Document performance issues. The manager should have objective documentation reflecting the dates and the results of the suboptimal employee job performance. For example, if the coding quality standard is to code all patient discharges with 95 percent accuracy and a coder's quality measures for the past two months are 92 percent and 88 percent accuracy rate, these employee performance standards should be documented. The coding manager should also have specific examples of coding errors or trends in the type of coding errors being made by the coder.

- *Step 2:* Develop an action plan incorporating SMART goals for improving an employee's job performance (Wayne State University 2015). Building on the example in Step 1, the coding manager should outline several performance goals in order to improve the employee's coding accuracy. These goals should include additional training and resources to assist the employee in achieving these performance improvement goals.

- *Step 3:* Review the performance plan with HR and the department director. After creating the PIP, the manager should review the actual plan with the department HIM director and the HR department. The HR department will provide guidance on the duration of the PIP and the next steps if the employee's performance does not improve.

- *Step 4:* Meet with the employee to review the PIP. A confidential meeting should be arranged with the employee to go over the job performance standards that are not being met and that resulted in the creation of the PIP. The manager should explain the suboptimal or deficient job performance and outline the specific performance improvement expectations. The manager should clearly and concisely delineate the time frame in which the employee has to meet these expectations. The employee should give feedback on the performance goals outlined within the PIP and add additional goals. The manager should provide training methods and tools that will assist the employee in improving job performance, define the communication process for the time frame of the PIP, and explain the next steps if the employee does not demonstrate improvement in job performance.

- *Step 5:* Follow-up with the employee. The manager should set up regular meeting times with the employee to ensure the employee is working toward the performance improvement goals. The manager should provide documentation of progress toward the performance improvement goals. For the example provided in Steps 1 and 2, the coder should have regular reports (daily or weekly) on coding accuracy rates and coding errors should be shared with the employee immediately.

- *Step 6:* PIP conclusion. The PIP will have a specific termination date and the job performance goals will need to be met at this time. If the employee successfully meets all the performance improvement goals, the manager and employee will sign off on the PIP and the results will be forwarded to the HR department to be stored in the employee's file. This process may be done manually or electronically depending on the HR performance management system used within the organization (How to Establish a Performance Improvement Plan 2015).

Improving employee performance is an important component of an HIM manager's job role. HIM managers should consistently review employee performance against job performance standards on a regular basis (daily, weekly, or monthly) and communicate these results to all employees via a standardized communication method such as a confidential email or weekly individual meetings. HIM managers and employees should work together to develop strategies for improving job performance both individually and as a workgroup.

Check Your **Understanding**

1. Discuss three ways performance appraisals are perceived as positive and three ways performance appraisals are perceived as negative.

2. Identify the six performance appraisal methods commonly used by HIM departments and explain the advantages and disadvantages of each.

3. Discuss best practices for performing a self-assessment appraisal.

4. Discuss best practices for giving a performance appraisal review.

5. Outline the six steps for initiating an employee PIP.

Case Study

Objectives

- Assess the factors that impact a long-term employee's job performance
- Evaluate a performance appraisal review meeting
- Identify methods for improving performance appraisal review outcomes

Instructions

Review the following case study and create a document that provides responses that correlate to the questions in terms of assessing an HIM coder's job performance.

Scenario

Margie has been a coder in the HIM department of a large acute-care facility for the past 10 years and prior to working at this organization, she coded for 15 years at a similarly sized acute-care facility. Throughout her coding tenure, Margie mostly coded outpatient encounters such as outpatient observations, outpatient surgeries, and Emergency Room Department visits. Two years ago, Margie was cross-trained to code inpatient discharges as well. At last year's performance appraisal, Margie received an overall score of 3.8 out of 5, which denotes that she "exceeds job performance expectations." This past performance appraisal cycle, the HIM coding area and Margie personally experienced the following changes:

- The hospital implemented a new EHR that required extensive training for all hospital employees.
- The coding area had some management turnover with the long-term coding manager retiring and the coding lead promoted to the coding manager position.
- The HIM department's coding productivity was updated to include computer-assisted coding and all coders went from using one monitor to dual monitors.
- Margie used to sit in a quiet office area with one other individual but the department was reconfigured and all coders were moved to a central location. The coding office is a large room with each coder occupying a "cubby-type" area with dividers between each desk. The noise in the open concept office tends to magnify even with the dividers.
- Margie's husband had some health issues as well, which caused Margie to be on family medical leave for six weeks.

It is that time of year for all performance appraisal reviews to be conducted and Margie has expectations that her performance evaluation will be similar to last year's. Margie's coding manager set up a time to go over Margie's review, Friday afternoon at 3:00 p.m. in the manager's office. Margie arrives promptly at the manager's office but has to sit outside the office for 10 minutes waiting for the coding manager to finish up a personal phone call. Margie enters the room and the coding manager has music playing from her iPhone and her computer is open with the email notification on. Margie sits down at the chair on the other side of the manager's desk and the coding manager hands Margie the evaluation and says, "review this please and let me know if you have any questions, I have to answer a few emails because it is Friday afternoon."

Margie reviews the evaluation and she is stunned by the final evaluation score that she is receiving this year. Her final score is a 2.8 out of 5 and she is being put on a PIP with no pay raise. There are items included in the evaluation that Margie had no idea had been a problem throughout the year. Margie's productivity and quality were marked below average and the statistics included in the review were ones that Margie had not seen all year. As Margie read the evaluation, the coding manager's phone kept ringing and the manager kept answering her emails. Margie was very upset and tried to address the evaluation with the coding manager, which in turn made the coding manager defensive. The coding manager was not open to discussing any of incidences noted in the evaluation and she stated that she did not have time to review Margie's monthly productivity and quality scores with her. As Margie typically does not like conflict, she signed the evaluation and PIP but she was very upset leaving the room. The coding manager did not seem to notice that Margie was upset and continued answering her emails.

Two months later: Margie accepted another job at a specialty hospital within the same geographic region of her facility and she resigned with a two-week notification.

Assumptions

- All performance appraisal reviews for the organization are performed at the end of the fiscal year.
- The healthcare facility requires periodic reviews of performance throughout the performance cycle but Margie did not receive any periodic feedback throughout the performance cycle.
- Margie did not get a chance to perform a self-evaluation or request 360 performance review from her peers.

Deliverables

1. Discuss two distinct items that might affect Margie's work performance. Explain in detail why you think these might cause Margie's job performance to vary from the previous year.
2. Identify three inappropriate occurrences that happened during the actual performance appraisal review meeting and how this meeting could be improved.
3. Identify three negative performance appraisal events that occurred throughout Margie's performance appraisal cycle and identify preventive methods so the same negative events do not occur next year.

Review Questions

1. Eleanor is a release of information clerk in the HIM department. Once a quarter she meets with her supervisor to review her productivity and progress toward her annual goals. This represents which phase in the performance appraisal life cycle?

   a. Annual review
   b. Periodic review
   c. Planning
   d. Training

2. Charles is a supervisor of the imaging section of the HIM department. In trying to update scanning productivity standards, Charles calls around to other area hospitals to ask what their scanning standards are. This is an example of what source of performance data?

   a. Benchmarking
   b. Job appraisal
   c. Observation
   d. Work sampling

3. In addition to calling other area hospitals, Charles also asked the current scanners to track their tasks on an activity log. Each scanner logs in the time it takes to scan a specific amount of records. This is an example of what source of performance data?

   a. Benchmarking
   b. Job appraisal
   c. Observation
   d. Work sampling

4. Elizabeth is single and has quite a few photos of her dog and two cats hung up where everyone can see them. Elizabeth's work environment influences her job performance by creating:

   a. Personal space
   b. Spatial density
   c. Workflow interdependence
   d. Workplace personalization

5. A sense of privacy in the work environment positively affects job performance by improving:

   a. Personal space
   b. Spatial density
   c. Workflow interdependence
   d. Workplace personalization

6. Angela's annual performance appraisal is scheduled for next month. She has been asked by her supervisor to provide the names of two peers and one person in another department with whom she regularly interacts. These individuals will contribute to Angela's evaluation. This is an example of what type of performance appraisal method?

   a. 360 performance appraisal
   b. Critical incident method
   c. Essay evaluation
   d. Graphic rating scale

7. As an HIM manager, Chelsea documents both positive and negative examples of her employees' work throughout the year. She refers back to these examples during annual evaluations. This is an example of what type of performance appraisal method?

   a. Forced ranking
   b. Critical incident method
   c. Graphic rating scale
   d. Management by objectives

8. The following statement—"emergency room records: 35 records coded per hour"—is an example of what type of performance indicator for a job performance standard?

   a. Fiscal
   b. Quality
   c. Quantity
   d. Sampling

9. The job performance standard "Inpatient records will be coded at 100 percent accuracy within one day of discharge" exhibits which of the SMART method attributes?

   a. Attainable and realistic
   b. Attainable and measurable
   c. Specific and measurable
   d. Realistic and measurable

10. Which of the following is an advantage to the graphic rating scale performance appraisal method?

    a. Involves peers and other colleagues in the appraisal process
    b. Scoring can be subjective and vary greatly from one supervisor to another
    c. Takes less time to complete than other method
    d. Training must be done for supervisors to use this method correctly

References

11 Performance Appraisal Methods. 2010. 4hrm.info Human Resources Management. www.4hrm.info/performance-appraisal-methods.

Arline, K. 2015 (January 26). Self-assessment: Tips for employees writing performance reviews. *Business News Daily.* http://www.businessnewsdaily.com/5379-writing-self-assessment.html.

Ashkanasy, N.M., O.B. Ayoko, and K.A. Jehn. 2014. Understanding the physical environment of work and employee behavior: An affective events perspective. *Journal of Organizational Behavior* 35(8):1169–1184.

Barnes, C.M. and F.P. Morgeson. 2007. Typical performance, maximal performance, and performance variability: Expanding our understanding of how organizations value performance. *Human Performance* 20(3):259–274.

Bowling, N., S. Khazon, R. Meyer, and C. Burrus. 2015. Situational strength as a moderator of the relationship between job satisfaction and job performance: A meta-analytic examination. *Journal of Business Psychology* 30:89–104.

Buhler, P. 1991. Evaluating an employee's performance. *SuperVision* 52(4):17.

Business Dictionary. 2015. http://www.businessdictionary.com.

Dartmouth College. 2015. Common Rater Errors. Human Resources of Dartmouth College. http://www.dartmouth.edu/~hrs/profldev/performance_management/rater_errors.html.

Fried, B.J. and M.D. Fottler. 2015. *Human Resources in Healthcare: Managing for Success*, 4th ed. Chicago: Health Administration Press: American College of Healthcare Executives.

Gerhart, B., S.L. Rynes, and I. Smithey Fulmer. 2009. Pay and performance: Individuals, groups, and executives. *The Academy of Management Annals* 3(1):251–315.

Han, J.H., K. Bartol, and S. Kim. 2015. Tightening up the performance–pay linkage: Roles of contingent reward leadership and profit-sharing in the cross-level influence of individual pay-for-performance. *Journal of Applied Psychology* 100(2):417–430.

How to Establish a Performance Improvement Plan. 2015. Society for Human Resources Management. http://www.shrm.org/templatestools/howtoguides/pages/performanceimprovementplan.aspx.

Hutchinson. 2014. *The Hutchinson Unabridged Encyclopedia with Atlas and Weather Guide*. Abington, UK: Helicon.

Lipman, V. 2012 (July 19). The Pros and Cons of Forced Rankings: A Manager's Perspective. *Forbes.* http://www.forbes.com/sites/victorlipman/2012/07/19/the-pros-and-cons-of-forced-rankings-a-managers-perspective/.

Merriam-Webster. 2015. http://www.merriam-webster.com/dictionary/.

Minbashian, A. and D. Luppino. 2014. Short-term and long-term variability in performance: An integrative model. *Journal of Applied Psychology* 99(5):898–914.

Performance Appraisal Methods. 2010. Human Resource Management. http://www.hrwale.com/performance-management/performance-appraisal-methods/.

Reb, J. and G.J. Greguras. 2010. Understanding performance ratings. *Journal of Applied Psychology* 95(1):213–220.

Rich, B., J. Lepine, and E. Crawford. 2010. Job engagement: Antecedents and effects on job performance. *Academy of Management Journal* 53(3):617–635.

Sturman, M. 2003. Searching for the inverted u-shaped relationship between time and performance: Meta-analyses of the experience/performance, tenure/performance, and age/performance relationships. *Journal of Management* 29(5):609–640.

USLegal, Inc. 2015. Probationary Employment Periods Law and Legal Definition. http://definitions.uslegal.com/p/probationary-employment-periods/.

Van Woerkhom, M. and M.C. Meyers. 2015. My strengths count! Effects of a strengths-based psychological climate on positive affect and job performance. *Human Resource Management* 54(1):81–103.

Wayne State University. 2015. S.M.A.R.T. Objectives. http://hr.wayne.edu/leads/phase1/smart-objectives.php.

Training and Development in Health Information Management

- Evaluate employee training and development models used in healthcare organizations
- Explain the benefits and components of a new employee orientation program
- Compare current methods in training and development that apply to health information management (HIM)
- Evaluate the impact of HIM employee training on performance appraisals
- Justify additional training needs based on emerging roles in HIM

ADDIE
Asynchronous
Audio conferencing
Auditory learners
Blended learning
Coaching
Continuing education (CE)
Credential
Cross-training

Department-level orientation
Development
Distance learning
Individual orientation
In-service education
Intranet
Job rotation
Job shadowing
Kinesthetic learners

License
Mentoring
On-the-job training (OTJ)
Organization-level orientation
Orientation
Role-playing
Self-directed learning
Simulation

Socialization
Succession planning
Synchronous
Training
Video conferencing
Visual learners
Web-based training
Webcast
Webinar

Amid the changes in healthcare today, it is important to commit time and resources to the training and development of personnel so everyone in the healthcare organization is prepared. Nothing has made this clearer than the recent transition from *International Classification of Diseases, Ninth Revision, Clinical Modification (ICD-9-CM)* to *International Classification of Diseases, Tenth Revision, Clinical Modification (ICD-10-CM)* and *International Classification of Diseases, Tenth Revision, Procedure Coding System (ICD-10-PCS)*. An entire workforce of HIM coding professionals had to learn a new coding classification system for both diagnosis and procedure coding. Some coding professionals had to relearn anatomy and physiology before they were ready to learn ICD-10-CM/PCS. Due to implementation delays, some people had to relearn what they had been taught already about the new coding system. Some coders found themselves in the position of training others, including their peers, supervisors, physicians, nurses, and other healthcare professionals. Some professionals needed in-depth knowledge of ICD-10-CM/PCS, others needed only to understand the basics. Policy and procedure manuals had to be rewritten; documentation guidelines had to be developed and communicated throughout the organization. The opportunities for training and developing were plentiful, and HIM managers needed to assume the role of teacher as they may not have had to before.

This chapter provides the fundamentals of staff training and development. There are many different definitions of both training and development. Some resources even use the terms interchangeably. In this chapter the terms are defined separately. **Training** is the set of activities and materials that provide the opportunity to acquire job-related skills, knowledge, and abilities; it is job-focused. **Development** is the career-focused process of progressing within one's profession or occupation. There may be overlap in these areas: job-related activities may also provide new knowledge that serves to advance an individual's career. A newly hired release-of-information (ROI) clerk attending Health Insurance Portability and Accountability Act of 1996 (HIPAA) training is also learning information that will help her to realize her ultimate career goal of becoming a privacy officer. Many of the concepts that apply to training (for example, learning styles) also apply to development.

There are five reasons why a healthcare organization provides training and development for its employees:

- Orient new employees to the organization
- Update employee skills to meet technological, organizational, and managerial changes
- Solve organizational problems such as personal conflicts or the impact of a restrictive legal environment
- Improve employee performance due to deficient job skills
- Prepare employees for promotion to support retention (Fottler et al. 1998)

This chapter covers orientation and training as well as staff development related to continuing education and career development. Training and development is often coordinated organizationwide through an education department or human resources (HR) department; but in a department or work section area, the HIM manager is responsible for training and development. HIM managers have the technical expertise, education, and practical experience to carry out necessary training, but they must also have the skills to perform needs assessments, understand learning styles, and choose appropriate training and development methods of instruction. This chapter discusses all of the necessary components of a training and development program.

Orientation and Training

Training and orientation focus on the skills necessary to be successful in the workplace. Support for training must start at the top of the organization. Most healthcare organization mission and vision statements speak to their commitment to quality patient care, and at the heart of quality patient care is a strong training program. Employees must be trained correctly from the start, through orientation, and must continue with on-the-job training and in-service education so learned skills are maintained, updated, and practiced.

New Employee Orientation

Specifically, **orientation** is a set of activities designed to familiarize new employees with their jobs, the organization, and its work culture. A positive orientation experience is important for any new hire. It is an opportunity for the organization to make a good first impression and at the same time provide a new employee with the tools to a successful tenure. Ideally, the orientation process begins with the offer of employment. At that time the new hire should be told when and where orientation will take place. This sets an expectation of learning right from the start and also makes the employee feel welcome. Orientation takes place on three levels: organizational, departmental, and individual (Patena and LeBlanc 2013).

Organization-level Orientation

Orientation on the organizational level is usually the first step in the new employee orientation process. **Organization-level orientation** is a large-scale introduction to the facility. All new hires are scheduled to attend orientation sessions as soon as possible after they start. The frequency of orientation depends on the size of the organization and the number of new hires. A small facility may hold an organizational orientation once a month, while a larger facility may hold orientation once every two weeks or even once a week if necessary. Some organizations accomplish orientation in one- or two-day sessions, while others spread the orientation over weeks or even months. The format for new employee orientation will vary according to the needs of the organization. It may take place in a group setting with all members present. This method is more personal and gives all new employees a chance to interact and meet people from other departments. In other cases, computer-based orientation may be used. While this is a less personal method, it works best when there is a lack of individuals to carry out orientation, or when it would be impractical to bring new employees on-site. Examples may be the hiring of remote workers or outsourced employees, especially from companies with overseas workers. A hybrid orientation is possible as well. In a hybrid setting, the majority of information is covered in a group setting, with employees responsible for covering some material on their own via computer-based programs. In addition to welcoming new employees to the organization, the purpose of orientation is to equip new hires with the information they need to be successful on the job. Each organization, at each level, will determine what material to cover in a new employee orientation; some examples of topics covered at the organizational level are:

- History of the organization
- Organization mission and vision statements
- Structure of the organization such as reporting and communication expectations
- Provision of name badges and paperwork completion
- Employment policies and procedures such as time and attendance, grievance, vacation and sick leave, parking, dress code, solicitation, infection control, and universal precautions
- Confidentiality such as computer security, passwords, and Internet access
- Safety such as fire, tornado, earthquake, and disaster preparedness
- Diversity
- Sexual harassment
- Benefits such as health insurance, life insurance, paid time off, and tuition reimbursement
- Tour of the facility

An invaluable tool of the organizational orientation is the employee handbook. This handbook contains the material covered during the orientation and serves as a reference for later, after the orientation program is over and the employee needs to be refreshed on the material covered.

Department-level Orientation

Once an employee has been introduced to the organization as a whole, the next level of orientation occurs at the department level. **Department-level orientation** should be provided to each new hire as soon as they begin employment. It is very tempting for HIM managers to delay, or skip entirely, a department orientation and put the new hire to work right away. Likely the position they filled has been open for some time and managers want the work to commence again immediately. But similar to organizational orientation, this is an opportunity for the department to put its best foot forward in welcoming the new hire. The good impression created at the organizational level can be quickly undone if a new employee is ignored or not educated to the ways of the department in which he or she will be spending their work day. Most department orientations use one-to-one sessions to cover the necessary information. Additional topics that need to be covered at the department level include:

- Tour of the department such as location of restrooms, cafeteria, entrances, and exits
- Introduction to co-workers
- Department mission and vision statements
- Hours of operation

- Structure of the department such as reporting and communication
- Department safety
- Department policies and procedures such as time clock, breaks, dress code, time off requests, and answering the phone
- Confidentiality such as signing a confidentiality agreement
- Operation of equipment such as phones, copy machines, and computers

A good practice is to immediately assign the new employee a "buddy" to guide them as he or she is oriented to the department. This buddy will invite the new co-worker to lunch, provide support as they train in the specifics of his or her new position, and explain the ins and outs of how the department works.

Departmental orientation may take place over a day or two, or it may be spread over a few weeks. Another best practice is to have the new employee rotate among each of the jobs in the HIM department observing how each position fits into the overall function of the HIM department. A new data quality specialist may spend a couple hours or even a half day each with scanning clerks, ROI specialists, transcriptionists, coders, and cancer registrars. Although time consuming, this allows the new employee to meet co-workers outside their work area and to see how each job in the HIM department impacts other jobs in the same department. Transcriptionists will understand why coders need their reports so quickly, and coders will understand the frustrations of scanning clerks. It is also important to include employees transferring into the department from elsewhere in the organization in any department orientation. An employee already familiar with the organization will not need the in-depth orientation that a new employee will, but they will need to know the specifics of his or her new department and work space. Consideration will also need to be given to off-site employees. Remote workers may be required to spend time on-site prior to working from home, and outsourced employees will have to know how the HIM department operates even though they are employed by a vendor and not the organization.

Individual Orientation

The final level of orientation occurs at the individual level. **Individual orientation**, or one-on-one training, may be done by the employee's direct supervisor or by the assigned buddy and overseen by the supervisor. Individual orientation covers those topics unique to the person's job in the department such as:

- Job description
- Job procedures or tasks demonstration
- Work hours
- Compensation issues not covered by the HR department such as incentive pay structure or merit pay requirements
- Productivity measures or performance standards
- Performance appraisal schedule and process
- Tour of work station including computer, desk, and how to raise and lower the chair
- Continuing education and career development opportunities

It is helpful for the HIM manager to create an orientation checklist for each employee. This allows monitoring of the new hire's progress through the levels of orientation and everyone involved will know when the orientation is complete. Some organizations require a checklist to be signed by both the manager and employee to indicate that each item was indeed covered, and that no questions remain. An orientation checklist will be different for each position. Some items on the checklist will apply to all employees such as attendance at organizational orientation or signing the confidentiality agreement, but most of the checklist will be specific to the needs of the individual. For example, a scanning clerk will need to know how to operate digital imaging equipment, but a second-shift supervisor will need to learn the payroll process.

Finally, the new employee orientation program at all levels should be evaluated by those using the program so that appropriate changes can be made as needed. Both supervisors and new hires should have an opportunity to provide feedback on the process and provide comments on what worked well and what could be changed. Feedback should be provided at the close of each separate orientation session (organizational, departmental, and individual) and then again a few weeks or months after the process to assess how successful the orientation program was in the long term. It may not be until a few months later that a new employee realizes that a topic was particularly helpful, or could have been covered in more detail. While each organization will tailor their orientation program to their own needs, the American Health Information Management Association (AHIMA) has provided some tips on how to plan for a successful orientation experience:

- Identify important organizational individuals such as the chief executive officer, chief financial officer, chief nursing officer, and chief of staff
- Reach out prior to orientation with information such as parking details, orientation schedules, or contact numbers
- Be sure to welcome new employees
- Do not introduce too much information into one day
- Connect paperwork with interactions with key stakeholders
- Do not focus too heavily on "not allowed" items
- Assign a work buddy (AHIMA 2013a)

Training Design

Once the orientation program is complete, the next step is to thoroughly train an employee in the skills, knowledge, and abilities necessary to do their job. This may be accomplished using on-the-job training, in-service education, off-site training, or distance learning, which are discussed later in this chapter. But regardless of the model chosen, all training (and development) programs must be carefully designed in order to be effective (Battles 2006). Training programs need structure in order to be measured against outcomes. One effective, step-by-step method of training program design is the ADDIE method. **ADDIE** is an acronym for the following steps: analysis, design, development, implementation, and evaluation. The ADDIE method is easy to understand and implement, so the method itself requires little training. The steps can be applied to many different types of training programs such as new employee orientation, on-the-job skills training, and in-service education for seasoned employees, making it especially useful in designing HIM training programs.

ADDIE: Analysis

The first step in the ADDIE method involves an analysis of the training needs. This is accomplished by conducting a needs assessment. As discussed in chapter 6, a needs assessment is a procedure performed by collecting and analyzing data to determine what is required, lacking, or desired by an employee, a group, or an organization. Similar to a successful orientation program, a needs assessment should be performed at the organizational, departmental, and individual levels. Data are collected to see what job skills are lacking, what problem-solving is desired by the group, or what new regulations require training to be met. Other areas that help to illustrate training needs are patient satisfaction surveys, job evaluations (chapter 7), performance appraisals (chapter 8), and implementation of new technology.

Once the needs have been identified, the analysis step also helps to identify the target audience as well as the overall goals for the training program. Clearly identified goals help to create assessment methods to use during the evaluation phase. If goals are defined, it should be clear at the end of the training sessions whether or not the goals were attained.

ADDIE: Design

Once the needs assessment has been completed and the goals have been determined, the next step is to design the training. Learning objectives are created so those being trained know what to expect. Employees will be able to tell if the proposed training is applicable to their jobs and worth their time. The SMART method (chapter 8) should be used to create learning objectives. Using the SMART method means that objectives will be specific, measurable, attainable, realistic, and timely. The objectives will be clear to both the trainer and the individuals being trained. It is during this phase that a training budget should be developed in connection with the SMART objectives. The budget will set parameters on how to use the objectives in the development phase.

ADDIE: Development

The development phase of the ADDIE method incorporates the data gathered in the analysis phase and the objectives created in the design phase to write the curriculum and prepare the training materials. When developing the curriculum a decision will need to be made as to whether the training expertise exists within the organization, or whether someone from the outside is best suited to do the training. The training materials are developed and tested. When developing training materials, an HIM manager does not have to create everything from scratch. Professional associations such as AHIMA provide up-to-date practice briefs and toolkits for training staff. If a new law is taking effect, a copy of the final regulation will provide a starting point for developing the curriculum. The next step is to determine how training materials will be presented to the participants. The method of delivery is chosen, after taking into account the advantages and disadvantages of the various delivery methods. Delivery methods are examined in more detail in the staff development section of this chapter.

ADDIE: Implementation

Implementation is where the actual training takes place. A training schedule is created and employees attend the sessions as required. Training may be done on-site in order to keep costs down and reach a number of employees over different days and shifts. Off-site training may be necessary if the resources are not available at the organization. It may be that specialized technology or subject matter experts are only available off-site. The assessment tool created earlier is deployed during the training sessions so data for evaluation are collected in a timely manner.

ADDIE: Evaluation

The last phase, evaluation, is a necessary but often overlooked step. Up to this point, time and money have been spent training employees based on a needs assessment and program design, but if no follow-up assessment of outcomes is done, all efforts could be in vain. If the desired outcomes are not reached, there is no point in continuing the training in the current form. Common evaluation methods are pre- and posttests. Knowledge or skill levels are tested prior to the training (pretest) and again when training is complete (posttest). Full evaluation does not end with the posttest assessment. Retention and effectiveness of the training should also be evaluated when the employee has had time to demonstrate the new learning on their job. Both the employee and their supervisor should contribute to this type of evaluation. If training was not effective, the process returns to the analysis phase. See figure 9.1 for a working example of the ADDIE method.

Figure 9.1. ADDIE: An example

Leslie is the assistant director of the HIM department at a large community hospital. A full electronic health record (EHR) was implemented 18 months ago.

Analysis: A recent employee satisfaction survey indicated that while HIM employees liked the EHR product and had adjusted to the implementation, many complained of back pain, eye strain, and repetitive motion injuries of the wrists. A review of time and attendance records verified that there was an increase in the number of sick days taken in the past 18 months. Leslie put forward the idea that ergonomic training would be beneficial to all members of the department.

Design: Leslie used the SMART approach to writing learning objectives that focused on correcting posture and adjusting desks, chairs, keyboards, and monitors to optimal alignment. She created a training budget to submit to the department director and it was approved.

Development: Leslie knew she was not a subject matter expert on ergonomics; in fact, she hoped to learn something to improve her own increasing back pain. She approached the rehabilitation services department in her own organization and connected with Janice, a physical therapist, who was willing to come to the department and provide ergonomic training. Janice had access to training materials from her professional association, which further reduced the cost and time to develop the curriculum.

Implementation: Leslie and Janice scheduled a 45-minute demonstration session to be supplemented with handouts for future reference. The session would be repeated five times over two shifts. Janice narrated a prerecorded slide deck presentation for any employees unable to attend the demonstration sessions to view on their own time. A posttest was given at the end of the training session to measure whether the learning objectives were met.

Evaluation: Leslie evaluated the posttests and was pleased to see that correct answers and positive comments indicated the ergonomics sessions were well-received by employees. Over the next six months, Leslie continued to monitor time and attendance records and noticed a three percent decrease in sick days.

Healthcare Training Methods

In addition to designing effective training, an HIM manager must be able to choose among different training methods. One single training method will not work for all employees and for all types of training. On-the-job training and in-service education are two healthcare training methods that provide employees with the opportunities to acquire and improve job-related skills.

On-the-job Training

On-the-job training (OTJ) is a method of training in which an employee learns necessary skills and processes by performing, under supervision, the functions of his or her position. Once a new hire has completed individual orientation, OTJ training is the next step in the process. On-the-job training is usually done by the employee's immediate supervisor or a senior employee in the same position, or a combination of both. In some cases, OTJ training might be done by an employee who is leaving the position. When designing an OTJ program, the first step is a needs assessment. Review the employee's prior education and experience and create a program that fills in the gaps. For example, a newly hired revenue cycle analyst who is a Registered Health Information Administrator (RHIA) graduate with no practical revenue cycle experience beyond what she learned in the classroom and during her professional practice experience will have different training needs than a newly hired revenue cycle analyst who moved from another state and has five years of revenue cycle experience. Most OTJ training is done on a one-to-one basis with the new employee first observing and then demonstrating the task. Assessment occurs throughout the process, and results are used to modify the training as necessary. Different methods of OTJ training include:

- **Job rotation:** A method in which workers are shifted periodically among different tasks. For example, an inpatient coder may spend three to six months coding cardiac cases, then rotate to trauma cases and then rotate to obstetrical cases. The employee may or may not return to their original job assignment. Job rotation increases the skills of the coder as well as their job satisfaction because they code a variety of records. The disadvantage is that there is a learning curve with each rotation that results in a loss of productivity until the employee is up to speed.

- **Cross-training:** A method in which employees learn a job other than their primary responsibility. An important distinction is that employees who are cross-trained are in the same pay grade. For example, an administrative assistant in the HIM department may be cross-trained as an administrative assistant in the business office. The purpose of cross-training is to provide coverage in times of extended absences or excessive workload. The employee will eventually return to their primary job.

- **Job shadowing:** A method in which one employee follows another employee to observe certain functions of their job. The intent of job shadowing is that the experienced employee educates the new employee on specific aspects of their job; for example, leading a team or giving a presentation. These are skills that the new employee may need to learn as part of their job and observing how an experienced employee handles a situation is an effective way to enhance a skill set.

- **Coaching:** A method in which an experienced person gives advice to a less-experienced worker on a formal or informal basis. A coach goes beyond training the new employee in the necessary skills needed for the job by also providing advice and support to boost morale and confidence. Coaching can be a short-term commitment, or last as long as the new employee and coach are with the organization.

OTJ training teaches a task by doing. In other words, the work is still being done during the training session, so there is less lost productivity. Employees receive instruction from an experienced employee and train in the actual work environment under normal working conditions. In this case, training is inexpensive and easy to arrange. Positive work relationships may develop as well (Fottler et al. 1998).

There are downsides to OTJ training. The employee doing the training may not want to do the training, or they may perform the job well but not have the ability to train others. Training may be rushed and critical elements of the job may be overlooked or not covered in detail, leading to costly errors (Fottler et al. 1998).

In-service Education

In-service education is different from on-the-job training. **In-service education** is training that teaches employees specific skills required to maintain or improve performance, usually internal to an organization. In-service education builds on the knowledge gained in orientation and OTJ training. Similar to OTJ training, in-service education is primarily done on-site by educators or managers. Larger facilities may have education departments that perform in-service education throughout the organization. For example, they may provide annual retraining to all employees on fire safety or provide basic education on teambuilding to a newly formed project group.

In-service education begins with a needs assessment. In an HIM department there may be Current Procedural Terminology (CPT) updates for coders or a new piece of equipment that all employees must be trained on how to use. A new clinical documentation improvement program may be scheduled for implementation. All of these items would require training to maintain or improve performance. After training is designed and implemented, evaluation should take place to assess whether learning was successful.

In-service education is an excellent opportunity for HIM professionals to educate other departments in the organization. HIM professionals are qualified to provide HIPAA in-service training sessions throughout the organization and coding updates to business office personnel and physician office staffs. Other opportunities include in-service training for nursing personnel on confidentiality and patient and community groups on the use of patient portals to access their health records.

Learning Styles

For any new employee orientation or subsequent training methods to be successful, an HIM manager must take into account the various learning styles of the adult. If an HIM manager understands their own learning style as well as the learning styles of employees, this knowledge can help choose the teaching methods that are going to be most effective. There are many types of learning styles. Most people are dominant in one kind of style, but exhibit traits in various learning styles. Three familiar types of sensory learning styles are visual (spatial), auditory, and kinesthetic (tactile).

Visual learners use the sense of sight to best learn new material. Most people are visual learners and prefer to read a textbook than listen to a lecture. They respond to charts, graphs, pictures, and videos. They prefer written instructions rather than being told how to do a task. Visual learners prefer a quiet environment for learning so they can concentrate on the material. They will often highlight or even color code their notes. When training a new chart completion analyst who is a visual learner, she will appreciate having access to updated policies and procedures and copies of written abstracting guidelines that provide future reference.

Auditory learners use the sense of hearing to best learn new material. Auditory learners prefer listening to a lecture and will record a lecture to listen to it again. They respond well to being told how to do things rather than reading about how to do things. Auditory learners might read material out loud, and they may prefer to listen to music while reading or working. When training a new chart completion analyst who is a auditory learner, she might prefer group discussions with other analysts to learn new skills.

Kinesthetic learners use the sense of touch to best learn new material. They favor a hands-on approach to learning so they can feel and manipulate the material. They prefer participating in a demonstration of the process rather than reading a textbook or listening to a lecture. When training a new chart completion analyst who is a kinesthetic learner, he or she will need to get up and move around every so often. Kinesthetic learners can get fidgety and lose concentration if asked to sit for too long. In addition, it may be beneficial to introduce the kinesthetic learner to the EHR chart completion tool and allow him or her to click through screens rather than read an instruction manual or listen to a lecture.

Training methods that combine visual, auditory, and kinesthetic learning styles will be most effective. When it comes to retention of material, most people remember 10 percent of what they hear, 20 percent of what they hear and see, and 90 percent of what they hear, see, and do (Fallon and McConnell 2014).

There are other learning styles besides sensory styles to consider when planning training activities. When determining the best methods to use for a training audience, identify the following types of additional learning styles:

- Relationship-oriented: People who favor this learning style focus on the individual first and data second. A good strategy for this learning style is to use stories to make points and convey new concepts.

- Bottom-line oriented: These people focus on data and facts first and the individual second. A good strategy for this learning style is to present information clearly and concisely without hesitation or indecisiveness.

- Logical: People who favor this learning style are most interested in facts and reasoned conclusions. A good strategy for this learning style is to include background information so that they feel they have all the data necessary for learning. Give them the time they need to gather the facts and process the information.

- Creative: These people make quick decisions and often change direction. A good strategy for this learning style is to use fast-paced and varied training methods to impart information. Do not provide too much technical information at one sitting (Bacik 2010).

Finally, there are many other aspects of the adult learner that impact his or her learning. Many of the characteristics stem from the desire for work-life balance. Adult learners appreciate knowing the purpose behind the learning. They need to know that the training is important to their job, and that the time spent in training will be worthwhile. They know their time is valuable and want training to happen quickly. Adult learners appreciate being able to control the pace of their learning and to be able to schedule their learning so it does not conflict with work or family life.

Check Your **Understanding**

1. What is the difference between employee training and employee development?
2. Explain the three levels of new employee orientation and give an example of information provided at each level.
3. What are the five components of the ADDIE method of training design?
4. Discuss the advantages and disadvantages to on-the-job training.
5. How is on-the-job training both similar and different to in-service education?
6. Explain the three sensory learning styles and provide examples of training methods best suited for each style.

Staff Development

Separate from employee training is staff development. As noted previously, staff development focuses on the career path of the individual rather than obtaining the skills and knowledge to perform the job activities. Staff development encompasses the continuing education necessary to maintain credentials as well as the planning necessary for an individual to progress to the next step in their career. HIM professionals are fortunate to have organizations like AHIMA that provide assistance to members who are interested in continuing their education and career development.

Continuing Education Methods

Many healthcare professionals hold some kind of credential or license to allow them to practice their profession and validate their learning. A **credential** is a formal agreement granting an individual permission to practice in a profession. A credential is usually conferred by a national professional organization dedicated to a specific area of healthcare practice. AHIMA grants credentials in health information management and coding as well as specialty credentials in data analysis, privacy and security, documentation improvement, and health technology. A **license** is a legal authorization granted by a state to an individual that allows the individual to provide healthcare services within a specific scope of services and geographical location. Both require an applicant to pass an examination to obtain the credential or license initially and then to participate in continuing education activities to maintain the credential or license thereafter. A healthcare professional must never stop learning. **Continuing education (CE)** is training that enables employees to remain current with advancing knowledge in their profession. Most professionals must earn a certain number of CE credits or units over a specific time frame, usually a year or two. Credits are generally awarded based on the time spent in a program; for example, a five-hour presentation will award five CE units. Continuing education training generally is the responsibility of the individual, especially when performed for credential or license maintenance, but CE activities may overlap with OTJ or in-service training activities. In fact, the definition of CE implies that all employees must participate in CE regardless of whether or not they hold a professional credential or license. External agencies also require that organizations offer continuing education programs to their employees to ensure that quality care is supported by continued learning in the field.

An HIM manager should set continuing education goals for all employees on an annual basis. This might be done during the performance appraisal (chapter 8), or at another time convenient for both the manager and employee. CE programs offered on-site will be job-focused. For example, a webinar on annual coding updates would be appropriate for HIM- and coding-credentialed employees as well as noncredentialed coders. A software upgrade to a cancer registry program may require an afternoon of training by the vendor for all users of the system regardless of whether they have a credential or not.

HIM managers should be aware of which employees in the department need continuing education to maintain a credential. It is unlikely that the number of required CE units can be obtained solely through work-related activities. Additional time off might be arranged, or a flexible schedule might be created so employees may attend off-site CE programs. Budget constraints may not permit an HIM manager to pay for all or even part of off-site CE programs, but allowing employees to use their paid time-off or to make up the time at a later date supports the efforts of the employee to maintain their credential.

When choosing a delivery method for CE activities, an HIM manager must be mindful of different factors: What is the purpose of the training? What is the level of education of the learners? How many people need to be trained? Where are they located—are they all in the same place or spread throughout the region or country? How many different sites are involved? Are special accommodations needed for employees with disabilities or language issues? CE activities often fall into the training category, so consideration of delivery methods also pertains to OTJ and in-service training. There are many types of delivery methods, but the most common are classroom learning, self-directed learning, simulation, seminars and workshops, and distance learning. In most cases, **blended learning**—a training strategy that uses a combination of techniques such as lecture, web-based training, or programmed text to appeal to a variety of learning styles and maximize the advantages of each training method—takes place.

Classroom learning, a traditional method of learning, is best used when the information to be delivered to a large group is factual in nature. It is relatively low-cost, as expenses are generally the time it takes to develop and present the program, and the time away from work for the attendees. No extensive travel expenses are present. The format for classroom learning is usually an instructor lecturing to the class, although videos may be used in a classroom setting to convey specific material to the group. Communication is primarily one-way—the instructor talking to the class—with opportunity for questions and discussion. An HIM manager might consider using a classroom delivery method to review annual coding updates with all coders in an organization.

Self-directed learning is an instructional method that allows participants to control their learning and progress at their own pace. This delivery method supports adult learners who wish to have some control over when and where their continuing education occurs. It is also relatively low-cost when compared to expenses to attend workshops or production costs for simulations. Self-directed learning works with both individuals and a large number of learners, especially if they are not located in the same place. A specific curriculum is presented and the learner progresses through the material at their own pace. There is usually some form of assessment at the end so that both completion and learning can be measured and recorded. The format for self-directed learning may be in the form of a textbook or workbook, or may be a computer-based program to present the material. A new graduate from an HIM program may use self-directed learning to prepare for their RHIA credential examination. An individual working in the HIM field may use self-directed learning to prepare for a privacy or data analyst credential examination. There are numerous exam review workbooks available and the individual works through each section of the review guide, taking the test at the end of each section. There are also examination prep courses for various credentials and mock credential examinations available for multiple credentials accessible online.

Simulation is a training technique for experimenting with real-world situations by means of a computerized model that represents the actual situation. The simulation is intended to give practical experience beyond what might occur in a classroom. It can be used in a group setting or with individuals, and when the computerized version is used it can be shared to several locations at once. Typically, a learner is presented with a scenario and then must figure out how to deal with the situation. The solution is analyzed and feedback is provided as to whether the learner acted appropriately, or if a better solution could have been reached. For example, an HIM supervisor may participate in a simulation in which he or she is presented with employee behavior or performance problems. In each case, the supervisor must react and decide what, if any, disciplinary action needs to be taken. Once a decision is made, the simulation program responds with feedback approving the decision or providing other suggestions as to how each situation could be handled differently. On a larger scale, simulation is also used for disaster preparedness continuing education that must be completed by healthcare organizations.

A variation of the simulation method is role-playing. **Role-playing** is a training method in which participants are required to respond to specific problems they may actually encounter in their jobs. In this case, the HIM supervisor may get to practice his or her interviewing skills by performing mock interviews or improve conflict resolution skills by acting out situations with angry physicians or frustrated patients.

Seminars and workshops are usually held off-site and are topic-specific. Many seminars are produced by professional associations (such as AHIMA) making them an excellent source for continuing education. For example, a seminar on clinical documentation improvement (CDI) may be attended by two of seven CDI specialists, who then bring back and share the material with the entire CDI section. There are benefits to off-site seminars and workshops:

- Training is cost-efficient on a large scale because groups, rather than individuals, are usually trained
- Trainers are likely to be more competent than on-site trainers who usually spend only a portion of their work time training
- More time is often spent on planning and organization
- Attendees learn in an environment free from the pressures and interruptions of the workplace
- Off-site seminars and workshops enable organizations with limited resources to train and develop employees without the expenses of a training staff and facilities (Fottler et al. 1998)

However, there are disadvantages associated with off-site seminars and workshops, too:

- Seminars are typically more expensive than on-site training and development
- There is lost productivity while employees are attending seminars
- Learning cannot be customized for each participant, so it may not address specific problems or situations (Fottler et al. 1998)

The final delivery method is distance learning. **Distance learning** is a learning delivery mode in which the instructor, classroom, and students are not all present in the same location at the same time. Distance learning should not be confused with self-directed learning. Self-directed learning allows the learner to progress at their own pace, on their own schedule. While learners may at times be able to proceed at their own pace, distance learning is not self-directed. Learners must still adhere to a schedule with deadlines and are not free to choose how quickly (or slowly) they will complete the learning curriculum. However, similar to self-directed learning, distance learning appeals to the adult learner who does not want to be constrained to a specific time or location. The technology necessary to carry out distance learning does add to the cost of the delivery method, but the technology cost may be less than the travel costs associated with bringing all participants together in integrated healthcare delivery systems that cover a large geographic area.

Distance learning takes place in different formats. **Audio conferencing** is a communication technique in which participants in different locations can learn together via telephone while listening to a presenter and looking at handouts or books. **Video conferencing** adds the ability to see the instructor and uses satellite, television, or computer capabilities. If the video conferencing uses the Internet for transmission, it is called a **webinar,** short for web-based seminar; or a **webcast,** in which a broadcast similar to a television show. Audio and video conferencing are **synchronous** (occurring at the same time), meaning that instructor and participants are present together for one- or two-way communication. This is beneficial as questions and answers are immediate. These methods also can be combined with other delivery methods such as classroom or simulation and the advantages of such methods can be realized at the same time.

Another distance learning method is web-based training. **Web-based training** is instruction via the Internet that enables individuals to learn in a structure that is self-paced while interacting and collaborating with other students and the instructor via a conferencing system. Web-based training can be synchronous or **asynchronous** (occurring at different times), meaning the instructor and students are not present at the same time. Web-conferencing is similar to audio or video conferencing, but uses the Internet as the communication medium. Webinars and webcasts, while originally presented in a synchronous mode, can be saved for future viewing, giving them an asynchronous quality. Some healthcare organizations deliver training and development programs via their own intranet. An **intranet** is a private information network that is similar to the Internet and whose servers are located inside a firewall or security barrier so that the general public cannot gain access to information housed within the network. This allows an organization to control who has access to the training and development material, and prevent unauthorized changes to the programs.

Web-based courses are available through the Internet or an organization's intranet. Courses offered via the Internet vary from short-term courses on a specific topic such as ICD-10-CM/PCS or privacy and security, to full online instruction for an associate's, bachelor's, master's, or even doctoral degree. The cost for short-term courses may be covered by the organization, especially if the course topic connects to their current job, but employees wishing to continue their education by obtaining another college degree generally must pay for the education themselves unless the organization has a tuition reimbursement benefit.

Career Development

Career development is activity that affects an employee's growth over his or her entire career. It is a highly unique endeavor, even though the process involves others. Career development means an employee is looking to the future and planning for his or her next job, and then the job after that. The objective of career development is "to expand the capabilities of staff beyond a narrow range of skills toward a more holistically prepared person" (Fottler et al. 1998). Two specific ways that an individual can meet this objective are mentoring and succession planning.

Mentoring

Mentoring is a type of coaching and training in which an individual (protégé) is matched with a more experienced individual (mentor) who serves as an advisor or counselor. Mentoring is generally a one-to-one experience, although a person may mentor more than one individual at a time. Although the mentor and protégé do not have to work for the same organization, for the purposes of this chapter on organizational training and development, the focus will be on the workplace mentoring that develops within the same organization. Mentoring focuses less on the protégé acquiring skills to do the job, but more on socializing them to the organization. **Socialization** is the process of influencing the behavior and attitudes of a new employee to adapt positively to the work environment. This means the mentor introduces the protégé to the culture of the organization. He or she stresses the mission and vision, values, and fit of the protégé to the organization. Initially, the mentor will give advice on job situations, help the protégé solve problems, and even provide the protégé with experiences to enhance his or her job training. For example, a new supervisor may be nervous about interviewing applicants for an open position. Their mentor could take the time to look over the list of questions, suggest lessons that were learned from his or her own interview experiences, or even role-play an interviewing situation. It is important that the mentor does not solve the problems or tell the protégé how to handle a situation, but aid them in reaching his or her own conclusions and course of action. As the relationship progresses, the mentor will shift focus to career development, perhaps giving advice on career options, assigning projects that help build new skills, and inviting the protégé to networking opportunities. For example, an HIM manager may be trying to decide what type of master's degree to pursue—a master's in business administration or a master's in health informatics. A mentor acts as a sounding board, offering advice and perspective that will help the manager make a decision.

A mentoring program is relatively inexpensive, as both mentor and protégé volunteer to participate. As much as the protégé benefits, there are positive reasons for the mentor to agree to become involved as well. Mentoring provides a sense of fulfillment and feeling of satisfaction for a senior employee who is looking for new challenges and work experiences, as well as helping them further refine and sharpen their management skills (Fallon and McConnell 2014). Successful mentoring programs exhibit these four characteristics:

- The mentor should be at least two pay grades above the protégé's pay level.
- Mentoring should consist of both career and personal development. The mentor-protégé relationship is most successful when it is one-on-one.
- The mentor or protégé should feel free to end the relationship if either one believes the relationship is no longer productive.
- There should be no pre-determined length to the mentor-protégé relationship and the level of involvement of both the mentor and protégé should be agreed upon by both parties (Fottler et al. 1998).

Succession Planning

Succession planning is a specific type of promotional plan in which senior-level position openings are anticipated and candidates are identified from within the organization; the candidates are given training through formal education, job rotation, and mentoring so they can eventually assume these positions. Succession planning has traditionally been practiced for senior-level management positions, but there is no reason the process cannot be instituted throughout the organization. Succession planning makes sense for a number of reasons. When individuals leave key positions due to promotion, retirement, extended illness, or separating from the organization, it is critical to have a backup in place so the work continues. If there is no one to succeed someone in a key position, it may require an expensive search to find a replacement. Succession planning also sends a positive message to employees that senior management is committed to promotion from within. A succession program also is a retention strategy (chapter 7), although there is no guarantee that the person being groomed to replace someone will stay with the organization while waiting for the succession to occur.

The steps in succession planning are formal education, job rotation, and mentoring. Formal education may mean obtaining a higher degree. An assistant director may need to obtain a bachelor's or master's degree to be considered as a replacement for a retiring department director. Short-term courses may be necessary to eliminate skill gaps such as privacy and security, public speaking and presentation, or project management. Completion of formal education may also result in the addition of an HIM credential such as certified in healthcare privacy and security (CHPS) or certified health data analyst (CHDA). Job rotation allows for an employee to learn new skills necessary at the next level. An HIM director who is developing an assistant director may assign a project or a presentation to improve practical skills in these areas. A director may arrange for job shadowing so that experience is gained outside the department. As discussed, mentoring is also an important aspect of any succession planning program.

Career Assistance

HIM professionals can rely on their professional association, such as AHIMA, to provide them with both CE opportunities as well as career development assistance. According to AHIMA:

> The new data age and innovations in technology are transforming HIM professionals' personal and professional lives. These changes are opening new doors to jobs and career paths that did not exist even a few years ago, while at the same time closing others. Being in a technology and information-driven profession means that individuals must expect continuous change in HIM practice and update their skills to stay relevant in today's healthcare system (AHIMA 2014).

The AHIMA Council on Education Excellence (CEE) developed competencies (appendix A) that address the learning and knowledge needs that HIM professionals will need to move forward in the profession. Even though the competencies are geared toward the education of HIM professionals in associate, baccalaureate, and graduate degree programs, AHIMA recommends that current HIM professionals review the competencies to assess gaps in knowledge and plan for the future. The CEE created a professional development inventory, which is a "self-assessment tool intended to allow current practicing HIM professionals to evaluate their own skills and knowledge in comparison to what is required for new program graduates (AHIMA 2014)." AHIMA offers self-directed learning materials for those who wish to obtain an AHIMA credential or add to their skill set. AHIMA also offers online courses in a variety of topic areas including coding basics, cancer registry, privacy and security, CDI, public speaking, business principles, and online education. Webinars are available that cover ICD-10-CM/PCS coding, health information exchange, and patient engagement. HIM departments may have training and development budgets to cover the cost of these materials, or AHIMA members may purchase them at reduced member prices.

AHIMA's Mentor Match program on Engage Online Communities is available only to AHIMA members. A potential protégé has the ability to search through a database of experienced mentors who are available to answer questions, provide insight, and offer guidance on advancing an HIM career. Mentors will find that their protégés are primarily new students and new AHIMA members (Engage AHIMA 2015). There is no fee for participation in the Mentor Match program outside of the regular association fees.

Additional free offerings from AHIMA include the Career Prep Workbook and the HIM Career Map. The AHIMA Career Prep Workbook assists with planning, preparing, and initiating a job search in the HIM industry.

The workbook provides tools on setting career goals, personal branding, resume writing, and interviewing (AHIMA 2015a).

AHIMA's HIM Career Map shows the path from entry-level through mid-level, advanced-level, to master-level positions in compliance or risk management, education or communication, informatics or data analytics, information technology or infrastructure, health records operation or administration, and revenue cycle management that includes coding and billing. The Career Map shows current careers such as ICD-10 educator, privacy officer, data quality manager, and clinical documentation improvement specialist as well as emerging careers such as research and development scientist, EHR implementation specialist, and chief learning officer (AHIMA 2015b). Users click on any one of the jobs listed to see the promotional and transitional pathways leading to other jobs on the map. For example, a data quality manager position shows a promotional path to an HIM manager or director or HIM position. A transitional path leads to a consultant career. In addition, each job expands to show a full position description, the job responsibilities and skills required, necessary training and education, salary data, and required work experience. There are also links to the AHIMA Career Assist Job Bank that shows open positions advertised by hospitals, healthcare systems, vendors, and universities. Some positions provide self-assessments so that members may determine where their strengths and opportunities for growth are, giving them the insight they need to prepare for a career move (AHIMA 2013b). The HIM Career Map is continually updated with new jobs, career paths, and salary information.

Check Your **Understanding**

1. What are the similarities and differences between a credential and a license?
2. Discuss the five learning delivery method and give an example of when each might be used for continuing education.
3. What are the advantages and disadvantages to obtaining continuing education at a seminar or workshop?
4. What are the benefits to a mentoring program?
5. Why is succession planning important to an HIM manager's roles and responsibilities?

Case Study

Objectives

- Outline a plan for performing a needs assessment for training and development purposes
- Identify and create a way to determine the sensory learning styles of employees
- Evaluate training models appropriate for use for department-wide topics
- Evaluate continuing education methods appropriate to use for specific HIM positions

Instructions

Review the scenario provided and develop a training and development plan to be submitted to the chief financial officer (CFO).

Scenario

Susan is the newly hired director of HIM at a rural 250-bed hospital. She was hired when the previous HIM director retired. During her interview, Susan was identified as being highly qualified and very enthusiastic about the HIM profession. Susan holds an RHIA credential and is working on her master's degree in organizational leadership. The previous director had been in place for over 25 years and her last two annual evaluations noted that she was not keeping pace with HIM industry standards. The HIM department has the following employees:

- Two transcriptionists with no credentials
- Two release-of-information (ROI) coordinators, one Registered Health Information Technician (RHIT) and one trained on the job
- Five coders, of which two hold RHITs, two with the Certified Coding Specialist (CCS) credential only, and one with the Certified Coding Associate (CCA) credential only
- One HIM supervisor who is RHIT-eligible, newly hired, with less than a year of management experience
- Four document imaging specialists with no credentials
- Two chart completion clerks with no credential
- One data quality specialist which is an open position, RHIT credential required

Susan has been directed by her boss, the CFO, to plan for specific positions in the department to be converted to remote positions because the hospital needs space to increase cardiac services. In the four months Susan has been leading the department, she has realized that there are serious knowledge gaps for many of the employees and many of them are not meeting monthly productivity or quality performance standards. Susan knows that there is a real risk to sending many of these individuals home to work because of the identified performance issues. She has decided a training and development plan will be necessary to prepare the majority of the workforce to work remotely.

Assumptions

- It is evident that the HIM employees are in need of training and development, but there is no departmental education plan in place and no record of any formal training or development programs offered in the last two years.
- There are acceptable productivity and quality performance standards in place for all of the positions, including the open position.
- There are no financial resources in the current budget to cover training and development activities, but the CFO indicated that he could make resources available on a limited basis.
- There is no education department but the HR department is able to assist with training needs.
- The CFO told Susan that she has six months to transition the employees to work remotely.
- The open data quality specialist position is a line item on the HIM budget that needs to be filled within the next month or the position is in jeopardy of being eliminated in the next fiscal year's budget process.

Deliverables

Create a training and development plan for the HIM department that includes the following items:

1. A method for assessing the needs and knowledge gaps for all HIM employees, including management positions. Design the assessment instrument.
2. A plan for identifying the sensory learning styles of the HIM department employees.
3. Develop a six-month training and development program for each of the employee categories listed previously. The plan should consist of the following:
   a. Identify at least two training topics that all employees have in common and a different training model to use for each of the two training topics.
   b. Create a CE plan for each credentialed position: ROI coordinator, coder, HIM supervisor, and data quality specialist. Include both on-site and off-site CE opportunities.
   c. Be mindful of budgetary constraints.
   d. A template is provided in figure 9.2 for guidance. A different template may be created.

Figure 9.2. Training and development template

Training and Development Plan Template

Department: Health Information Management

Date:

Position	Training needs	Continuing education needs	Method of delivery	Budget impact

© AHIMA

Review Questions

1. Jason reads the annual coding updates and records them onto his MP3 player and listens to them while driving to work. He feels this additional step makes him a more successful coder. Jason is most likely what type of sensory learner?

    a. Auditory
    b. Kinesthetic
    c. Tactile
    d. Visual

2. A hospital system in Oregon has recently purchased several small hospitals scattered throughout Alaska. When it comes time to review and discuss coding updates for CPT and ICD-10-CM/PCS, the best delivery method to use to reach all coders is:

    a. Classroom lecture
    b. Distance learning
    c. Self-directed learning
    d. Simulations

3. A successful on-the-job training program begins with:

    a. Choosing the right person to do the training
    b. Performing a needs assessment
    c. Reviewing the job description and job specifications
    d. Writing competency statements

4. During new employee orientation, Jennifer, the assistant director of HIM, demonstrates how to use the copier and fax machine, instructs new employees on how to clock in and out, and introduces them to their new co-workers. This orientation is taking place at what level?

    a. Administrative
    b. Clinical
    c. Departmental
    d. Organizational

5. Each year when coding updates are published, Amy plans a training program for coders, business office employees, and physician office personnel involved in coding and billing. It generally takes her three weeks to complete the training of all necessary personnel. Which method of employee training is being described?

    a. Continuing education
    b. In-service education
    c. On-the-job training
    d. Orientation training

6. In the HIM department at Memorial Hospital, scanning documentation specialists perform three main functions: preparation of documents to be scanned, scanning, and quality checking. Each scanning specialist spends one month doing a specific function, then moves to perform another function for the next month. This is an example of what type of on-the-job training?

    a. Coaching
    b. Cross-training
    c. Job rotation
    d. Job shadowing

7. A needs assessment is done during which phase of the ADDIE method of training design?

    a. Analysis
    b. Design
    c. Development
    d. Implementation

8. Distance learning may include all of the following delivery methods except:

    a. Audio conferencing
    b. Computer-based training
    c. Video conferencing
    d. Web-based courses

9. Julie is a coder but would like to someday be a privacy officer. Tracey, the privacy officer at her hospital, has agreed to help Julie on her career path. Tracey has suggested that Julie begin to look at master's degree programs and has taken her to a local association meeting where she can begin to network with other privacy officers. This is an example of:

    a. Continuing education
    b. Job rotation
    c. Mentoring
    d. Succession planning

10. Dana, the director of HIM at a large community hospital, is going to retire next year. She believes that her assistant director, Karen, would be a great choice to replace her. Dana has begun taking Karen to her meetings to introduce her and acclimate her to the responsibilities Dana has on various committees in the hospital. Dana has also given Karen the task of orientating the new medical residents to HIPAA and the EHR so that she can improve her presentation skills. This is an example of:

a. Continuing education
b. Job rotation
c. Mentoring
d. Succession planning

References

American Health Information Management Association. 2015a. Career Prep Workbook. http://www.ahima.org/careers/careerprep?tabid=workbook.

American Health Information Management Association. 2015b. HIM Career Map. http://hicareers.com/CareerMap/.

American Health Information Management Association. 2014. Professional Development Inventory. http://www.ahima.org/competency.

American Health Information Management Association. 2013a. Recruitment, Selection, and Orientation for CDI Specialists. *Journal of AHIMA* 84(7): 58–62.

American Health Information Management Association. 2013b. Career Assist Job Bank. http://careerassist.ahima.org/home/index.cfm?site_id=681.

Bacik, S. 2010. Smart Training on Privacy and Security. *Journal of AHIMA* 81(4).

Battles, J.B. 2006. Improving patient safety by instructional systems design. *Quality & Safety in Health Care* 15(Suppl 1):i25–i29.

Engage AHIMA. 2015. About Mentor Match. http://engage.ahima.org/mentoring/mentormatchfaqs.

Fallon, L. and C. McConnell. 2014. *Human Resource Management in Health Care*. Burlington: Jones and Bartlett.

Fottler, H., S. Hernandez, and C. Joiner, eds. 1998. *Essentials of Human Resource Management in Health Service Organizations*. Albany: Delmar.

Patena, K. R. and M. M. LeBlanc. 2013. Human Resources Management and Employee Training and Development. Chapter 24 in *Health Information Management: Concepts, Principles, and Practice*. 4th ed. Edited by K.M Latour, S. E. Maki, and P. K. Oachs. Chicago: AHIMA.

Organizational Structure of Health Information Management

- Evaluate health information management's (HIM's) organizational model based on influence and structure
- Assess HIM's future role in healthcare based on industry guidance
- Discuss how to leverage HIM's role within the healthcare community
- Discuss the impact of a healthcare organization's committee structure in relation to HIM
- Examine the American Health Information Management Association's (AHIMA's) strategic plan and professional competencies to maintain relevancy as an HIM professional

Chain of command
Committee
Computer-assisted
    coding (CAC)
External forces

Internal forces
Line management/
    hierarchical
    organizational model

Nonhierarchical
    organizational
    model
Organizational chart

Population health
Span of control

The health information management (HIM) landscape is changing at a fast pace. HIM students and practitioners need to keep pace with the changes that are significantly impacting the HIM field. HIM professionals need to be cognizant of the environmental factors that are affecting the profession and learn how to adapt to these changes. The largest single change for the HIM professional is the implementation of health information technology and the bearing this technology has on the tasks and job roles needed in healthcare organization. This chapter provides guidance in assessing a healthcare organization's landscape in relation to internal and external influences and how these influences impact the HIM department's organization model. Health information professionals also need to be aware of the committee structure that exists within the healthcare organization and how these committees can impact the management of HIM departments. This chapter also discusses the external influences as related to government initiatives that directly impact the management of health information. The next section of the chapter discusses competitors for HIM roles and how HIM professionals can stay current and relevant in today's competitive healthcare market. The last section addresses the American Health Information Management (AHIMA) educational curriculum competencies that can be assessed using the AHIMA Professional Development Inventory and how this inventory provides HIM professionals with a working career tool.

Healthcare Organizational Models and Health Information Management

The healthcare organizational structures where HIM professionals are employed differ from organization to organization. Organizational structure is the "hierarchical arrangement of the lines of authority, communications, rights and duties of an organization" (Business Dictionary 2015). HIM is an organizational department "without walls" and is becoming decentralized in healthcare organizations. The introduction of healthcare technology has allowed those HIM jobs that were bound by paper records and the physical location of these records to now be performed in different locations throughout a healthcare organization and even within employees' homes. The visible walls that were once evident in all HIM departments are no longer tethered to the physical location of paper health records. Healthcare professionals can be found within information technology, quality, financial services, revenue cycle, compliance, and utilization review departments (Butler 2015). Within larger healthcare organizations, HIM professionals may manage the information, coding, and billing and general operations for particular clinical divisions such as cardiology and home health. Alternatively, larger healthcare corporations may purchase or acquire many different healthcare organizations and these organizations elect to centralize all HIM functions. These trends within healthcare are dramatically changing the paradigm for many HIM professionals as the traditional HIM department no longer exists. The key to surviving as an HIM professional in any of these venues is identifying the role of the job tasks being performed and how they relate to the overall healthcare operations.

It is important that HIM professionals understand the organization models that are apparent in most healthcare organizations. The organizational model of the healthcare organization provides a framework for the facility's management structure and provides guidance to the HIM professional as to where he or she fits within the facility. Organizational models are depicted in healthcare organizations as visual organizational charts. An **organizational chart** is a graphic representation of an organization's formal reporting structure; it aids in understanding the reporting relationships and functional responsibilities throughout the healthcare organization (AHIMA 2014). A healthcare organization will have a large organizational chart that represents all departments throughout the facility. Each department will have an organizational chart showing reporting relationships and functional responsibilities specific to the tasks performed within this area. Organizational charts typically represent two distinct organizational models within healthcare organizations—hierarchical (line management) and nonhierarchical. Some healthcare organizations use a mix of both models and frequently healthcare organizations transition from the use of a line management or hierarchical to a nonhierarchical model. As healthcare organizational models shift, HIM managers need to adapt to new reporting structures and provide guidance for HIM staff in this transition. The two distinct organizational models will be outlined as well as strategic guidance for transitioning from one model to another.

Line Management or the Hierarchical Organizational Model

Line management or hierarchical organizational structure clearly defines the **chain of command** (a hierarchical reporting structure within an organization) within and outside of HIM departments and is hierarchical from the executive to front-line level. Line management is the traditional and least complex management structure in which top management has total and direct authority and employees report to only one supervisor. Managers in this type of organizational structure have direct responsibility to give orders to their subordinates. Line management structures are usually organized along functional lines, although they increasingly undertake a variety of cross-functional duties such as employee development or strategic direction. The lowest managerial level in an organization following the line management structure is supervisory management (Sikora and Ferris 2014).

Hierarchical organizations tend to be stable and predictable as work rules are documented and strictly enforced. Classical management styles are deployed in these organizations and career progression is linear. The span of control is clearly defined in line management organizations and decision making is centralized with each manager. **Span of control** is the area of activity and number of duties and employees for which an individual or organization is responsible (Business Dictionary.com 2015).

Span of control is a concept of classical organization theory that suggests managers are capable of supervising only a limited number of employees. Difficulties occur in linear models as organizations grow and become more complex. The lines of communication widen and it becomes increasingly more difficult for these organizations to respond to the changing dynamics required in today's healthcare environment.

Nonhierarchical Organizational Model

Nonhierarchical organizations are emerging as a healthcare organizational model because they allow for more responsiveness within a changing healthcare environment. Nonhierarchical organizations are relatively flat with very few layers and each layer reports to a single individual. The term nonhierarchical reflects that there is no true line or hierarchy to reporting within the organization. Nonhierarchical organizations reflect a combination of interconnected horizontal networks. The nonhierarchical organizational structure combines aspects of functional and divisional hierarchies to create a rather complex structure where an employee may report to one or more managers. The management within a nonhierarchical organization is decentralized where the authority to make decisions will be spread throughout the organization rather than vested in one individual (Uhlig 2015).

Figures 10.1 and 10.2 are a graphic depiction of the two different organizational models. Defining reporting relationships is essential for all HIM managers and employees. Unclear lines of authority or links to the overall

Figure 10.1. HIM hierarchical or line management organizational chart

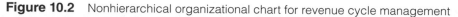

© AHIMA

Figure 10.2 Nonhierarchical organizational chart for revenue cycle management

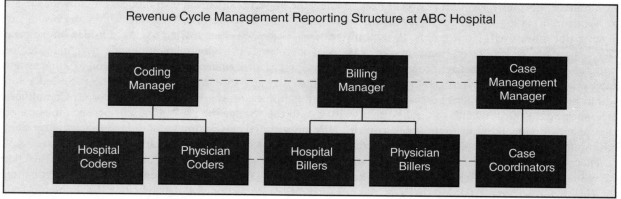

© AHIMA

healthcare operations can cause confusion in the HIM department. Figure 10.1 depicts a typical line or hierarchical organization structure in an HIM department where each manager is responsible for the tasks performed by his or her workgroup. The HIM director is ultimately responsible for ensuring all the tasks in the HIM department are performed as directed by the mission and vision of the department. Figure 10.2 depicts a nonhierarchical organizational chart in regards to revenue cycle management within a healthcare organization. In this example, there are several different areas (hospital coding, physician coding, billing, case management) that all work together to perform the work necessary to manage the revenue in the healthcare organization. The responsibility for performance outcomes in nonhierarchical models is shared by all managers at the same level.

Transitioning from a Line Management or Hierarchical Organization Model to a Nonhierarchical Organizational Model

Typically the executive leadership in a healthcare organization decides on the organizational structure but HIM professionals may have a chance to provide input regarding the structure as mergers, acquisitions, and combining of related services occurs within a facility. HIM professionals should be judicial in setting the organizational model for a department as change may be difficult for many individuals and the rationale for the change must be justified and communicated (as discussed in chapter 4). The most important element when transitioning between organizational models is to provide facts and data that support the need for the change and keep all individuals involved in the decision-making processes (Price 2011). Overall, the keys to success for transitioning from a line management or hierarchical model to a nonhierarchical organizational model include building strategic relationships throughout the organization rather than just reporting relationships and developing solid collaboration skills that can be applied within the HIM team as well as throughout the organization (as reflected in chapters 3 and 4). An HIM manager can develop an innovative culture that fosters employees who can work in a complex, flexible, and adaptable work environment (Klenke 2011).

A specific HIM example of the need to transition to a nonhierarchical model is when coding is moved into the revenue cycle management division, which may be comprised of coding, patient financial services, professional billing, and case management. The managers within this department become a horizontal interconnected network where responsibility for managing the cash flow within the healthcare organization is shared by all entities within this department. Figure 10.2 reflects what the organizational chart will resemble in a nonhierarchical structure such as the revenue cycle management functions.

HIM professionals need to be familiar with the type of organizational structure in which they are employed. Learning how to adapt to different organizational structures is essential for surviving or thriving within a healthcare organization. HIM plays an integral role in the overall functions of a healthcare organization so knowing the reporting relationships that exist within the organization is essential for creating a collaborative work environment with other departments.

Committees

As discussed previously, HIM professionals need to know the impact of organizational models and how they relate to health information operations. They also need to know how the committee structure within the healthcare organization affects HIM operations. A **committee** is a "body of persons delegated to consider, investigate, take action on, or report on some matter" (Merriam-Webster 2015). Committees provide a framework for interdisciplinary teams to manage process outcomes, assess quality, offer guidance in ethical decision making, review appropriate consumption of resources, and provide administrative guidance for healthcare operations. Silos develop within healthcare organizations because of the specialized nature each department or area performs. Committees help mitigate the effect of silos on healthcare operations and they bridge the gaps that occur between medical or clinical and administrative or support departments. HIM does not rely on committees for day-to-day management but committees can provide support for the overall operations in the healthcare organization.

There are committees that are a requirement of accrediting bodies such as the Joint Commission, Health Facilities Accreditation Program (HFAP), Det Norske Veritas Healthcare, Inc. (also known as National Integrated Accreditation for Health Care Organizations [NIAHO]), Commission on Accreditation for Rehabilitation Facilities (CARF),

Accreditation Association for Ambulatory Health Care (AAAHC), Accreditation Commission for Health Care (ACHC), and other accrediting bodies specific to the particular categories of healthcare organizations. Committees also are required for providing information and guidance to governmental entities and licensure organizations in terms of healthcare operations. Examples of governmental entities are the Centers for Medicaid and Medicare Services (CMS), Department of Public Health, and the Agency for Healthcare Research and Quality.

Committees are a part of the formal structure of a healthcare organization with assigned distinct purposes and functions. The formality of the committee structure affords healthcare organizations the ability to require committees to be accountable for their actions. Table 10.1 reflects typical committees that function within a healthcare organization and outlines the functions HIM might perform for each of these committees. This is not an exhaustive list of committees and the names of committees may vary from organization to organization, but the functions that each of these committees provide for the healthcare organizations are relatively standardized throughout the healthcare industry.

Table 10.1 Committee structure within a healthcare organization

Name of committee	Functions of committee	Interdisciplinary team members	HIM functions
Accreditation committee	Oversight of accreditation and licensure surveys for the healthcare organization, performs mock surveys and identifies gaps in actual performance to optimal performance in relation to accreditation standards	Representatives from a variety of clinical and nonclinical departments	Involved in mock surveys and providing policies and procedures pertaining to HIM
Ethics committee	Joint Commission requires a means for addressing troubling medical care issues and this must be managed either through an ethics committee or ethics consultant	Representatives from a variety of clinical departments, legal counsel, and outside representatives	Provides access to the appropriate health record documentation required in the committee decision-making process
Infection control	Reviews infection rate trends, benchmarks healthcare organization infection data against similar organizations, develops and implements infection control policies and procedures	Nurses, physicians, clinical laboratory, and pharmacy staff	Provides reports on infection rates based on coded data
Medical executive committee	Oversight of the medical staff, upholds and reviews medical staff bylaws	Physician representatives from all medical and surgical specialties	Provides statistics on physician chart completion rates, verbal orders, and so on
Patient care or patient safety committee	Oversight of patient outcomes, monitors national trends regarding patient safety, and implements initiatives to improve patient safety	Physicians, nurses, other clinical caregivers, and quality improvement staff	Provides reports on patient outcomes based on coded or abstracted data
Pharmacy and therapeutics committee	Reviews drug usage, creates policy and procedures in relation to particular drugs and therapies, and evaluates the use of technology for dispensing and prescribing drugs	Pharmacists, physicians, and nurses	Provides statistics on drug reactions, overdosing and underdosing as identified by coded data
Quality management committee	Reviews all incident reports on a regular basis, initiates hospital-wide quality improvement initiatives	Quality management staff: nurses, physicians, and other clinical and nonclinical members as appropriate; HIM may be on this team	Provides reports on pre- and post-quality initiatives outcomes

(*Continued*)

Table 10.1   Committee structure within a healthcare organization (*Continued*)

Name of committee	Functions of committee	Interdisciplinary team members	HIM functions
Sentinel events committee	Committee called upon when a sentinel event occurs; performs extensive research on the incident, makes recommendations and process changes so that the incident does not occur again, provides a report to the accrediting body	Nurses, physicians, and any other appropriate individuals as related to the particular incident	Ensures the committee has access to the documentation required for assessing the incident
Surgical case review, tumor board or cancer committee	Reviews particular surgical cases and the pathology associated with the surgeries, performs as an advisory body to the attending physician	Physicians, HIM professionals, or the cancer registrar	Provides reports on newly reported malignancies, number of surgical operations per physician, and so on
Utilization review committee	Oversight of the utilization of hospital services in relation to patient admissions	Utilization review staff, physicians, nurses	Provides statistical reports on utilization of services, case mix index, admission denials, and so on

Smaller healthcare organizations such as physician office practices or clinics, small community hospitals, critical access hospitals, behavioral health organizations, home health, hospice and long-term care facilities will have one or two committees that perform the multiple functions for that entity. In larger healthcare organizations each of these committees represented in table 10.1 will be standalone committees. Ad hoc task forces are groups formed for a specific task or objective, and are assembled as needed. These task forces or committees perform the tasks assigned and then disband when the work is done (Business Dictionary 2015).

HIM professionals play an important role within healthcare organizational committees as *custodians of the health records*. They not only represent the needs of the HIM department but also provide a role in patient advocacy ensuring the healthcare organization is always acting in the best interest of the patient in terms of managing protected health information (PHI). HIM professionals will not be on all of the committees listed within table 10.1 but it is important to understand the functions that each of the committees' perform so when health records issues arise, concerns can be triaged to the appropriate committee. The next sections address the purposes and structure of these committees.

Purposes of Committees

Committees may be temporary or permanent. The purposes and uses of committees in general are to engage a multidisciplinary group of healthcare individuals in decision-making processes that impact a multitude of services within a healthcare organization. Patient care outcomes are dependent on a variety of healthcare individuals working together. Discussions and decisions about healthcare operations need to be made outside of the patient care settings, and committees are where this type of coordination can occur in a very neutral manner. Committees also play a role in ensuring that all departments within a healthcare organization have a mechanism to collaborate regarding healthcare operations.

Committee Structure

The structure for most committees includes an appointed chair of the committee and often this role is rotated throughout the membership of the committee annually. New committee members should be oriented to the committee by the committee chair or another returning committee member. Agendas and minutes of the committee meetings are created and used as a guide for managing each committee meeting. These documents are saved in an appropriate manner and are accessible to the committee members and the healthcare organization's executive team. Agendas are created based on the functions of the committee and the required committee activities to be performed on a regular basis. Some of the committees may discuss issues that have protected status such as physician peer review committees, so the minutes from these meetings should be retained in a confidential manner.

A few of the committees listed in table 10.1 are discussed in further detail delineating the purpose of the committee, typical committee membership, and committee functions and HIM's role in the functions of the committee.

Accreditation Committee

The purpose of the accreditation committee is to provide oversight and guidance in preparation for accreditation and licensure surveys. The major functions of this committee include assuring that hospital policies and procedures are in alignment with accreditation standards, reviewing accrediting or licensing body standards for updates, communicating changes to the standards to the healthcare organization, performing ongoing mock accreditation surveys, and hosting the accreditation team as it arrives on-site for a review. A larger healthcare organization will have a standalone accreditation committee but smaller organizations or alternative healthcare settings may fold accreditation and licensing preparation into the organizational management structure. HIM will participate in accreditation mock surveys and develop policies and procedures in relation to the management and access of health information throughout the organization.

Quality Management Committee

The quality management committee reviews all incident reports on a regular basis and initiates hospital-wide quality improvement initiatives based on incident report data and patient safety outcomes. The committee will be comprised of management staff: nurses, physicians, and other clinical and nonclinical members as appropriate. The quality management committee may be combined with the patient safety committee in many organizations. HIM may provide a committee member and reports on pre- and post-quality improvement initiatives.

Specific Health Information Management Committees

The HIM department may also have several committees within the department that allow employees from differing areas to interact with one another and to work on departmental issues. Typical HIM department committees are:

- Employee activities committee. This committee will provide support for ongoing employee social activities throughout the department such as planning potlucks, managing the office coffee pot and snacks, providing policies for when flowers should be sent to employees (for congratulations or consolation), and organizing parties for employee life events such as wedding showers and baby showers. Sometimes this committee also works through suggestions for department improvements and communicates employee requests for department improvements to management.

- Health information professionals week committee. Health information professionals (HIP) week is a nationally recognized week (usually celebrated the third week of March) honoring HIM professionals who work in a variety of healthcare settings. The HIP week theme is developed by AHIMA and AHIMA provides a variety of tools for HIM professionals to employ for marketing the week in the healthcare organization and to the public.

- Performance improvement committees. This committee can help organize and manage a variety of performance initiatives that cross multiple areas of the HIM department. A project manager or facilitator who is trained in the use of the performance improvement tools may be assigned to this committee.

- HIM committee. This is a hospital-wide committee that is required by The Joint Commission and is usually chaired or co-chaired by the HIM director. This committee provides healthcare organizational support in terms of managing all aspects of health information including approval of documentation templates, paper forms management, physician chart completion issues, record and retention policies, and copy and paste policies. It is very important that the HIM director keeps the HIM committee well informed on the issues impacting health information throughout the organization.

- Specific HIM workgroup committees. These teams may meet on a regular basis to discuss specific job tasks, provide training and ongoing education, and develop team cohesiveness. An example of an HIM workgroup that might meet on a regular basis is the coding team. This team would meet to discuss specific coding issues and provide coding education on clinical or process topics impacting the coding area.

Additional committees may be assembled when needs arise within the department that are applicable for discussion in a committee structure. For example, if issues occur within a department that have to do with dress code, an ad hoc committee could be assembled and a new dress code could be developed for the department. The size and complexity of the HIM department will impact the type and number of committees that need to be in place.

Limitations and Disadvantages to Committees

Committees provide an important role in the management of healthcare operations but there are some limitations and disadvantages to committees. The committee structure and activities in the healthcare organization must be supported by the executive management team in order for this model to be constructive. The time to make decisions within a committee is slow as group deliberation and participation is required in all decision-making activities. If a decision needs to be made quickly on patient care, the committee structure is not the right venue for this action. The members of each committee should take their roles seriously and perform due diligence prior to each committee meeting by reading the previous meeting's minutes, performing any required homework, reviewing the agenda, and arriving to the meeting on time. Ill-prepared committee members can significantly impede the decision-making process with the committee meeting.

Each committee member should engage in discussions at the meeting and strive to limit any sidebar discussions. Outside of the committee, committee members should only share final outcomes or committee decisions that are necessary for healthcare operations. Personal issues or individual stances shared within the committee structure should remain confidential. A committee should review its purpose and function on a regular basis, assess membership, and revise as necessary.

All committee members should be versed on the mission and vision of the committee and play a key role in ensuring that the committee functions are carried out appropriately. Committee structure is an effective way of managing complex healthcare organizational issues and HIM professionals should be aware of the role that it plays in regards to this model.

Check Your **Understanding**

1. How is HIM moving away from a traditional structure to an HIM without walls concept?
2. What purposes do committees serve in the overall functioning of a healthcare organization?
3. Discuss the disadvantages to the committee structure in a healthcare organization.

External and Internal Influences on Health Information Management

HIM managers are responsible for assessing the internal and external forces that affect performance and appropriately address these forces when considering the type of organizational model that fits best for the department. **External forces** are the influences, resources, and activities that exist outside of the healthcare organization but significantly impact and affect HIM. **Internal forces** are the areas of focus the manager needs to address on a daily basis so the HIM department performs at its peak level. Table 10.2 outlines the typical external and internal forces that impact HIM. Reflecting on internal and external forces allows the HIM manager to make operational decisions in line with the organizational model. HIM managers will need to embrace the following strategies in order to mitigate the effects of these influences on the day-to-day operations:

- Provide better opportunities for "integration of healthcare information across the continuum of care
- Develop processes and systems that promote the understanding and use of health information by patients and families

Table 10.2.   Forces impacting HIM

External forces	Internal forces
Governmental agencies such as Centers for Medicare and Medicaid Services (CMS), Agency for Healthcare Research and Quality (AHRQ), Office of the National Coordinator (ONC), and the National Quality Forum (NQF)	Budgeting, such as the impact that new healthcare delivery models afford to healthcare organizations
State regulations such as departments of public health	Staffing, such as the need for experienced HIM individuals
Privacy and security of PHI such as patient access to PHI via patient portals	Training and development, such as ongoing training needs for current HIM staff to meet challenges of the changing HIM work environment
Changing workforce demographics such as an aging workforce with limited numbers of younger individuals ready to assume vacated roles	Management of HIM functions and services, such as quality coding, turnaround times for release of information and transcription as it relates to either internal processes or the use of outsourced services for these functions
New models of healthcare delivery such as Accountable Care Organizations (ACOs) and Patient Centered Medical Homes	Effective and secure use of health information technology such as PHI accessibility
Changes in health insurance such as an increase of the number of individuals who have insurance	Changing organizational models from line management to nonhierarchical in order to keep pace with the changes in healthcare

- Reframe the way coded data and information is used to obtain payment in a system that rewards quality and efficiency of services over the traditional emphasis on the quantity of services (Desai 2015)

Professional organizations and competition for HIM roles are discussed as follows.

Professional Organizations

HIM has access to a variety of professional organizations that can offer assistance and support to HIM professionals depending on the job roles that might require additional support outside of the traditional HIM field. Table 10.3 on the following page lists the professional organizations that many HIM professionals are members of or interact with on a regular basis. This is not an exhaustive list of organizations but rather the more common organizations that impact many HIM professionals. AHIMA is the leading source of HIM knowledge and it is a respected authority for rigorous education and training. AHIMA is the premier association to which HIM professionals should belong in order to benefit from the multitude of resources available. AHIMA is working to advance the implementation of electronic health records by leading key initiatives and advocating for consistent standards. AHIMA keeps HIM professionals informed on healthcare industry trends and provides members the resources in order to develop the knowledge, skills, and abilities necessary to manage these changes. The AHIMA Body of Knowledge is the official repository of peer-reviewed information created by HIM professionals. The AHIMA Body of Knowledge contains the most current and relevant articles, white papers, conference proceedings, and practice briefs supporting HIM initiatives. AHIMA provides the oversight of HIM certifications like Registered Health Information Technician (RHIT) and Registered Health Information Administrator (RHIA) by monitoring continuing education (CE) compliance. AHIMA provides opportunities for HIM professionals to gain additional credentials that provide credence to advanced skills such as Certified Coding Associate (CCA), Certified Coding Specialist (CCS), Certified Coding Specialist—Physician-based (CCS-P),Certified Health Data Analyst (CHDA), Certified in Healthcare Privacy and Security (CHPS), Certified Documentation Improvement Practitioner (CDIP), and Certified Health Technology Specialist (CHTS) (AHIMA 2015).

Table 10.3. Professional organizations influencing HIM professionals

Name of organization	Organizational purpose	Membership	Impact on HIM
American Association for Professional Coders (AAPC)	"Provides education and professional certification to physician-based medical coders. Provides student training, certification, and ongoing education, networking, and job opportunities. Provides certification for the entire business side of healthcare. (AAPC 2015).	Physician-based medical coders and billers	HIM professionals may employ AAPC certified coders to perform physician billing within either a physician practice or for hospital-based physician billing.
American College of Healthcare Executives (ACHE)	International professional society of more than 40,000 healthcare executives who lead hospitals, healthcare systems, and other healthcare organizations. Provides access to networking, education and career development. Established to further advance healthcare management excellence through education and research (ACHE 2015).	Healthcare executives	HIM professionals who lead at upper levels within a healthcare organization may be members of this organization. This is a professional society that provides support for those HIM professionals who perform in executive roles within healthcare organizations.
Association of Clinical Documentation Improvement Specialists (ACDIS)	"A community in which CDI professionals share the latest tested tips, tools, and strategies to implement successful CDI programs and achieve professional growth" (ACDIS 2015).	Healthcare professionals involved within CDI initiatives such as nurses, physicians, and HIM professionals.	This association provides support for HIM professionals that work in the role as clinical documentation improvement specialists and offers a credential that can be obtained as proof of knowledge regarding clinical documentation improvement.
American Hospital Association (AHA)	"Represents and serves all types of hospitals, healthcare networks, and their patients and communities." Provides education for healthcare leaders and is a source of information on healthcare issues and trends (AHA 2015).	Healthcare organizations	HIM professionals can access the information provided by this association if their healthcare organization is a member.
American Health Information Management Association (AHIMA)	"AHIMA's primary goal is to provide the knowledge, resources, and tools to advance health information professional practice and standards for the delivery of quality healthcare" (AHIMA 2015).	HIM students and professionals Corporate membership includes other alliance organizations and vendors Membership levels: active, student, cooperate, and emeritus	AHIMA is the premier organization for providing current HIM knowledge. Provides oversight of HIM credentials and offers opportunities for additional credentialing opportunities.

(Continued)

Table 10.3. Professional organizations influencing HIM professionals (*Continued*)

Name of organization	Organizational purpose	Membership	Impact on HIM
American Medical Association (AMA)	"Provides a vision for a healthier nation by advocating on behalf of physicians and patients to address their day-to-day needs and works to shape a healthier future for patients" (AMA 2015).	Physicians, residents, medical students	AMA is responsible for maintaining the CPT code set. HIM professionals may obtain CPT code books from AMA. HIM professionals may solicit advice from AMA regarding CPT coding issues.
American Medical Informatics Association (AMIA)	"Center of action for more than 4,000 healthcare professionals, informatics researchers, and thought-leaders in biomedicine, healthcare and science" (AMIA 2015).	Physicians, nurses, dentists, pharmacists, and other clinicians Researchers and educators Biomedical and health science librarians Advanced students pursuing a career in informatics Scientists and developers Government officials and policymakers Consultants and industry professionals	HIM professionals may belong to this organization as many HIM roles are turning into health informatics rather than just health information roles.
Health Information Management Systems Society (HIMSS)	"Global, cause-based, not-for-profit organization focused on better health through information technology (IT). HIMSS leads efforts to optimize health engagements and care outcomes using information technology" (HIMSS 2015).	Physicians, nurses, IT professionals, HIM professionals, IT vendors	HIM professionals who fill more IT or technical roles in healthcare may join this organization for additional information and support.
Medical Group Management Association (MGMA)	"Provides the essential education, legislative information, data, and career resources to help improve patient services and operational efficiencies." Examples of information provided by MGMA: online practice management solutions, online networking, benchmarking data, access to certification programs, webinars, and advice on legislative and regulatory issues (MGMA 2015)	Medical practice administrators and healthcare executives	HIM professionals who manage physician practices may be members of this association. HIM professionals will glean information and support that is specific to medical group management when they join this association.

(*Continued*)

Table 10.3. Professional organizations influencing HIM professionals (*Continued*)

Name of organization	Organizational purpose	Membership	Impact on HIM
National Association for Healthcare Quality (NAHQ)	"Provides education, leadership development opportunities, and products to support healthcare quality professionals" (NAHQ 2015).	Healthcare professionals involved in quality initiatives such as nurses and physicians	HIM professionals involved in quality improvement job roles may belong to this organization; the organization can provide knowledge and support in regards to healthcare quality for those HIM professionals performing quality roles.
National Cancer Registrars Association (NCRA)	"Serves as the education, credentialing, and advocacy resource for cancer data professionals" (NCRA 2015).	Cancer registry professionals	Many HIM professionals fill job roles as cancer registrars. The credential that this organization provides is a requirement for maintaining cancer registries within healthcare organizations.

Professional organizations do not provide overall governance for HIM operations but they do provide guidance and support for interested, qualified individuals in terms of offering best practices, lobbying and advocacy for the profession, and advanced credentials.

Competitors for Health Information Management Roles

When discussing the professional organizations impacting the HIM profession it is easy to see how many different professions can be allies as well as competitors for the same healthcare job tasks and roles in healthcare organizations. With the advent of health information technology, HIM roles have dramatically changed—these changes evolved quickly and it allowed others who are more proficient with the technology components to step in and perform jobs normally suited for HIM professionals. Many of the components of implementation of health information technology require technical information services skills such as those dealing with hardware, software, and interfaces. There are other components that require HIM skills such as designing documentation templates that meet accreditation and licensure guidelines, designing reports that can extract appropriate health information for release of information activities, and coding and billing workflow activities. HIM professionals need to step up and advocate for the skills and job roles that are appropriate for the HIM profession so others do not assume HIM roles within healthcare organizations.

Check Your **Understanding**

1. Explain the difference between internal and external forces and how they affect the HIM department.
2. What are three governmental entities that are external forces and how do they influence HIM?
3. Choose three professional organizations that impact HIM and discuss their purpose, membership, and bearing on HIM.
4. Why are there so many competitors for HIM roles?

Staying Relevant as an Health Information Management Professional

It is important to stay current and relevant as an HIM professional because there are many individuals outside of HIM who are waiting or actively competing for typical HIM job roles. There will be an increased need for HIM professionals to perform in the following areas: coding skills (CDI, revenue cycle, and registry), data and information governance skills, and leadership skills. HIM professionals will require further education, analytical and critical thinking skills, and additional clinical knowledge (Desai 2015). A new HIM graduate has the advantage of being exposed to new HIM curriculum competencies that address emerging workforce issues. As an example, information technology professionals are assuming roles of extracting and reporting on coded dated because of their information technology background but they have no knowledge of what this data means. An HIM professional with some additional information technology skills in data mining and reporting would be more suited for this position as he or she would be more knowledgeable as to what the data means. Practicing HIM professionals have the advantage of work experience although many have a limited scope of the different types of health information roles emerging in today's healthcare environment due to limited job duties and tasks within their own healthcare organizations. How does the practicing HIM professional become knowledgeable about current workforce trends? How does the new graduate gain the practical experience to enter into the HIM job pool? Guidance for both of these groups of HIM professionals will be described in the following section.

AHIMA's Strategic Plan and Vision

AHIMA's primary goal is to provide the knowledge, resources, and tools to advance health information professional practice and standards for the delivery of quality healthcare. The AHIMA Board of Directors along with the AHIMA House of Delegates and Envisioning Collaborative developed five strategic goals that provide guidance for health information practitioners when managing health information in today's healthcare environment. These strategic goals can be utilized by any HIM professional and within any healthcare organization. A link to the strategic plan is in figure 10.3 (found before the chapter case study). The five strategic goals address:

- Public good: HIM professionals need to empower consumers to optimize their health through management of their personal information
- Information governance: HIM professionals need to be recognized as the experts in health information governance and should share the knowledge with others in their healthcare organizations
- Informatics: HIM professionals should assist healthcare organizations in transforming data into health intelligence
- Innovation: HIM professionals should increase thought leadership and evidence-based HIM research in their healthcare organizations
- Leadership: HIM professionals should assist in developing HIM leaders across all healthcare sectors (AHIMA 2015)

Embracing these five concepts as an HIM professional can provide a foundation to build a current and relevant knowledge base. Ensuring these goals are considered in daily activities and that the work performed strives to incorporate these strategic initiatives provides a current and relevant foundation for any HIM professional. Table 10.4 on the following page outlines some practical guidance for HIM professionals to incorporate these goals into daily operations. Being able to perform some of these activities as an HIM professional may require additional research but this in turn will provide relevance to the individual.

Some of the suggested activities for incorporating the AHIMA strategies into daily operations require HIM professionals to obtain further education or training. These activities also require the HIM professional to step out of traditional HIM roles and engage with others throughout the healthcare organization or community. The HIM professionals in a healthcare organization should be viewed as the leaders in managing health information at all levels.

Table 10.4. Applying AHIMA strategic goals to HIM daily operations

AHIMA strategic goal	Practical guidance for daily HIM operations
Public good	Engage in ongoing healthcare consumer education in regards to the use of the healthcare organization's patient portal or development of a personal health record (PHR).
	Develop educational handouts for healthcare consumers that describe how to log into the patient portal or how to create a PHR.
	Educate the community about gaining access to their PHI, release of information authorizations, and so on.
	Provide educational sessions at the local senior center, nursing home, or community center on the importance of managing health information.
Information governance	Read the AHIMA white paper on information governance and share this with your executive management team within the healthcare organization (link in figure 10.3).
	Volunteer to lead an information governance taskforce or workgroup within your organization.
	Step up and volunteer to be on the information governance team, if one has already formed.
	Lead by example within the HIM department by developing policies and procedures outlining information governance performed within HIM.
Informatics	Create reports on HIM coded data that are relevant to the healthcare organization such as case mix index, service line statistics and data, severity of illness, and risk of mortality for particular units, or departments.
	Develop mapping tools for classification systems and terminologies that assist the healthcare organization to understand current and legacy data.
	Review externally reported data for data quality and data integrity.
	Take a course on statistical analysis or data analytics to advance your skills.
	Partner with the local health information exchange organization to analyze and evaluate community or regional health information data.
Innovation	Help all HIM professionals within your department to be out-of-the box thinkers.
	Partner with health IT vendors to develop products that meet the high standards required for the management of health information.
	Engage in research activities or performance improvement initiatives that result in better management of health information.
Leadership	Demonstrate ethical leadership within the HIM department and throughout the healthcare organization.
	Educate others within the healthcare organization about the skills of HIM professionals and the role that HIM plays in healthcare outcomes.
	Volunteer to participate or lead within your regional, state, or national association.
	Volunteer to present at colleges and universities on hot topics in HIM such as HIPAA, ethics, information technology, and coding.
	Volunteer to present at other professional associations to share HIM topics.

AHIMA Health Information Management Educational Curriculum Competencies in Practice

It is the responsibility of an HIM manager to maintain his or her own skills as well as develop his or her employees' skills. In 2014, the AHIMA Council on Education in Excellence developed educational competencies that address the learning and knowledge needs for HIM professionals (see appendix A). These competencies will be required for all accredited educational programs beginning in 2017 but it is recommended that individuals and educational curriculums incorporate these standards as soon as possible (AHIMA 2015). These same competencies can be used to assess gaps in knowledge for current practicing HIM professionals by employing a competency checklist tool developed by the AHIMA Council on Excellence in education (AHIMA 2014). The competencies are divided into six domains that include:

- Domain I. Data content, structure, and standards (information governance)
- Domain II. Information protection: access, disclosure, archival, privacy, and security
- Domain III. Informatics, analytics, and data use
- Domain IV. Revenue management
- Domain V. Compliance
- Domain VI. Leadership

These six domains are divided into subdomain topics and the levels of expected learning differ between associate, baccalaureate, and graduate degree programs. It is recommended that HIM professionals review the curriculum appropriate to their level of learning and in relation to HIM career aspirations. Chapter 9 discusses the use of the AHIMA Career Map in relation to training and development needs for HIM professionals (link to the map in figure 10.3). The HIM educational curriculum competences can assist HIM professionals in connecting the career progression with learning needs (AHIMA Foundation 2013).

The Council on the Excellence in Education developed an AHIMA Professional Development Inventory that can be utilized by HIM professionals to assess gaps in knowledge. This tool is developed using the HIM educational curriculum competencies and it can be located using the link in figure 10.3 (AHIMA 2014). This guide also provides an extensive list of resources that can be consulted for gaining additional knowledge. Guidance for completing the inventory is included within the tool. A practicing HIM professional needs to assess current HIM knowledge for each domain and subdomain of the curriculum competencies and identify whether he or she is unskilled, a novice, or a master of that particular topic. The next step is to evaluate what level of knowledge attainment this same individual wishes to attain—unskilled, novice, or master—based on identified career goals. For example, a CCS who is also an RHIT might have a career goal of a coding manager. At this time in regards to Domain I—Classification Systems this individual can mark "master" for current knowledge and also "master" for goal knowledge but for Domain IV—Leadership roles, the individual will need to mark "unskilled" and "master" for goal knowledge. This individual has clearly identified an area where he or she needs to develop additional skills in order to attain a coding manager position.

Emerging Roles in Health Information Management

The HIM emerging job roles are limitless as many of the skills and talents exhibited by HIM professionals span a wide variety of knowledge. The foundational curriculum competencies provide a baseline for new HIM graduates as well as a guide for practicing HIM professionals. Mastery of all competencies is not possible for any one individual because of the wide array of knowledge competencies identified for HIM professionals. HIM professionals need to develop a career plan and develop skills based on a career trajectory as discussed in chapter 9.

One emerging role that is best suited to the skill set of HIM professionals is enterprise information management (EIM) and governance. "EIM aligns people, processes, data, and technology with information policies and practices throughout an entire healthcare organization" (Kloss 2013). Traditional health information record practices need to be expanded to encompass management as an asset throughout the healthcare organization. A broader range of knowledge is required for embarking on an EIM manager role as skills should include a combination of the following items:

- Leadership skills in gaining collaboration and cooperation from others in terms of managing and governing enterprise information
- Privacy and security issues associated with EIM need to be addressed on a larger scale as there are compliance issues and risks within enterprise-wide data
- Understanding and applying the concepts of data quality and integrity for enterprise-wide data is essential
- Development of clear and concise data dictionaries for managing enterprise-wide information are imperative
- Creation of information policies and standards that can be utilized by healthcare organizations to meet operational needs will be key to effective EIM (Kloss 2013)

Population health information management (PHIM) is another job role that fits the skills and talents inherent to HIM professionals. **Population health** is the capture and reporting of healthcare data that is used for public health purposes. It allows the healthcare provider to report infectious diseases, immunizations, cancer, and other reportable conditions to public health professionals. A strategic initiative of PHIM should include optimal clinical documentation along with accurate and compliant coding using appropriate classification systems and terminologies. The data created from this initiative will allow data from diverse sources to be extrapolated and aggregated to create information and knowledge related to the management of population health. The management of the immense amount of data that is collected from diverse entities in managing population health requires HIM expertise. HIM professionals excelling in PHIM will be able to innovatively assist organizations in developing EHRs that collect longitudinal data regarding public health issues as well as creatively assess patient demographics and coded data to aid clinicians in studying population health (Cassidy 2013).

The emergence of **computer-assisted coding (CAC)** technologies will change the role of the traditional coding professional as well. CAC is the process of extracting and translating diagnostic and procedural information from electronic health records into ICD and CPT evaluation and management codes for billing and coding purposes. HIM coding professionals will need to develop skills to assess automated coding workflows as electronic documentation is captured, stored, and transformed into coded data. Coding professionals will also need to understand the mapping between a natural language process (NLP) and classification systems that occurs within the CAC. Coders will need to have in-depth knowledge of the structure and content of electronic health record documentation and what source documents are used during the CAC process. Two new job titles that may emerge with the use of CAC will be the clinical coding editor and the clinical coding analyst. The skills required by these new coding professionals will specifically require skills in automated coding workflow design and critical thinking skills to discern if code selection by the tool provides a clear clinical depiction of the documentation (AHIMA 2011).

A vast array of job roles that are emerging within HIM departments are focused around data analytics and data informatics. The HIM educational curriculum competencies clearly outline the skills needed to approach these new job roles. The titles for these new data analytics and informatics jobs greatly vary depending on the type of healthcare organization. Data mapping is another fast growing field that clearly matches the attention to detail skills as well as knowledge of classification systems and terminologies that HIM professionals possess. HIM professionals need to develop the skills to undertake these job roles so that others outside of the HIM realm do not jump in and take them over. Job roles are changing for HIM professionals as quickly as health information technology is advancing. HIM professionals not only need to keep pace with the new skill sets required for performing emerging roles, but they also need to ensure that their HIM team develops these skills as well. Continuing education and advanced formal education needs to be embraced by all HIM professionals in order to keep pace with the healthcare industry (Dimick 2012).

Summary

This book has taken HIM professionals on an entry-level journey into the world of management. Chapter one provided management and leadership theories as a foundation for developing an HIM management and leader style. Chapter two discussed the basic management functions and how they relate to health information management tasks. Chapter three addressed cultural diversity, teams, and motivating an HIM workforce. Chapter four outlined the necessary skills required to handle the ever-changing healthcare environment. Chapter five provided the HIM manager with fundamental issues associated with legal aspects of healthcare management. Chapter six dove into creating job descriptions and job roles in HIM that are current and relevant to today's workforce. Chapter seven provided guidance for the HIM manager in terms of recruiting and staffing the HIM department. Chapter eight addressed the controlling function of management through development of job standards that are effective in managing HIM performance. Chapter nine wrapped up the management functions by reviewing the best practices for HIM employee training and development. The tenth and final chapter of this text reflects on how changing organizational structures impact HIM and how the HIM department is actually becoming a department within walls or boundaries.

Figure 10.3. Links to AHIMA tools for HIM

2014–2017 AHIMA Strategic Plan: http://library.ahima.org/xpedio/groups/public/documents/ahima/bok1_050165.pdf

AHIMA Career Map: http://hicareers.com/CareerMap/

AHIMA Information Governance White Paper: http://www.ahima.org/IGwhitepaper

AHIMA Professional Development Inventory: http://www.ahima.org/competency

---

© AHIMA

Check Your **Understanding**

1. Define AHIMA's five strategic goals.
2. Choose three of AHIMA's strategic goals and discuss how an HIM professional can incorporate them into daily operations.
3. Describe two emerging HIM job roles.

Case Study

Objectives

- Examine the AHIMA strategic plan and professional competencies to maintain relevancy as an HIM professional
- Develop a 5-year career development plan

Instructions

Complete an AHIMA professional inventory for an HIM professional and develop a career plan based on individual career needs. The AHIMA professional development inventory can be accessed via the link in figure 10.3 and the career plan template is provided as follows.

Scenario

Mary Beth Jones, RHIA, is an HIM director at a small rural community healthcare facility. She has been in the HIM field for approximately 15 years and realizes that even though her facility is pretty progressive for its size and location, she may not be keeping pace with the type of skills that are required for the future HIM workforce. Her husband may be transferred within the year to a more suburban city in another state that has a lot of opportunities for an HIM professional. Mary Beth is worried that she may not be as marketable as some of her peers. She has talked with one of the faculty members from where she attained her bachelor's degree and this individual recommended that Mary Beth use the AHIMA competency assessment tool to assess her gaps in her knowledge. The faculty member also suggested that Mary Beth consider attaining a master's degree in health informatics or HIM.

Mary Beth's current skill set is as follows:

- Her first position was as cancer registrar. She was a certified registrar for three years.
- Her second position was coding at a large physician practice for one and a half years.
- Her third position was the supervisor of the outpatient coding area, which included physician billing, outpatient surgery and observation coding, and all clinical coding. She was in this position for four years.
- She did not work for one and a half years after the birth of her third child.
- She was promoted to director of HIM five years ago. The projects she has completed include:
  - While on the project team for implementation of an ambulatory EHR, she helped the design team with the build for the inpatient EHR that will go-live in six months
  - She outsourced medical transcription
  - She developed a coding workforce that works remotely
  - She was an AHIMA-approved ICD-10 trainer and she performed, in conjunction with the coding manager, all the coding training in preparation for ICD-10
  - She has not done much with reporting or data analytics and relies heavily on her data quality manager to run most of these reports
  - Her healthcare organization has not embraced information governance

Assumptions

- Mary Beth is willing to do what it takes to get her learning on target with the HIM workforce.
- Mary Beth will be moving in the next year and she may need additional skills prior to obtaining another job as outlined by her career goals.
- Mary Beth wants to remain in management and she would like to be the assistant director or director at a large urban or suburban healthcare organization.

Deliverables

1. Create a five-year career plan for Mary Beth using the template provided. Include three strategic goals that Mary Beth should work on within her current facility to demonstrate relevancy in the HIM profession and for each of these strategic goals identify three operational goals similar to those in table 10.4.

2. Identify two internal forces impacting HIM (table 10.2) and provide two resources from the AHIMA Body of Knowledge that Mary Beth can consult to gain additional knowledge.

3. Identify two external forces impacting HIM (table 10.2) and provide two resources from the AHIMA Body of Knowledge that Mary Beth can consult to gain additional knowledge.

4. Create two personal goals for Mary Beth in regards to long-term career development.

Career Plan Template

AHIMA strategy	Operational goal	Start date	End date	Comments
1.	1-1 1-2 1-3			
2.	2-1 2-2 2-3			
3.	3-1 3-2 3-3			
Internal forces impacting HIM				
1.	1-1 1-2			
2.	2-1 2-2			
External forces impacting HIM				
1.	1-1 1-2			
2.	2-1 2-2			
Personal goals	1			
	2			

Review Questions

1. Which of the following is not an internal force impacting HIM?

   a. Budget
   b. Span of control
   c. Staffing
   d. State regulations

2. Which of the following is not an external force impacting HIM?

   a. Patient portals
   b. Privacy of personal health information (PHI)
   c. Training and development
   d. Changes in workforce demographics

3. Emily is a coder who reports directly to the assistant director of HIM. The assistant director reports directly to the director of HIM. This reporting structure illustrates which organizational model?

   a. Interconnected management
   b. Line management
   c. Horizontal network
   d. Nonhierarchical organization

4. Which of the following committees is responsible for overseeing medical staff activity within an organization?

   a. Accreditation Committee
   b. Medical Executive Committee
   c. Patient Care Committee
   d. Pharmacy and Therapeutics

5. Jon is an HIM professional interested in healthcare informatics and biomedical issues. Which of the following professional organizations would Jon be most likely to join to further his career in these areas?

   a. AMIA
   b. HIMSS
   c. NCRA
   d. NAHQ

6. Charlotte is scheduled to give a presentation to a senior citizen's group at the local community center. Charlotte is meeting which of AHIMA's strategic goals?

   a. Information governance
   b. Innovation
   c. Leadership
   d. Public good

7. Michelle was recently elected to the position of president-elect in her state HIM association. Michelle is meeting which of AHIMA's strategic goals?

   a. Informatics
   b. Information governance
   c. Leadership
   d. Public good

8. Allison's position at the Department of Public Health requires that she perform coding and data analysis on infectious disease reporting forms. As an HIM professional, Allison is involved in what emerging role?

   a. Computer-assisted coding
   b. Enterprise information management
   c. Information governance
   d. Population health

9. Creation of a drug formulary for organizational use is the responsibility of which committee?

   a. Infection Control Committee
   b. Pharmacy and Therapeutics Committee
   c. Quality Management Committee
   d. Sentinel Events Committee

10. This area within AHIMA contains published articles, convention proceedings, and practice briefs that all members may access for continuing education and research needs:

   a. Body of Knowledge
   b. Council on Educational Excellence
   c. House of Delegates
   d. Professional Development Inventory

References

American Association of Professional Coders (AAPC). 2015. https://www.aapc.com/.

American Health Information Management Association. 2015. http://www.ahima.org.

American Health Information Management Association. 2014. AHIMA Professional Development Inventory. http://www.ahima.org/competency.

American Health Information Management Association. 2011. CAC 2010–11 Industry Outlook and Resources Report. http://library.ahima.org/xpedio/groups/public/documents/ahima/bok1_048947.pdf.

AHIMA Foundation. 2013. http://www.ahimafoundation.org/downloads/pdfs/2014%20Side-by-Side_Curriculum_Map.pdf.

American College of Healthcare Executives (ACHE). 2015. http://www.ache.org.

American Hospital Association (AHA). 2015. http://www.aha.org.

American Medical Association (AMA). 2015. http://www.ama-assn.org.

American Medical Informatics Association (AMIA). http://www.amia.org.

Association of Clinical Documentation Improvement Specialists (ACDIS). 2015. http://www.hcpro.com/acdis/.

Business Dictionary. 2015. http://www.businessdictionary.com.

Butler, M. 2015. Mind the gap: HIM rushes to bridge educational and professional gaps caused by a quickly advancing industry. *Journal of AHIMA* 86(2):20–24.

Cassidy, B.S. 2013. The next HIM frontier: Population health information management presents a new opportunity for HIM. *Journal of AHIMA* 84(8):40–46.

Desai, A. 2015. Scanning the HIM environment: AHIMA's 2015 report offers insight on emerging industry trends and challenges. *Journal of AHIMA* 86(5):38–43.

Dimick, C. 2012. Health information management 2025: Current "health IT revolution" drastically changes HIM in the near future. *Journal of AHIMA* 83(8):24–31.

Health Information Management Systems Society (HIMSS). 2015. http://www.himss.org.

Klenke, K. 2011. Keeping Control in Nonhierarchical Organizations. Chapter in *Business: The Ultimate Resource,* 3rd ed. London: A&C Black.

Kloss, L. 2013. Redefining the Role of Health Information Management in the New World of Information Governance. Iron Mountain. http://www.ironmountain.com/Knowledge-Center/Reference-Library/View-by-Document-Type/White-Papers-Briefs/R/Redefining-the-Role-of-Health-Information-Management-in-the-New-World-of-Information-Governance.aspx

Medical Group Management Association (MGMA). 2015. http://www.mgma.org.

Merriam-Webster. 2015. http://www.merriam-webster.com/

National Association for Healthcare Quality (NAHQ). 2015. http://www.nahq.org.

National Cancer Registrars Association (NCRA). 2015. http://www.ncra-us.org.

Price, C. 2011. Reorganizing the Company without Destroying It. Chapter in *Business: The Ultimate Resource,* 3rd ed. London: A & C Black.

Sikora, David M. and G. R. Ferris. 2014. Strategic human resource implementation: The critical role of line management. *Human Resource Management Review.* 24(2): 271–281.

Uhlig, D. 2015. Hierarchical Leadership vs Nonhierarchical Leadership. *Houston Chronicle.* http://smallbusiness.chron.com/hierarchical-leadership-vs-nonhierarchical-leadership-35422.html.

Side by Side Progression Map of Health Information Management Curricula

Concepts to be interwoven throughout all levels of the curricula include:
- CRITICAL THINKING: For example the ability to work independently, use judgment skills effectively, be innovative by thinking outside of the box
- PERSONAL BRANDING: For example personal accountability, reliability, self-sufficiency

Associate Degree	Bloom's Level	Baccalaureate Degree	Bloom's Level	Graduate Degree	Bloom's Level
Domain I. Data Content, Structure & Standards (Information Governance)					
Definition: Academic content related to diagnostic and procedural classification and terminologies; health record documentation requirements; characteristics of the healthcare system; data accuracy and integrity; data integration and interoperability; respond to customer data needs; data management policies and procedures; information standards.					
Subdomain I.A Classification Systems					
1. Apply diagnosis/procedure codes according to current guidelines	3	1. Evaluate, implement and manage electronic applications/systems for clinical classification and coding	5	1. Interpret terminologies, vocabularies and classification systems	5
2. Evaluate the accuracy of diagnostic and procedural coding	5	2. Identify the functions and relationships between healthcare classification systems	3	2. Construct examples of mapping of clinical vocabularies and terminologies to appropriate classification systems	6

Associate Degree	Bloom's Level	Baccalaureate Degree	Bloom's Level	Graduate Degree	Bloom's Level
3. Apply diagnostic and procedural groupings	3	3. Map terminologies, vocabularies and classification systems	4		
4. Evaluate the accuracy of diagnostic/procedural groupings	5	4. Evaluate the accuracy of diagnostic/procedural coding	5		
Subdomain I.B. Health Record Content and Documentation					
1. Analyze the documentation in the health record to ensure it supports the diagnosis and reflects the patient's progress, clinical findings, and discharge status	4	1. Verify that documentation in the health record supports the diagnosis and reflects the patient's progress, clinical findings, and discharge status	4	1. Examine required documentation and record structures	4
2. Verify the documentation in the health record is timely, complete, and accurate	4	2. Compile organization-wide health record documentation guidelines	6		
3. Identify a complete health record according to, organizational policies, external regulations, and standards	3	3. Interpret health information standards	5		
4. Differentiate the roles and responsibilities of various providers and disciplines, to support documentation requirements, throughout the continuum of healthcare	5				
Subdomain I.C. Data Governance					
1. Apply policies and procedures to ensure the accuracy of health data	3	1. Format data to satisfy integration needs	4	1. Evaluate data integration needs	5
		2. Construct and maintain the standardization of data dictionaries to meet the needs of the enterprise	6	2. Propose data interoperability and sharing policies, structures, methods	6
		3. Demonstrate compliance with internal and external data dictionary requirements	3	3. Recommend data standard policies for interoperability and sharing	5
		4. Advocate information operability and information exchange	5		
Subdomain I.D. Data Management					
1. Collect and maintain health data	2	1. Analyze information needs of customers across the healthcare continuum	4	1. Develop data management policies	6

Associate Degree	Bloom's Level	Baccalaureate Degree	Bloom's Level	Graduate Degree	Bloom's Level
2. Apply graphical tools for data presentations	3	2. Evaluate health information systems and data storage design	5	2. Evaluate data from varying sources to create meaningful presentations	5
		3. Manage clinical indices/databases/registries	5	3. Design patient-centered health information systems	6
		4. Apply knowledge of database architecture and design to meet organizational needs	3	4. Manage virtual network communications	5
		5. Evaluate data from varying sources to create meaningful presentations	5		
Subdomain I.E Secondary Data Sources					
1. Identify and use secondary data sources	3	1. Validate data from secondary sources to include in the patient's record, including personal health records	3	1. Compile data from secondary sources	6
2. Validate the reliability and accuracy of secondary data sources	3				
Domain II. Information Protection: Access, Disclosure, Archival, Privacy & Security					
Definition: Understand healthcare law (theory of all healthcare law to exclude application of law covered in Domain V); develop privacy, security, and confidentiality policies, procedures and infrastructure; educate staff on health information protection methods; risk assessment; access and disclosure management.					
Subdomain II.A. Health Law					
1. Apply healthcare legal terminology	3	1. Identify laws and regulations applicable to health care	3	1. Create regulatory policies based on health laws	6
2. Identify the use of legal documents	3	2. Analyze legal concepts and principles to the practice of HIM	4		
3. Apply legal concepts and principles to the practice of HIM	3				
Subdomain II.B. Data Privacy Confidentiality and Security					
1. Apply confidentiality, privacy and security measures, policies and procedures for internal and external use/exchange to protect electronic health information	3	1. Analyze privacy, security and confidentiality policies and procedures for internal and external use and exchange of health information	4	1. Design a privacy and security infrastructure	6
2. Apply retention and destruction policies for health information	3	2. Recommend elements included in the design of audit trails and data quality monitoring programs	5		

Associate Degree	Bloom's Level	Baccalaureate Degree	Bloom's Level	Graduate Degree	Bloom's Level
3. Apply system security policies according to departmental and organizational data/information standards	3	3. Collaborate in the design and implementation of risk assessment, contingency planning, and data recovery procedures	4		
		4. Analyze the security and privacy implications of mobile health technologies	4		
		5. Develop educational programs for employees in privacy, security, and confidentiality	6		
Subdomain II.C. Release of Information					
1. Apply policies and procedures surrounding issues of access and disclosure of protected health information	3	1. Create policies and procedures to manage access and disclosure of personal health information	6	1. Mitigate access and disclosure risks	5
		2. Protect electronic health information through confidentiality and security measures, policies and procedures	3		
Domain III. Informatics, Analytics and Data Use					
Definition: Creation and use of Business health intelligence; select, implement, use and manage technology solutions; system and data architecture; interface considerations; information management planning; data modeling; system testing; technology benefit realization; analytics and decision support; data visualization techniques; trend analysis; administrative reports; descriptive, inferential and advanced statistical protocols and analysis; IRB; research; patient-centered health information technologies; health information exchange; data quality					
Subdomain III.A. Health Information Technologies					
1. Utilize software in the completion of HIM processes	3	1. Utilize technology, for data collection, storage, analysis, and reporting of information	3	1. Evaluate use of data capture technologies	5
2. Explain policies and procedures of networks, including intranet and Internet to facilitate clinical and administrative applications	2	2. Assess systems capabilities to meet regulatory requirements	5	2. Construct information systems capabilities	6
		3. Recommend device selection based on workflow, ergonomic and human factors	5	3. Design user-centric interfaces and portals	6
		4. Take part in the development of networks, including intranet and Internet applications	4	4. Propose the use of artificial intelligence applications	6

Associate Degree	Bloom's Level	Baccalaureate Degree	Bloom's Level	Graduate Degree	Bloom's Level
		5. Evaluate system architecture, database design, data warehousing	5	5. Evaluate systems life cycle concepts	5
		6. Create the electronic structure of health data to meet a variety of end user needs	6	6. Lead the implementation of health information systems	6
				7. Construct information architectural models	6
Subdomain III.B. Information Management Strategic Planning					
1. Explain the process used in the selection and implementation of health information management systems	2	1. Take part in the development of information management plans that support the organization's current and future strategy and goals	4	1. Create information systems to ensure compliance	6
2. Utilize health information to support enterprise wide decision support for strategic planning	3	2. Take part in the planning, design, selection, implementation, integration, testing, evaluation, and support of health information technologies	4	2. Propose policy development and advocacy	6
				3. Develop strategic initiatives for information management systems and regulatory policies	6
				4. Appraise benefit realization of information technologies	5
				5. Engage key stakeholders in information systems planning	5
Subdomain III.C. Analytics and Decision Support					
1. Explain analytics and decision support	2	1. Apply analytical results to facilitate decision-making	3	1. Design data sources for intelligence extraction	6
2. Apply report generation technologies to facilitate decision-making	3	2. Apply data extraction methodologies	3	2. Create business intelligence through data analytics	6
		3. Recommend organizational action based on knowledge obtained from data exploration and mining	5	3. Create data visualization techniques	6
		4. Analyze clinical data to identify trends that demonstrate quality, safety, and effectiveness of healthcare	4		

Associate Degree	Bloom's Level	Baccalaureate Degree	Bloom's Level	Graduate Degree	Bloom's Level
		5. Apply knowledge of database querying and data exploration and mining techniques to facilitate information retrieval	3		
		6. Evaluate administrative reports using appropriate software	5		
Subdomain III.D. Health Care Statistics					
1. Utilize basic descriptive, institutional, healthcare statistics	3	1. Interpret inferential statistics	5	1. Interpret inferential statistics	5
2. Analyze data to identify trends	4	2. Analyze statistical data for decision making	4	2. Create statistical business models to leverage enterprise wide information assets	6
Subdomain III.E. Research Methods					
1. Explain common research methodologies and why they are used in healthcare	2	1. Apply principles of research and clinical literature evaluation to improve outcomes	3	1. Analyze principles of research and clinical literature evaluation to improve outcomes	4
		2. Plan adherence to Institutional Review Board (IRB) processes and policies	3	2. Comply with research administrative processes and policies	5
				3. Create an evidence based practice body of knowledge	6
Subdomain III.F. Consumer Informatics					
1. Explain usability and accessibility of health information by patients, including current trends and future challenges	2	1. Educate consumers on patient-centered health information technologies	3	1. Compare personalized medicine models	5
Subdomain III.G. Health Information Exchange					
1. Explain current trends and future challenges in health information exchange	2	1. Collaborate in the development of operational policies and procedures for health information exchange	4	1. Lead the development of policies for health information exchange (HIE)	6
		2. Conduct system testing to ensure data integrity and quality of health information exchange	6		
		3. Differentiate between various models for health information exchange	5		

Associate Degree	Bloom's Level	Baccalaureate Degree	Bloom's Level	Graduate Degree	Bloom's Level
Subdomain III.H. Information Integrity and Data Quality					
1. Apply policies and procedures to ensure the accuracy and integrity of health data both internal and external to the health system	3	1. Discover threats to data integrity and validity	3	1. Assess data integrity	5
		2. Implement policies and procedures to ensure data integrity internal and external to the enterprise	3	2. Oversee policies and technologies to protect data integrity	5
		3. Apply quality management tools	3	3. Conduct and direct quality assessment studies	6
		4. Perform quality assessment including quality management, data quality, and identification of best practices for health information systems	4		
		5. Model policy initiatives that influence data integrity	3		
Domain IV. Revenue Management					
Definition: Healthcare reimbursement; revenue cycle; chargemaster; DOES NOT INCLUDE COMPLIANCE regulations and activities related to revenue management (coding compliance initiatives, fraud and abuse, etc.) AS THESE ARE COVERED IN DOMAIN V.					
Subdomain IV.A. Revenue Cycle and Reimbursement					
1. Apply policies and procedures for the use of data required in healthcare reimbursement	3	1. Manage the use of clinical data required by various payment and reimbursement systems	5	1. Develop enterprise-wide strategic and operational planning models for revenue cycle management	6
2. Evaluate the revenue cycle management processes	5	2. Take part in selection and development of applications and processes for chargemaster and claims management	4	2. Forecast on-going regulatory impact on revenue cycle and enterprise-wide reimbursement	6
		3. Apply principles of healthcare finance for revenue management	3	3. Formulate healthcare reimbursement models	6
		4. Implement processes for revenue cycle management and reporting	3	4. Oversee revenue cycle program	5

Associate Degree	Bloom's Level	Baccalaureate Degree	Bloom's Level	Graduate Degree	Bloom's Level
Domain V. Compliance					
Definition: COMPLIANCE activities and methods for all health information topics. For example, how to comply with HIPAA, Stark Laws, Fraud and Abuse, etc.; coding auditing; severity of illness; data analytics; fraud surveillance; clinical documentation improvement.					
Subdomain V.A. Regulatory					
1. Analyze policies and procedures to ensure organizational compliance with regulations and standards	4	1. Appraise current laws and standards related to health information initiatives	5	1. Integrate data analytics for regulatory compliance measures	6
2. Collaborate with staff in preparing the organization for accreditation, licensure, and/or certification	4	2. Determine processes for compliance with current laws and standards related to health information initiatives and revenue cycle	5	2. Formulate organizational compliance programs and policies	6
3. Adhere to the legal and regulatory requirements related to the health information management	3			3. Analyze standards and regulations in healthcare and how they drive and/or constrain operations	4
Subdomain V.B. Coding					
1. Analyze current regulations and established guidelines in clinical classification systems	4	1. Construct and maintain processes, policies, and procedures to ensure the accuracy of coded data based on established guidelines	6	1. Analyze current regulations and established guidelines in clinical classification systems and computer assisted coding applications	4
2. Determine accuracy of computer assisted coding assignment and recommend corrective action	5	2. Manage coding audits	5		
		3. Identify severity of illness and its impact in healthcare payment systems	3		
Subdomain V.C. Fraud Surveillance					
1. Identify potential abuse or fraudulent trends through data analysis	3	1. Determine policies and procedures to monitor abuse or fraudulent trends	5	1. Develop forensic models for fraud surveillance and improvement measures	6
Subdomain V.D. Clinical Documentation Improvement					
1. Identify discrepancies between supporting documentation and coded data	3	1. Implement provider querying techniques to resolve coding discrepancies	3	1. Formulate enterprise-wide CDI strategic and operational methods	6

Associate Degree	Bloom's Level	Baccalaureate Degree	Bloom's Level	Graduate Degree	Bloom's Level
2. Develop appropriate physician queries to resolve data and coding discrepancies	6	2. Create methods to manage Present on Admission, hospital acquired conditions, and other CDI components	6		
Domain VI. Leadership					
Definition: Leadership models, theories, and skills; critical thinking; change management; workflow analysis, design, tools and techniques; human resource management; training and development theory and process; strategic planning; financial management; ethics and project management					
Subdomain VI.A Leadership Roles					
1. Summarize health information related leadership roles	2	1. Take part in effective negotiating and use influencing skills	4	1. Create health information related public policy	6
2. Apply the fundamentals of team leadership	3	2. Discover personal leadership style using contemporary leadership theory and principles	3	2. Evaluate executive decision-making	5
3. Organize and facilitate meetings	3	3. Take part in effective communication through project reports, business reports and professional communications	4	3. Build and maintain strategic business alliances, networks, and partnerships	6
		4. Apply personnel management skills	3		
		5. Take part in enterprise-wide committees	4		
		6. Build effective teams	6		
Subdomain VI.B. Change Management					
1. Recognize the impact of change management on processes, people and systems	2	1. Interpret concepts of change management theories, techniques and leadership	5	1. Master concepts of change management theories	6
Subdomain VI.C. Work Design and Process Improvement					
1. Utilize tools and techniques to monitor, report, and improve processes	3	1. Analyze workflow processes and responsibilities to meet organizational needs	4	1. Integrate data analytics to enhance workflow design and process improvement	6
2. Identify cost-saving and efficient means of achieving work processes and goals	3	2. Construct performance management measures	6	2. Design process improvement research methods and models	6
3. Utilize data for facility-wide outcomes reporting for quality management and performance improvement	3	3. Demonstrate workflow concepts	3		

Associate Degree	Bloom's Level	Baccalaureate Degree	Bloom's Level	Graduate Degree	Bloom's Level
Subdomain VI.D. Human Resources Management					
1. Report staffing levels and productivity standards for health information functions	3	1. Manage human resources to facilitate staff recruitment, retention, and supervision	5	1. Leverage human capital	5
2. Interpret compliance with local, state, and federal labor regulations	5	2. Ensure compliance with employment laws	5		
3. Adhere to work plans, policies, procedures, and resource requisitions in relation to job functions	3	3. Create and implement staff orientation and training programs	6		
		4. Benchmark staff performance data incorporating labor analytics	4		
		5. Evaluate staffing levels and productivity, and provide feedback to staff regarding performance	5		
Subdomain VI.E. Training and Development					
1. Explain the methodology of training and development	2	1. Evaluate initial and on-going training programs	5	1. Design enterprise-wide training and development research models and methods	6
2. Explain the return on investment for employee training and development	2				
Subdomain VI.F. Strategic and Organizational Management					
1. Summarize a collection methodology for data to guide strategic and organizational management	2	1. Identify departmental and organizational survey readiness for accreditation, licensing and/or certification processes	3	1. Create integrative health information analytics for effective enterprise-wide strategic planning	6
2. Understand the importance of healthcare policy-making as it relates to the healthcare delivery system	2	2. Implement a departmental strategic plan	3	2. Design enterprise-wide strategic planning research models and methods	6
3. Describe the differing types of organizations, services, and personnel and their interrelationships across the health care delivery system	2	3. Apply general principles of management in the administration of health information services	3	3. Propose innovative, draft healthcare policies which could directly or indirectly impact the national or global healthcare delivery system	6

Associate Degree	Bloom's Level	Baccalaureate Degree	Bloom's Level	Graduate Degree	Bloom's Level
4. Apply information and data strategies in support of information governance initiatives	3	4. Evaluate how healthcare policy-making both directly and indirectly impacts the national and global healthcare delivery systems	5	4. Compare the differing types of organizations, services, and personnel and their interrelationships across the health care delivery system	5
5. Utilize enterprise-wide information assets in support of organizational strategies and objectives	3	5. Identify the differing types of organizations, services, and personnel and their interrelationships across the health care delivery system	3	5. Engage key stakeholders in information governance initiatives	5
		6. Collaborate in the development and implementation of information governance initiatives	4	6. Leverage enterprise-wide information assets to enable achievement of organizational strategies and objectives	5
		7. Facilitate the use of enterprise-wide information assets to support organizational strategies and objectives	4		
Subdomain VI.G. Financial Management					
1. Plan budgets	3	1. Evaluate capital, operating and/or project budgets using basic accounting principles	5	1. Govern information assets	6
2. Explain accounting methodologies	2	2. Perform cost-benefit analysis for resource planning and allocation	4		
3. Explain budget variances	2	3. Evaluate the stages of the procurement process	5		
Subdomain VI.H. Ethics					
1. Comply with ethical standards of practice	5	1. Comply with ethical standards of practice	5	1. Create an ethical business culture	6
2. Evaluate the consequences of a breach of healthcare ethics	5	2. Evaluate the culture of a department	5	2. Design ethical research models	6
3. Assess how cultural issues affect health, healthcare quality, cost, and HIM	5	3. Assess how cultural issues affect health, healthcare quality, cost, and HIM	5	3. Evaluate ethical training and compliance programs and measures	5
4. Create programs and policies that support a culture of diversity	6	4. Create programs and policies that support a culture of diversity	6	4. Assess how cultural issues affect health, healthcare quality, cost, and HIM	5
				5. Create programs and policies that support a culture of diversity	6

Associate Degree	Bloom's Level	Baccalaureate Degree	Bloom's Level	Graduate Degree	Bloom's Level
Subdomain VI.I. Project Management					
1. Summarize project management methodologies	2	1. Take part in system selection processes	4	1. Assess project management tools	5
		2. Recommend clinical, administrative, and specialty service applications	5	2. Develop collaborative alliances and partnerships to effectively manage complex projects	6
		3. Apply project management techniques to ensure efficient workflow and appropriate outcomes	3	3. Evaluate applied research tools and methods to integrate best practices in project planning and management	5
		4. Facilitate project management by integrating work efforts	4		
Subdomain VI.J. Vendor/Contract Management					
1. Explain Vendor/Contract Management	2	1. Evaluate vendor contracts	5	1. Master critical negotiation skills	6
		2. Develop negotiation skills in the process of system selection	6	2. Design comparative research models for vendor solutions	6
Subdomain VI.K. Enterprise Information Management					
1. Apply knowledge of database architecture and design	3	1. Manage information as a key strategic resource and mission tool	5	1. Design enterprise-wide strategic planning and information management tools and resources for mission-critical business decisions	6
				2. Integrate business intelligence using appropriate analytic tools and methods	6
				3. Develop enterprise-wide information business plans, strategic forecasts, and operational plans	6
Supporting Body of Knowledge (Pre-requisite or Evidence of Knowledge)					
Pathophysiology and Pharmacology		Pathophysiology and Pharmacology		Pathophysiology and Pharmacology	
Anatomy and Physiology		Anatomy and Physiology		Anatomy and Physiology	
Medical Terminology		Medical Terminology		Medical Terminology	
Computer Concepts and Applications		Computer Concepts and Applications		Computer Concepts and Applications	
		Statistics		Statistics	

BLOOM'S TAXONOMY—REVISED FOR AHIMA CURRICULA MAPPING

Taxonomy Level	Category	Definition	Verbs
1	Remember	Recall facts, terms, basic concepts of previously learned material	Choose, Define, Find
2	Understand	Determine meaning and demonstrate clarity of facts and ideas	Collect, Depict, Describe, Explain, Illustrate, Recognize, Summarize
3	Apply	Use differing methods, techniques and information to acquire knowledge and/or solve problems	Adhere To, Apply, Demonstrate, Discover, Educate, Identify, Implement, Model, Organize, Plan, Promote, Protect, Report, Utilize, Validate
4	Analyze	Contribute to the examination of information in part or aggregate to identify motives and causes	Analyze, Benchmark, Collaborate, Examine, Facilitate, Format, Map, Perform, Take part In, Verify
5	Evaluate	Make judgments in support of established criteria and/or standards	Advocate, Appraise, Assess, Compare, Comply, Contrast, Determine, Differentiate, Engage, Ensure, Evaluate, Interpret, Leverage, Manage, Mitigate, Oversee, Recommend
6	Create	Generate new knowledge through innovation and assimilation of data and information	Build, Compile, Conduct, Construct, Create, Design, Develop, Forecast, Formulate, Govern, Integrate, Lead, Master, Propose

The layout for the levels and categories was adapted from Lorin W. Anderson and David R. Krathwohl's *A Taxonomy For Learning, Teaching, and Assessing,* Abridged edition, Allyn and Bacon, Boston, MA 2001.

Appendix

B

Examples of Job Descriptions

Example Job Description 1

Health Information Management (HIM) Data Analyst

I. Data Analyst

Initial Date: 01/01/2015

Review Date: 06/01/2015

Job Title: Data Analyst

Department: Health Information Management

Reporting Relationship: Reports to Data Quality Manager, Health Information Management; no direct reports

Pay Grade: Exempt, Grade VI

Job Purpose: Provide expertise to acquire, manage, manipulate, and analyze data and reports.

Job Responsibilities and Tasks:

1. Daily Operations
   - Identify data problematic areas and conduct research to determine the best course of action.
   - Analyze and problem solve issues with current and planned systems as they relate to the integration and management of patient data (for example, review for accuracy record merge and unmerge processes).
   - Analyze reports of data duplicates or other errors to provide ongoing, appropriate interdepartmental communication and monthly or daily data reports (for example, related to the electronic master patient index).
   - Monitor for timely and accurate completion of select data elements (for example, physician verbal orders).
   - Identify, analyze, and interpret trends or patterns in complex datasets.
   - Monitor data dictionary statistics.
2. Data Capture
   - Develop and maintain databases and data systems necessary for projects and department functions, in collaboration with others.
   - Acquire and abstract primary or secondary data from existing internal or external data sources.
   - Develop and implement data collection systems and other strategies that optimize statistical efficiency and data quality, in collaboration with others.
   - Perform data entry, either manually or using scanning technology, when needed or required.

3. Data Reporting
   - Interpret data and develop recommendations based on findings, in collaboration with others.
   - Develop graphs, reports, and presentations of project results.
   - Perform basic statistical analyses for projects and reports.
   - Create and present quality dashboards.
   - Generate routine and ad hoc reports.

Job Requirements and Specifications:
   - Technical expertise regarding data models and database design development
   - Understanding of XML and SQL
   - Proficiency in MS Word, Excel, Access, and PowerPoint
   - Experience using SAS, SPSS, or other statistical package is desirable for analyzing large datasets
   - Programming skills preferred; adept at queries and report writing
   - Knowledge of statistics, at least to the degree necessary in order to communicate easily with statisticians
   - Experience in data mining techniques and procedures particularly knowing when to use these techniques and procedures
   - Ability to present complex information in an understandable and compelling manner

HIA Job Competencies:

Domain I. Data Content Structure and Standards

Subdomain 1.C. Data Governance

1. Format data to satisfy integration needs—Level of Learning: Analyzing
2. Construct and maintain the standardization of data dictionaries to meet the needs of the enterprise—Level of Learning: Creating
3. Demonstrate compliance with internal and external data dictionary requirements—Level of Learning: Apply

Subdomain 1.D. Data Management

1. Analyze information needs of customers across the healthcare continuum—Level of Learning: Analyzing
2. Evaluate health information systems and data storage design—Level of Learning: Evaluating
3. Manage clinical indices, databases, and registries—Level of Learning: Evaluating
4. Apply knowledge of database architecture and design to meet organizational needs—Level of Learning: Applying
5. Evaluate data from varying sources to create meaningful presentations—Level of Learning: Evaluating

Subdomain I.E. Secondary Data Sources

1. Validate data from secondary sources to include the patient's record, including personal health records—Level of Learning: Applying

Domain III. Informatics, Analytics, and Data Use

1. Utilize technology for data collection, storage, analysis, and reporting of information—Level of Learning: Applying
2. Assess system capabilities to meet regulatory requirements—Level of Learning: Evaluating
3. Evaluate system architecture, database design, data warehousing—Level of Learning: Evaluating
4. Create the electronic structure of health data to meet a variety of end user needs—Level of Learning: Creating

Subdomain III.B. Information Management Strategic Planning

1. Take part in the development of information management plans that support the organization's current and future strategy and goals—Level of Learning: Analyzing
2. Take part in the planning, design, selection, implementation, integration, testing, evaluation, and support of health information technologies—Level of Learning: Analyzing

Subdomain III.C. Analytics and Decision Support.

1. Apply analytical results to facilitate decision making—Level of Learning: Applying
2. Apply data extraction methodologies—Level of Learning: Applying
3. Recommend organizational action based on knowledge obtained from data exploration and mining—Level of Learning: Evaluating
4. Analyze clinical data to identify trends that demonstrate quality, safety, and effectiveness of healthcare—Level of Learning: Analyzing
5. Apply knowledge of database querying and data exploration and mining techniques to facilitate information retrieval—Level of Learning: Applying
6. Evaluate administrative reports using appropriate software—Level of Learning: Evaluating

Subdomain III.D. Healthcare Statistics

1. Interpret inferential statistics—Level of Learning: Evaluating
2. Analyze statistical data for decision making—Level of Learning: Analyzing

Job Qualifications:

- Bachelor's degree in information management, healthcare information management or informatics, computing, mathematics, statistics, or related field
- Credentials preferred: RHIA
- Healthcare background or experience
- At least one year of previous data analyst experience
- Ability to work with a team in a collaborative manner

Job Context:

- Ability to work in an office environment and perform repetitive computer tasks related to data manipulation
- Potential to work from home one or two days per week

Example Job Description 2

I. Terminology Mapping Specialist

II. Clinical Data Mapping

Initial Date: 01/01/2015

Review Date: 06/01/2015

Job Title: Terminology Mapping Specialist

Department: Health Information Management

Reporting Relationship: Reports to Director of Health Information Management and Information Services; no direct report

Pay Grade: Exempt, Grade VI

Job Purpose: The terminology mapping specialist is responsible for developing and maintaining accurate and compliant administrative code set(s) mappings to the electronic health record (EHR) interface terminology, which is comprised of SNOMED CT and Intelligent Medical Objects. The code sets include but are not limited to *International Classification of Diseases, Tenth Revision, Clinical Modification (ICD-10-CM)*; and *International Classification of Diseases, Tenth Revision, Procedure Coding System (ICD-10-PCS)*, Current Procedural Terminology (CPT)-4, and Healthcare Common Procedure Coding System (HCPCS). This position contributes to terminology modeling projects and clinical code set(s) mapping within the healthcare organization.

Job Responsibilities and Tasks:

- Assign or review administrative code set mappings for interface terminology in accordance with production and release schedule updates from the electronic health record.
- Align terminologies utilized within the electronic record to appropriate semantic terminologies mapped within the interface.
- Adhere to nationally recognized correct coding guidelines for ICD-10-CM/PCS, CPT-4, and HCPCS.
- Act as an internal resource for administrative coding mapping issues and questions that arise throughout the healthcare organization.
- Support product release schedules through resolving identified coding issues within the electronic health record mapping.
- Contribute to the development of terminology and coding editorial policies and procedures.
- Provide education to clinical staff and others within the healthcare organization regarding the mapping of clinical terminologies.

Job Requirements and Specifications:

- Knowledge of SQL a plus
- Medical terminology experience preferred
- Detail-oriented
- Self-motivated
- Strong analytic skills
- Excellent written and oral communication skills
- Ability to work collaboratively and independently in a deadline-driven environment
- Stay current in industry activities focused on administrative code sets

HIA Competencies—Graduate Level:

Subdomain I.A. Classification Systems

1. Interpret terminologies, vocabularies and classification systems—Learning Level: Evaluating
2. Construct examples of mapping clinical vocabularies and terminologies to appropriate classification systems—Level of Learning: Creating

Subdomain I.B. Health Record Content and Documentation

1. Examine required documentation and record structures—Level of Learning: Applying

Subdomain I.C. Data Governance

1. Evaluate data integration needs—Level of Learning: Analyzing

Subdomain I.D. Data Management

1. Develop data management (mapping) policies—Level of Learning: Creating

Job Qualifications:

- ICD-10-CM/PCS, CPT, and HCPCS coding experience required
- Associate degree in HIT or bachelor's degree in HIM with the RHIA, RHIT, CCS, or CCS-P or CPC credentials required
- Master's degree in health informatics preferred
- Five or more years of coding experience in a variety of healthcare settings preferred
- Experience with an electronic health record preferred

Job Context:

- Offers a casual dress work environment, healthy living initiatives, and a strong benefits package including medical, dental, vision, 403B, and paid time off
- Opportunity to work from home after 3 months probationary period

Example Job Description 3

Job Title: Release of Information Specialist

Department: Health Records and the Health Information Management Department

Supervisor's Title: Release of Information Manager

General Summary

Purpose: To provide coverage for release of health information functions, including written and verbal requests for health information. Duties include: opening mail, verification of proper authorization, using Master Patient Index to obtain medical record numbers, using chart location system to locate paper charts, using EHR system to locate electronic health information, copying health information, billing for copies of health information when applicable, entering all releases into correspondence tracking system, answering telephone calls related to the release of information function and numerous other small associated duties.

Policy Setting Responsibilities: The person in this job is responsible for providing input into policies and procedures associated with the job's purpose and essential responsibilities.

Decision-Making Authority: Routine decisions include: verification of appropriate authorization, prioritizing requests, problem solving record locations, problem solving in customer service for internal and external departmental personnel.

Supervisory Responsibility: No formal supervisory responsibility.

Patient Care Provider Responsibility: None

Essential Responsibilities:

Responsibility A	Processes incoming requests for the release of information area with 98% accuracy.	Time% 15%	Relative Importance 5
Task #1: Opens and date stamps 100% of all requests received each day. Task #2: Screens each request for release of information requirements and verifies proper authorization. Task #3: Utilizes the facility computer system to obtain medical record numbers and dates of service. Task #4: Enters medical record number, name, requestor, requestor type, date received, and other data items into correspondence tracking system.			

Responsibility B	Identifies locations and retrieves medical records needed to complete release of information request with 98% accuracy.	Time% 20%	Relative Importance 5
Task #1: Locates patient charts, utilizing the chart tracking system. Task #2: Locates older charts on microfilm using the microfilm system. Task #3: Locates and obtains records from other departments not housed in the health record or HIM department			

Responsibility C	Tracks medical records during release of information request processing with 98% accuracy.	Time% 5%	Relative Importance 4
Task #1: Transfers location of chart in the chart location system. Task #2: Returns all health records to correct location.			

Responsibility D	**Processes authorizations or subpoenas with 98% accuracy.**	**Time%** 25%	**Relative Importance** 5

Task #1: Determines information requested on authorization.
Task #2: Communicates with requestor regarding possible charges.
Task #3: Photocopies requested information.
Task #4: Calculates invoice and determines whether prepayment is required.
Task #5: Determines disposition/mails out copies (pick-up/mail/overnight.)
Task #6: Completes request in the correspondence tracking system, entering date processed, documents sent, etc.

Responsibility E	**Processes STAT requests and walk-in requests the same day with 98% accuracy.**	**Time%** 10%	**Relative Importance** 4

Task #1: Stat requests are completed according to the need of the patient for patient care purposes.
Task #2: Assist walk-in requestors in filling out "Authorization for release of confidential Medical information."

Responsibility F	**Processes problem requests.**	**Time%** 5%	**Relative Importance** 4

Task #1: Researches request.
Task #2: Returns request with letters stating reason for return.
Task #3: Sends final notices on requests pending more than two months.
Task #4: Cancels unpaid prepayment requests after thee to four months.

Responsibility G	**Answers phone calls related to release of information.**	**Time%** 20%	**Relative Importance** 4

Task #1: Assists requestors with verbal continuity of care requests.
Task #2: Assists callers concerning status of requests.

Required Knowledge and Skills

Component	Description
Knowledge	Working knowledge of health record functions to include chart order or assembly, terminal digit order filing and record flow of department. Required for completely satisfactory performance in this job is knowledge of medical record format, computerized registration inquiry process and back-up manual registration system, as well as admissions process. Working knowledge of computerized access systems.
Skills	Required for completely satisfactory performance in this job is the ability to communicate effectively, provide good customer service, problem solve routine medical record issues, prioritize tasks, be punctual and dependable regarding work tasks, work independently, and pay attention to detail. Must utilize well-organized work habits along with good written and verbal communication skills, utilize electronic messaging, and perform accurate data entry, verification, updating. Computer skills proficiency required.
Formal education and experience	The formal education normally associated with completely satisfactory performance in this job is a high school diploma or the equivalent. A minimum of two years of experience in medical record department or equivalent is required.

Working Conditions

Conditions, which differ from the normal work environment, include stress when communicating with parents, patients, physicians, attorneys, telephones constantly ringing, meeting deadlines, and frequent distractions.

The above statements are intended to describe the essential responsibilities being performed by people assigned to this job. They are not intended to be an exhaustive list of the responsibilities assigned to these people.

Approved by

NAME:

TITLE:

Source: AHIMA. 2013. Release of Information Toolkit. Chicago: AHIMA. http://library.ahima.org/xpedio/groups/secure/documents/ahima/bok1_050184.pdf.

AHIMA Code of Ethics

American Health Information Management Association Code of Ethics

Preamble

The ethical obligations of the health information management (HIM) professional include the safeguarding of privacy and security of health information; disclosure of health information; development, use, and maintenance of health information systems and health information; and ensuring the accessibility and integrity of health information.

Healthcare consumers are increasingly concerned about security and the potential loss of privacy and the inability to control how their personal health information is used and disclosed. Core health information issues include what information should be collected; how the information should be handled, who should have access to the information, under what conditions the information should be disclosed, how the information is retained and when it is no longer needed, and how is it disposed of in a confidential manner. All of the core health information issues are performed in compliance with state and federal regulations, and employer policies and procedures.

Ethical obligations are central to the professional's responsibility, regardless of the employment site or the method of collection, storage, and security of health information. In addition, sensitive information (that is, genetic, adoption, drug, alcohol, sexual, health, and behavioral information) requires special attention to prevent misuse. In the world of business and interactions with consumers, expertise in the protection of the information is required.

Purpose of the American Health Information Management Association Code of Ethics

The HIM professional has an obligation to demonstrate actions that reflect values, ethical principles, and ethical guidelines. The American Health Information Management Association (AHIMA) Code of Ethics sets forth these values and principles to guide conduct. The code is relevant to all AHIMA members and CCHIIM credentialed HIM professionals [hereafter referred to as certificants], regardless of their professional functions, the settings in which they work, or the populations they serve. These purposes strengthen the HIM professional's efforts to improve overall quality of healthcare.

The AHIMA Code of Ethics serves seven purposes:

- Promotes high standards of HIM practice.
- Identifies core values on which the HIM mission is based.

- Summarizes broad ethical principles that reflect the profession's core values.
- Establishes a set of ethical principles to be used to guide decision-making and actions.
- Establishes a framework for professional behavior and responsibilities when professional obligations conflict or ethical uncertainties arise.
- Provides ethical principles by which the general public can hold the HIM professional accountable.
- Mentors practitioners new to the field to HIM's mission, values, and ethical principles.

The code includes principles and guidelines that are both enforceable and aspirational. The extent to which each principle is enforceable is a matter of professional judgment to be exercised by those responsible for reviewing alleged violations of ethical principles.

The Code of Ethics and How to Interpret the Code of Ethics

Principles and Guidelines

The following ethical principles are based on the core values of the American Health Information Management Association and apply to all AHIMA members and certificants. Guidelines included for each ethical principle are a non-inclusive list of behaviors and situations that can help to clarify the principle. They are not meant to be a comprehensive list of all situations that can occur.

I. *Advocate, uphold, and defend the individual's right to privacy and the doctrine of confidentiality in the use and disclosure of information.*

A health information management professional **shall:**

1.1. Safeguard all confidential patient information including, but not limited to, personal, health, financial, genetic, and outcome information.

1.2. Engage in social and political action that supports the protection of privacy and confidentiality, and be aware of the impact of the political arena on the health information issues for the healthcare industry.

1.3. Advocate for changes in policy and legislation to ensure protection of privacy and confidentiality, compliance, and other issues that surface as advocacy issues and facilitate informed participation by the public on these issues.

1.4. Protect the confidentiality of all information obtained in the course of professional service. Disclose only information that is directly relevant or necessary to achieve the purpose of disclosure. Release information only with valid authorization from a patient or a person legally authorized to consent on behalf of a patient or as authorized by federal or state regulations. The minimum necessary standard is essential when releasing health information for disclosure activities.

1.5. Promote the obligation to respect privacy by respecting confidential information shared among colleagues, while responding to requests from the legal profession, the media, or other non-healthcare related individuals, during presentations or teaching and in situations that could cause harm to persons.

1.6. Respond promptly and appropriately to patient requests to exercise their privacy rights (that is, access, amendments, restriction, confidential communication, and such.). Answer truthfully all patients' questions concerning their rights to review and annotate their personal biomedical data and seek to facilitate patients' legitimate right to exercise those rights.

II. *Put service and the health and welfare of persons before self-interest and conduct oneself in the practice of the profession so as to bring honor to oneself, peers, and to the health information management profession.*

A health information management professional **shall:**

2.1. Act with integrity, behave in a trustworthy manner, elevate service to others above self-interest, and promote high standards of practice in every setting.

2.2. Be aware of the profession's mission, values, and ethical principles, and practice in a manner consistent with them by acting honestly and responsibly.

2.3. Anticipate, clarify, and avoid any conflict of interest, to all parties concerned, when dealing with consumers, consulting with competitors, in providing services requiring potentially conflicting roles (for example, finding out information about one facility that would help a competitor), or serving the Association in a volunteer capacity. The conflicting roles or responsibilities must be clarified and appropriate action taken to minimize any conflict of interest.

2.4. Ensure that the working environment is consistent and encourages compliance with the AHIMA Code of Ethics, taking reasonable steps to eliminate any conditions in their organizations that violate, interfere with, or discourage compliance with the code.

2.5. Take responsibility and credit, including authorship credit, only for work they actually perform or to which they contribute. Honestly acknowledge the work of and the contributions made by others verbally or written, such as in publication.

A health information management professional **shall not**:

2.6. Permit one's private conduct to interfere with the ability to fulfill one's professional responsibilities.

2.7. Take unfair advantage of any professional relationship or exploit others to further one's own personal, religious, political, or business interests.

III. *Preserve, protect, and secure personal health information in any form or medium and hold in the highest regards health information and other information of a confidential nature obtained in an official capacity, taking into account the applicable statutes and regulations.*

A health information management professional **shall**:

3.1. Safeguard the privacy and security of written and electronic health information and other sensitive information. Take reasonable steps to ensure that health information is stored securely and that patients' data are not available to others who are not authorized to have access. Prevent inappropriate disclosure of individually identifiable information.

3.2. Take precautions to ensure and maintain the confidentiality of information transmitted, transferred, or disposed of in the event of termination, incapacitation, or death of a healthcare provider to other parties through the use of any media.

3.3. Inform recipients of the limitations and risks associated with providing services via electronic or social media (that is, computer, telephone, fax, radio, and television).

IV. *Refuse to participate in or conceal unethical practices or procedures and report such practices.*

A health information management professional **shall**:

4.1. Act in a professional and ethical manner at all times.

4.2. Take adequate measures to discourage, prevent, expose, and correct the unethical conduct of colleagues. If needed, utilize the Professional Ethics Committee Policies and Procedures for potential ethics complaints.

4.3. Be knowledgeable about established policies and procedures for handling concerns about colleagues' unethical behavior. These include policies and procedures created by AHIMA, licensing and regulatory bodies, employers, supervisors, agencies, and other professional organizations.

4.4. Seek resolution if there is a belief that a colleague has acted unethically or if there is a belief of incompetence or impairment by discussing one's concerns with the colleague when feasible and when such discussion is likely to be productive.

4.5. Consult with a colleague when feasible and assist the colleague in taking remedial action when there is direct knowledge of a health information management colleague's incompetence or impairment.

4.6. Take action through appropriate formal channels, such as contacting an accreditation or regulatory body and/or the AHIMA Professional Ethics Committee if needed.

4.7. Cooperate with lawful authorities as appropriate.

A health information management professional **shall not:**

4.8. Participate in, condone, or be associated with dishonesty, fraud and abuse, or deception. A non-inclusive list of examples includes:

— Allowing patterns of optimizing or minimizing documentation and/or coding to impact payment
— Assigning codes without physician documentation
— Coding when documentation does not justify the diagnoses or procedures that have been billed
— Coding an inappropriate level of service
— Miscoding to avoid conflict with others
— Engaging in negligent coding practices
— Hiding or ignoring review outcomes, such as performance data
— Failing to report licensure status for a physician through the appropriate channels
— Recording inaccurate data for accreditation purposes
— Allowing inappropriate access to genetic, adoption, health, or behavioral health information
— Misusing sensitive information about a competitor
— Violating the privacy of individuals

Refer to the AHIMA Standards for Ethical Coding for additional guidance.

4.9. Engage in any relationships with a patient where there is a risk of exploitation or potential harm to the patient.

V. *Advance health information management knowledge and practice through continuing education, research, publications, and presentations*.

A health information management professional **shall:**

5.1. Develop and enhance continually professional expertise, knowledge, and skills (including appropriate education, research, training, consultation, and supervision). Contribute to the knowledge base of health information management and share one's knowledge related to practice, research, and ethics.

5.2. Base practice decisions on recognized knowledge, including empirically based knowledge relevant to health information management and health information management ethics.

5.3. Contribute time and professional expertise to activities that promote respect for the value, integrity, and competence of the health information management profession. These activities may include teaching, research, consultation, service, legislative testimony, advocacy, presentations in the community, and participation in professional organizations.

5.4. Engage in evaluation and research that ensures the confidentiality of participants and of the data obtained from them by following guidelines developed for the participants in consultation with appropriate institutional review boards.

5.5. Report evaluation and research findings accurately and take steps to correct any errors later found in published data using standard publication methods.

5.6. Design or conduct evaluation or research that is in conformance with applicable federal or state laws.

5.7. Take reasonable steps to provide or arrange for continuing education and staff development, addressing current knowledge and emerging developments related to health information management practice and ethics.

VI. *Recruit and mentor students, staff, peers, and colleagues to develop and strengthen professional workforce*.

A health information management professional **shall:**

6.1. Provide directed practice opportunities for students.

6.2. Be a mentor for students, peers, and new health information management professionals to develop and strengthen skills.

6.3. Be responsible for setting clear, appropriate, and culturally sensitive boundaries for students, staff, peers, colleagues, and members within professional organizations.

6.4. Evaluate students' performance in a manner that is fair and respectful when functioning as educators or clinical internship supervisors.

6.5. Evaluate staff's performance in a manner that is fair and respectful when functioning in a supervisory capacity.

6.6. Serve an active role in developing HIM faculty or actively recruiting HIM professionals.

A health information management professional **shall not:**

6.7. Engage in any relationships with a person (that is, students, staff, peers, or colleagues) where there is a risk of exploitation or potential harm to that other person.

VII. *Represent the profession to the public in a positive manner.*

A health information management professional **shall:**

7.1. Be an advocate for the profession in all settings and participate in activities that promote and explain the mission, values, and principles of the profession to the public.

VIII. *Perform honorably health information management association responsibilities, either appointed or elected, and preserve the confidentiality of any privileged information made known in any official capacity.*

A health information management professional **shall:**

8.1. Perform responsibly all duties as assigned by the professional association operating within the bylaws and policies and procedures of the association and any pertinent laws.

8.2. Uphold the decisions made by the association.

8.3. Speak on behalf of the health information management profession and association, only while serving in the role, accurately representing the official and authorized positions of the association.

8.4. Disclose any real or perceived conflicts of interest.

8.5. Relinquish association information upon ending appointed or elected responsibilities.

8.6. Resign from an association position if unable to perform the assigned responsibilities with competence.

8.7. Avoid lending the prestige of the association to advance or appear to advance the private interests of others by endorsing any product or service in return for remuneration. Avoid endorsing products or services of a third party, for-profit entity that competes with AHIMA products and services. Care should **also** be exercised in endorsing any other products and services.

IX. *State truthfully and accurately one's credentials, professional education, and experiences.*

A health information management professional **shall:**

9.1. Make clear distinctions between statements made and actions engaged in as a private individual and as a representative of the health information management profession, a professional health information association, or one's employer.

9.2. Claim and ensure that representation to patients, agencies, and the public of professional qualifications, credentials, education, competence, affiliations, services provided, training, certification, consultation received, supervised experience, and other relevant professional experience are accurate.

9.3. Claim only those relevant professional credentials actually possessed and correct any inaccuracies occurring regarding credentials.

9.4. Report only those continuing education units actually earned for the recertification cycle and correct any inaccuracies occurring regarding CEUs.

X. *Facilitate interdisciplinary collaboration in situations supporting health information practice.*

A health information management professional **shall:**

10.1. Participate in and contribute to decisions that affect the well-being of patients by drawing on the perspectives, values, and experiences of those involved in decisions related to patients.

10.2. Facilitate interdisciplinary collaboration in situations supporting health information practice.

10.3. Establish clearly professional and ethical obligations of the interdisciplinary team as a whole and of its individual members.

10.4. Foster trust among group members and adjust behavior in order to establish relationships with teams.

XI. *Respect the inherent dignity and worth of every person.*

A health information management professional **shall:**

11.1. Treat each person in a respectful fashion, being mindful of individual differences and cultural and ethnic diversity.

11.2. Promote the value of self-determination for each individual.

11.3. Value all kinds and classes of people equitably, deal effectively with all races, cultures, disabilities, ages and genders.

11.4. Ensure all voices are listened to and respected.

The Use of the Code

Violation of principles in this code does not automatically imply legal liability or violation of the law. Such determination can only be made in the context of legal and judicial proceedings. Alleged violations of the code would be subject to a peer review process. Such processes are generally separate from legal or administrative procedures and insulated from legal review or proceedings to allow the profession to counsel and discipline its own members although in some situations, violations of the code would constitute unlawful conduct subject to legal process.

Guidelines for ethical and unethical behavior are provided in this code. The terms "shall" and "shall not" are used as a basis for setting high standards for behavior. This does not imply that everyone "shall" or "shall not" do everything that is listed. This concept is true for the entire code. If someone does the stated activities, ethical behavior is the standard. The guidelines are not a comprehensive list. For example, the statement "safeguard all confidential patient information to include, but not be limited to, personal, health, financial, genetic, and outcome information" can also be interpreted as "shall not fail to safeguard all confidential patient information to include personal, health, financial, genetic, and outcome information."

A code of ethics cannot guarantee ethical behavior. Moreover, a code of ethics cannot resolve all ethical issues or disputes or capture the richness and complexity involved in striving to make responsible choices within a moral community. Rather, a code of ethics sets forth values and ethical principles, and offers ethical guidelines to which a HIM professional can aspire and by which actions can be judged. Ethical behaviors result from a personal commitment to engage in ethical practice.

Professional responsibilities often require an individual to move beyond personal values. For example, an individual might demonstrate behaviors that are based on the values of honesty, providing service to others, or demonstrating loyalty. In addition to these, professional values might require promoting confidentiality, facilitating interdisciplinary collaboration, and refusing to participate in or conceal unethical practices. Professional values could require a more comprehensive set of values than what an individual needs to be an ethical agent in one's own personal life.

The AHIMA Code of Ethics is to be used by AHIMA members and certificants, consumers, agencies, organizations, and bodies (such as licensing and regulatory boards, insurance providers, courts of law, government agencies, and other professional groups) that choose to adopt it or use it as a frame of reference. The AHIMA Code of Ethics reflects the commitment of all to uphold the profession's values and to act ethically. Individuals of good character who discern moral questions and, in good faith, seek to make reliable ethical judgments must apply ethical principles.

The code does not provide a set of rules that prescribe how to act in all situations. Specific applications of the code must take into account the context in which it is being considered and the possibility of conflicts among the code's values, principles, and guidelines. Ethical responsibilities flow from all human relationships, from the personal and familial to the social and professional. Further, the AHIMA Code of Ethics does not specify which values, principles, and guidelines are the most important and ought to outweigh others in instances when they conflict.

Code of Ethics 2011 Ethical Principles

Ethical Principles: The following ethical principles are based on the core values of the American Health Information Management Association and apply to all AHIMA members and certificants.

A health information management professional shall:

1. *Advocate, uphold, and defend the individual's right to privacy and the doctrine of confidentiality in the use and disclosure of information.*

2. *Put service and the health and welfare of persons before self-interest and conduct oneself in the practice of the profession so as to bring honor to oneself, their peers, and to the health information management profession.*

3. *Preserve, protect, and secure personal health information in any form or medium and hold in the highest regards health information and other information of a confidential nature obtained in an official capacity, taking into account the applicable statutes and regulations.*

4. *Refuse to participate in or conceal unethical practices or procedures and report such practices.*

5. *Advance health information management knowledge and practice through continuing education, research, publications, and presentations.*

6. *Recruit and mentor students, peers, and colleagues to develop and strengthen professional workforce.*

7. *Represent the profession to the public in a positive manner.*

8. *Perform honorably health information management association responsibilities, either appointed or elected, and preserve the confidentiality of any privileged information made known in any official capacity.*

9. *State truthfully and accurately one's credentials, professional education, and experiences.*

10. *Facilitate interdisciplinary collaboration in situations supporting health information practice.*

11. *Respect the inherent dignity and worth of every person.*

Acknowledgment

Adapted with permission from the Code of Ethics of the National Association of Social Workers.

Resources

National Association of Social Workers. Code of Ethics. 1999. Available online on the NASW website.

AHIMA. Code of Ethics, 1957, 1977, 1988, 1998, and 2004.

AHIMA. Standards for Ethical Coding. 2008. Available in the AHIMA Body of Knowledge.

Harman, L.B., ed. *Ethical Challenges in the Management of Health Information,* 2nd ed. Sudbury, MA: Jones and Bartlett, 2006.

McWay, D.C. *Legal and Ethical Aspects of Health Information Management,* 3rd ed. Clifton Park, NY: Cengage Learning, 2010.

Revised & adopted by AHIMA House of Delegates—(October 2, 2011)

Copyright ©2011 by the American Health Information Management Association

AHIMA Standards of Ethical Coding

Standards of Ethical Coding

Coding professionals should:

1. Apply accurate, complete, and consistent coding practices for the production of high-quality healthcare data.

2. Report all healthcare data elements (that is, diagnosis and procedure codes, present on admission indicator, discharge status) required for external reporting purposes (that is, reimbursement and other administrative uses, population health, quality and patient safety measurement, and research) completely and accurately, in accordance with regulatory and documentation standards and requirements and applicable official coding conventions, rules, and guidelines.

3. Assign and report only the codes and data that are clearly and consistently supported by health record documentation in accordance with applicable code set and abstraction conventions, rules, and guidelines.

4. Query provider (physician or other qualified healthcare practitioner) for clarification and additional documentation prior to code assignment when there is conflicting, incomplete, or ambiguous information in the health record regarding a significant reportable condition or procedure or other reportable data element dependent on health record documentation (that is, present on admission indicator).

5. Refuse to change reported codes or the narratives of codes so that meanings are misrepresented.

6. Refuse to participate in or support coding or documentation practices intended to inappropriately increase payment, qualify for insurance policy coverage, or skew data by means that do not comply with federal and state statutes, regulations, and official rules and guidelines.

7. Facilitate interdisciplinary collaboration in situations supporting proper coding practices.

8. Advance coding knowledge and practice through continuing education.

9. Refuse to participate in or conceal unethical coding or abstraction practices or procedures.

10. Protect the confidentiality of the health record at all times and refuse to access protected health information not required for coding-related activities (examples of coding-related activities include completion of code assignment, other health record data abstraction, coding audits, and educational purposes).

11. Demonstrate behavior that reflects integrity, shows a commitment to ethical and legal coding practices, and fosters trust in professional activities.

Revised and approved by the House of Delegates, September 2008.

Resources

AHIMA Code of Ethics: http://www.ahima.org/about/ethics.asp

ICD-9-CM Official Guidelines for Coding and Reporting: http://www.cdc.gov/nchs/datawh/ftpserv/ftpicd9/ icdguide07.pdf.

AHIMA's position statement on Quality Health Data and Information: Available at http://www.ahima.org/dc/ positions.

AHIMA's position statement on Uniformity and Consistency of Healthcare Data (DRAFT).

AHIMA Practice Brief titled "Managing an Effective Query Process": http://www.ahima.org/ infocenter/briefs.asp.

How to Interpret the Standards of Ethical Coding

The following ethical principles are based on the core values of the American Health Information Management Association and the AHIMA Code of Ethics and apply to all coding professionals. Guidelines for each ethical principle include examples and situations that can help to clarify the principle. They are not meant as a comprehensive list of all situations that can occur.

1. *Apply accurate, complete, and consistent coding practices for the production of high-quality healthcare data.*

   Coding professionals and those who manage coded data shall:

   1.1. Support selection of appropriate diagnostic, procedure, and other types of health service related codes (that is, present on admission indicator, discharge status).

   Example:

   Policies and procedures are developed and used as a framework for the work process, and education and training are provided on their use.

   1.2. Develop and comply with comprehensive internal coding policies and procedures are consistent with official coding rules and guidelines and reimbursement regulations and policies, and prohibit coding practices that misrepresent the patient's medical conditions and treatment provided or are not supported by the health record documentation.

   Example:

   Code assignment resulting in misrepresentation of facts carries significant consequences.

   1.3. Participate in the development of institutional coding policies and ensure that coding policies complement, and do not conflict with, official coding rules and guidelines.

   1.4. Foster an environment that supports honest and ethical coding practices resulting in accurate and reliable data.

   Coding professionals **shall not:**

   1.5. Participate in improper preparation, alteration, or suppression of coded information.

2. *Report all healthcare data elements (that is, diagnosis and procedure codes, present on admission indicator, discharge status) required for external reporting purposes (that is, reimbursement and other administrative uses, population health, public data reporting, quality and patient safety measurement, research) completely and accurately, in accordance with regulatory and documentation standards and requirements and applicable official coding conventions, rules, and guidelines.*

   Coding professionals **shall:**

   2.1. Adhere to the ICD coding conventions, official coding guidelines approved by the Cooperating Parties,1 the CPT rules established by the American Medical Association, and any other official coding rules and guidelines established for use with mandated standard code sets.

Example:

Appropriate resource tools that assist coding professionals with proper sequencing and reporting to stay in compliance with existing reporting requirements are available and used.

2.2. Select and sequence diagnosis and procedure codes in accordance with the definitions of required data sets for applicable healthcare settings.

2.3. Comply with AHIMA's standards governing data reporting practices, including health record documentation and clinician query standards.

3. *Assign and report only the codes that are clearly and consistently supported by health record documentation in accordance with applicable code set conventions, rules, and guidelines.*

   Coding professionals **shall:**

   3.1. Apply skills, knowledge of currently mandated coding and classification systems, and official resources to select the appropriate diagnostic and procedural codes (including applicable modifiers), and other codes representing healthcare services (including substances, equipment, supplies, or other items used in the provision of healthcare services).

   Example:

   Failure to research or confirm the appropriate code for a clinical condition not indexed in the classification, or reporting a code for the sake of convenience or to affect reporting for a desired effect on the results, is considered unethical.

4. *Query provider (physician or other qualified healthcare practitioner) for clarification and additional documentation prior to code assignment when there is conflicting, incomplete, or ambiguous information in the health record regarding a significant reportable condition or procedure or other reportable data element dependent on health record documentation (that is, present on admission indicator).*

   Coding professionals **shall:**

   4.1. Participate in the development of query policies that support documentation improvement and meet regulatory, legal, and ethical standards for coding and reporting.

   4.2. Query the provider for clarification when documentation in the health record that impacts an externally reportable data element is illegible, incomplete, unclear, inconsistent, or imprecise.

   4.3. Use queries as a communication tool to improve the accuracy of code assignment and the quality of health record documentation, not to inappropriately increase reimbursement or misrepresent quality of care.

   Example:

   Policies regarding the circumstances when clinicians should be queried are designed to promote complete and accurate coding and complete documentation, regardless of whether reimbursement will be affected.

   Coding professionals **shall not:**

   4.4. Query the provider when there is no clinical information in the health record prompting the need for a query.

   Example:

   Query the provider regarding the presence of gram-negative pneumonia on every pneumonia case, regardless of whether there are any clinical indications of gram-negative pneumonia documented in the record.

5. *Refuse to change reported codes or the narratives of codes so that meanings are misrepresented.*

   Coding professionals **shall not:**

   5.1. Change the description for a diagnosis or procedure code or other reported data element so that it does not accurately reflect the official definition of that code.

Example:

The description of a code is altered in the encoding software, resulting in incorrect reporting of this code.

6. *Refuse to participate in or support coding or documentation practices intended to inappropriately increase payment, qualify for insurance policy coverage, or skew data by means that do not comply with federal and state statutes, regulations, and official rules and guidelines.*

Coding professionals **shall:**

6.1. Select and sequence the codes such that the organization receives the optimal payment to which the facility is legally entitled, remembering that it is unethical and illegal to increase payment by means that contradict regulatory guidelines.

Coding professionals **shall not:**

6.2. Misrepresent the patient's clinical picture through intentional incorrect coding or omission of diagnosis or procedure codes, or the addition of diagnosis or procedure codes unsupported by health record documentation, to inappropriately increase reimbursement, justify medical necessity, improve publicly reported data, or qualify for insurance policy coverage benefits.

Examples:

A patient has a health plan that excludes reimbursement for reproductive management or contraception; so rather than report the correct code for admission for tubal ligation, it is reported as a medically necessary condition with performance of a salpingectomy. The narrative descriptions of both the diagnosis and procedures reflect an admission for tubal ligation and the procedure (tubal ligation) is displayed on the record.

A code is changed at the patient's request so that the service will be covered by the patient's insurance.

Coding professionals **shall not:**

6.3. Inappropriately exclude diagnosis or procedure codes in order to misrepresent the quality of care provided.

Examples:

Following a surgical procedure, a patient acquired an infection due to a break in sterile procedure; the appropriate code for the surgical complication is omitted from the claims submission to avoid any adverse outcome to the institution.

Quality outcomes are reported inaccurately in order to improve a healthcare organization's quality profile or pay-for-performance results.

7. *Facilitate interdisciplinary collaboration in situations supporting proper coding practices.*

Coding professionals **shall:**

7.1. Assist and educate physicians and other clinicians by advocating proper documentation practices, further specificity, and re-sequence or include diagnoses or procedures when needed to more accurately reflect the acuity, severity, and the occurrence of events.

Example:

Failure to advocate for ethical practices that seek to represent the truth in events as expressed by the associated code sets when needed is considered an intentional disregard of these standards.

8. *Advance coding knowledge and practice through continuing education.*

Coding professionals **shall:**

8.1. Maintain and continually enhance coding competency (that is, through participation in educational programs, reading official coding publications such as the Coding Clinic for ICD-9-CM, and maintaining professional certifications) in order to stay abreast of changes in codes, coding guidelines, and regulatory and other requirements.

9. *Refuse to participate in or conceal unethical coding practices or procedures.*

   Coding professionals **shall:**

   9.1. Act in a professional and ethical manner at all times.

   9.2. Take adequate measures to discourage, prevent, expose, and correct the unethical conduct of colleagues.

   9.3. Be knowledgeable about established policies and procedures for handling concerns about colleagues' unethical behavior. These include policies and procedures created by AHIMA, licensing and regulatory bodies, employers, supervisors, agencies, and other professional organizations.

   9.4. Seek resolution if there is a belief that a colleague has acted unethically or if there is a belief of incompetence or impairment by discussing their concerns with the colleague when feasible and when such discussion is likely to be productive. Take action through appropriate formal channels, such as contacting an accreditation or regulatory body and/or the AHIMA Professional Ethics Committee.

   9.5. Consult with a colleague when feasible and assist the colleague in taking remedial action when there is direct knowledge of a health information management colleague's incompetence or impairment.

   Coding professionals **shall not:**

   9.6. Participate in, condone, or be associated with dishonesty, fraud and abuse, or deception. A non-exhaustive list of examples includes:

   — Allowing inappropriate patterns of retrospective documentation to avoid suspension or increase reimbursement

   — Assigning codes without supporting provider (physician or other qualified healthcare practitioner) documentation

   — Coding when documentation does not justify the diagnoses and/or procedures that have been billed

   — Coding an inappropriate level of service

   — Miscoding to avoid conflict with others

   — Adding, deleting, and altering health record documentation

   — Copying and pasting another clinician's documentation without identification of the original author and date

   — Knowingly reporting incorrect present on admission indicator

   — Knowingly reporting incorrect patient discharge status code

   — Engaging in negligent coding practices

10. *Protect the confidentiality of the health record at all times and refuse to access protected health information not required for coding-related activities (examples of coding-related activities include completion of code assignment, other health record data abstraction, coding audits, and educational purposes).*

    Coding professionals **shall:**

    10.1. Protect all confidential information obtained in the course of professional service, including personal, health, financial, genetic, and outcome information.

    10.2. Access only that information necessary to perform their duties.

11. *Demonstrate behavior that reflects integrity, shows a commitment to ethical and legal coding practices, and fosters trust in professional activities.*

    Coding professionals **shall:**

    11.1. Act in an honest manner and bring honor to self, peers, and the profession.

    11.2. Truthfully and accurately represent their credentials, professional education, and experience.

11.3. Demonstrate ethical principles and professional values in their actions to patients, employers, other members of the healthcare team, consumers, and other stakeholders served by the healthcare data they collect and report.

[1]The Cooperating Parties are the American Health Information Management Association, American Hospital Association, Centers for Medicare and Medicaid Services, and National Center for Health Statistics.

Source: AHIMA House of Delegates. 2008 (Sept.) "AHIMA Standards on Ethical Coding."

Case Studies in Health Information Management

Case Study 1: Mergers and Acquisitions

Objectives

- Evaluate the centralization of health information management (HIM) services as required by the acquisition of one hospital by a larger hospital.
- Develop mission and vision statements for the new University Health Systems (UHS) HIM department.
- Create a new organizational chart for the new UHS HIM department.
- Assess the impact of centralizing HIM functions between the two merged HIM departments utilizing Kotter's change model.
- Analyze the coding job descriptions and develop one job description that covers all coding job tasks and incorporates appropriate coding job productivity and quality standards.
- Develop an orientation checklist that will be utilized by all HIM employees to orient them to the new UHS HIM department.

Instructions

Review the case study below and complete the deliverables utilizing content available within the chapters of the text. The following chapters may be used: chapter 4, chapter 6, chapter 9, and chapter 10.

Scenario

Sarah, HIM director at University Hospital was recently informed by her boss, the chief financial officer (CFO), that the healthcare organization acquired a local hospital, Memorial Community Hospital. This acquired hospital is located 25 miles away from University Hospital. Most of the HIM functions from Memorial Community Hospital will be centralized into University Hospital by the end of the fiscal year. Functions such as coding, transcription, chart completion, and data quality review will be moved and centralized to the main hospital campus; an HIM satellite station will stay open on the Memorial Community Hospital site to deal with release of information (ROI) requests. Patient care services will remain the same at Memorial Community Hospital to serve the population that currently utilizes this facility for care.

The name of the new, combined organization is University Health Systems (UHS). The UHS Executive Management Team shared the mission and vision of the newly merged healthcare organization.

UHS Mission Statement: UHS will provide quality, cost-effective, collaborative, and integrative healthcare services to its surrounding community with an emphasis on compassion and education.

UHS Vision Statement: UHS will be the healthcare system of choice for both consumers and providers.

University Hospital's HIM Organizational Structure

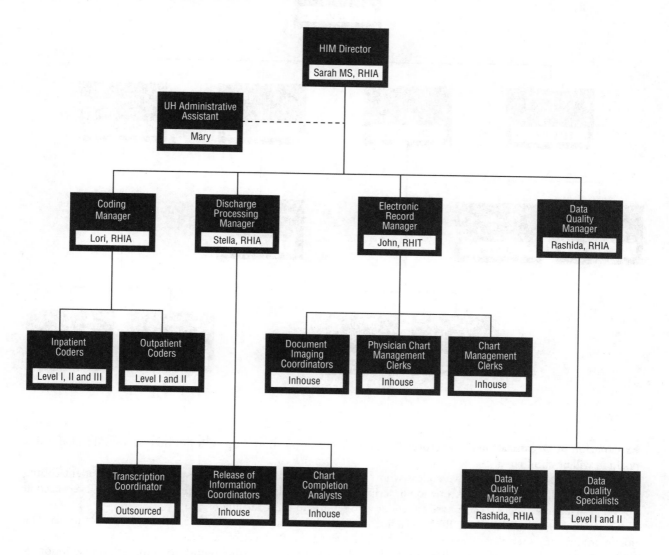

Explanation of Organizational Structure: The discharge processing manager has two chart completion analysts and eight ROI coordinators who report to her. The transcription coordinator does not have any direct reports but she coordinates all of the outsourced transcription and reports to the discharge processing manager.

The electronic record manager has eight chart management clerks, three document imaging coordinators and two physician chart management clerks who report to him.

The data quality manager has four data quality specialists who report to her. They perform data integrity tasks for the entire HIM Department.

The coding manager has eight inpatient coders and eight outpatient coders who report to her.

University Hospital Coding Productivity and Quality Standards:
Inpatient Coders—4 charts per hour with 95 percent accuracy
Outpatient Coders—6 charts per hour with 95 percent accuracy

Memorial Community Hospital Organizational Structure

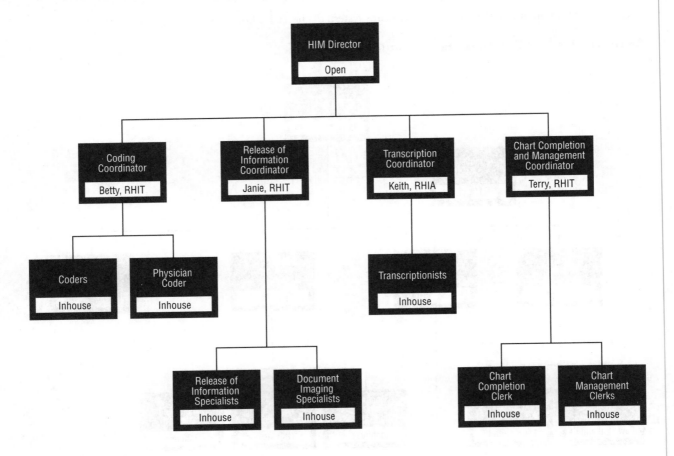

Explanation of Organizational Structure: The HIM manager position is open. It has not yet been decided if this position will be eliminated.

The coding coordinator has five coders who report to her and perform both inpatient and outpatient coding tasks. These coding positions have one job description that only has one level as opposed to multiple levels used at University Hospital. There is one physician coder who reports to this coordinator.

The ROI coordinator has three ROI specialists and two documenting imaging specialists who report to her. The document imaging specialists also perform copying of records for ROI as time allows.

The transcription coordinator has three medical transcriptionists who report to him. All transcription is performed within the hospital.

The chart completion and management coordinator has two chart completion clerks and three chart management clerks who report to her. The chart completion clerks perform chart analysis and the chart management clerks retrieve medical records for ROI coordinators and for other areas within the health system.

Memorial Community Hospital Coding Productivity and Quality Standards
Coder—Codes both inpatient and outpatient records 5 charts per hour with 98 percent accuracy
Physician Coder—Codes all physician services and 10 charts per hour with 98 percent accuracy

Assumptions

- The HIM manager position at Memorial Community Hospital is open so the HIM director for this new, combined department will be Sarah, MS, RHIA—HIM director of University Health Systems.
- As an electronic health record (EHR) is utilized by the combined UHS, all HIM functions, except for ROI at the satellite office at the Memorial Community Hospital site, will be centralized within the HIM department at University Hospital. Memorial Community Hospital HIM employees will physically move to University Hospital except for four employees who will remain at an HIM Release of Information Satellite Center. The new UHS HIM department has been allotted additional space to accommodate all the employees who will be moving.
- UHS will no longer provide physician coding services.
- Memorial Community Hospital has not been utilizing an EHR; they use a document imaging product with some paper records. Memorial Community Hospital will convert to the EHR with integration of the document imaging into the EHR. Paper records will remain at the Memorial Community Hospital site.
- Outpatient services will continue to be provided at the Memorial Community Hospital site. There will be additional space for physician offices but HIM will not manage these records.

Deliverables

1. Create new mission and vision statements for the combined HIM department.
2. Develop an updated organizational chart that combines all the functions of both departments into a centralized UHS HIM department. Provide a brief written description of the new organizational chart. Include the rationale to align the jobs as depicted by the new organizational chart. Make sure to identify the HIM management team in this description and decide whether or not an additional HIM manager is needed within the new organizational structure.
3. Use Kotter's change management model (chapter 4) to discuss what the HIM management team (identified above) will mostly like face in regards to centralization of the HIM services. Create an outline describing each step of Kotter's change management module and how the merging of these two HIM departments will be impacted. Make sure that the outline includes a brief description of the type of behaviors that may be exhibited by employees within each step of the module and how management will communicate changes through each step of the model.
4. Develop one job description that combines the different coding job roles identified at both hospitals above into one position that has two different levels: I and II. Utilize one of the job description templates provided within appendix B of this text as a guide when creating the new job description. Make sure to include updated standards for coding quality and productivity within the job description.
5. Develop an orientation checklist (chapter 9) that will be utilized by all HIM employees to orient them to the new UHS merged HIM department.

Case Study 2: The Remote Health Information Management Department

Objectives

- Assess the strengths, weaknesses, opportunities and threats associated with developing a remote HIM department.
- Report on the best practices for managing HIM functions remotely.
- Create a procedure for evaluating the quality and quantity of work performed by remote workers.
- Create a training session to prepare HIM employees to successfully work remotely.

Instructions

Review the case scenario below and complete the required deliverables utilizing content from the following chapters: chapter 2, chapter 8, chapter 9.

Scenario

The HIM department at University Hospital is running out of space for all of its employees. The department is not physically located on the same property as the main hospital so many functions within the department are managed at a remote site. Lindsey, the director of HIM, has been networking with some of her HIM colleagues and found that many have their employees work remotely. Lindsey reports to the chief financial officer (CFO) who feels that Lindsey should perform a thorough analysis of all the job functions prior to assigning all of her workforce to work from home. The CFO also feels that further research should be performed by Lindsey in regards to the best practices associated with a remote HIM workforce. The current functions performed by the HIM department are outlined below along with general information about the typical tasks for each function and the number of staff performing the tasks.

HIM Current Functions

HIM Function	Location	Typical Tasks	Staff Performing Tasks
HIM staff management	In-house	Manages day to day functions of the tasks outlined below. • Communicates with employees via email and in person meetings. • Utilizes electronic systems for managing and assigning work performed by employees.	HIM director HIM manager HIM coding manager
Coding	In-house All coders currently work onsite. The number of coding staff has grown by about 30% over the last year so desk space is at a premium.	Code all inpatient and outpatient encounters utilizing the her. All coding lists are managed electronically by coding staff and the coding manager.	Inpatient and outpatient coders (10 total) report to the coding manager.
Transcription	Outsourced	Reports are electronically interfaced into the EHR by the transcription vendor	The transcription coordinator reviews interface logs to ensure the appropriate transfer of data takes place between the transcription company and the EHR. Reports to the HIM manager.

HIM Function	Location	Typical Tasks	Staff Performing Tasks
Release of information (ROI)	In-house	ROI coordinators perform the ROI function utilizing the EHR. There are still some paper records on site and at remote storage. ROI coordinators retrieve information as needed and make paper or electronic copies. ROI staff also manage the patient information desk and handle in-person and phone requests.	ROI coordinators (5 total) report to the HIM manager
Chart completion	In-house	All chart completion processes are managed utilizing electronic worklists. Chart completion analysts contact physicians regarding online chart completion via a work basket.	Chart completion analysts (2 total) report to the HIM manager
Data quality	In-house	Duplicate record clean up. Coding quality analysis. Interface management of scanned documents. All of these tasks are performed utilizing electronic worklists.	Data quality specialists (6 total) 2 report to the HIM coding manager 4 report to the HIM manager
Document imaging and chart management	In-house	All imaging of documents that cannot be created electronically are performed by the document imaging staff. Chart management clerks pull paper records and charts for ROI and for caregivers as requested. The portion of paper records on site has decreased over the past few years.	Document imaging coordinators (2 total) and chart management clerks (3 total) report to the HIM manager

Assumptions

- The information services department is willing to set up the appropriate health information systems so that work can be performed safely and securely at home for the selected HIM employees.
- The CFO will support Lindsey's decision for a remote HIM workforce as long as she performs a SWOT analysis (chapter 2) and a thorough research of best practices.

Deliverables

1. Perform a SWOT analysis that outlines the appropriate items for creating a remote HIM department. An example is provided in chapter 2.

2. Create a report (no more than two pages) to the CFO that outlines which HIM functions could be managed from home and which functions will need to stay located within the HIM office. Research the best practices associated with the functions that are selected to be managed from home and explain how to incorporate these practices into managing a remote workforce. Evaluate whether or not HIM management staff can work

remotely as well and if so, outline the portion of time each manager may work at home. Provide appropriate references for the researched articles.

3. Choose one HIM function mentioned above and develop a procedure for evaluating the quality and quantity of work performed by a remote workforce. This procedure will include the tools that will be utilized to evaluate the quality and quantity of work, the frequency of monitoring the work, and outcomes if employees are performing below agreed upon job standards of quality and quantity. Use the job procedure template in chapter 2.

4. Develop a training session that prepares the selected HIM employees to work from home. Create an outline of all the items that need to be included within the training session based on the best practices found when researching managing remote workers. Utilize a presentation product and create slides for the presentation based on the outline. The presentation should utilize good slide format with a title and five to six bullet items on each slide. The second slide of the presentation should include learning objectives for the audience. The presentation should include no more than 10 to 12 slides with a summary slide that allows for questions. The final slide in the presentation should include references.

Case Study 3: Health Information Management Department Technology Needs

Objectives

- Evaluate whether an application specialist should be located within the HIM department or the information services department.
- Outline the proposed critical conversation needed between two different managers based on the scenario provided.
- Select an appropriate job analysis method for a new position.
- Create a new job title and job summary for a new HIM position.
- Develop interview questions to be used during the interview process for a new HIM position.
- Evaluate the candidate pool for the new HIM position based on appropriate candidate selection criteria.

Instructions

Review the case study and develop the deliverables outlined below utilizing content from the following chapters: chapter 4, chapter 5, chapter 6, chapter 7.

Scenario

The EHR was implemented by University Hospital two years ago and management of the HIM information systems was provided by the information services department. The individual that has been performing information technology (IT) functions in regards to the HIM systems is leaving the hospital and the HIM director, Kate, feels this is an opportunity to move the position into the HIM department. The director of IT, Richard, feels they are doing a competent job and the position should stay within IT. The HIM information systems maintained are as follows:

- Digital transcription
- Encoder and abstracting
- ROI
- Computer assisted coding

Kate feels these applications would be better serviced by an HIM professional who has IT experience along with HIM knowledge. Also, HIM productivity has been impacted because of the physical location of the IT department and the lack of quick response from the assigned IT specialist when the HIM department has issues with the systems.

Assumptions

- All HIM applications must be managed by the same individual. It is more important that the individual who manages the applications have a familiarity with HIM processes rather than IT experience.
- The outcome of the critical conversation between Kate and Richard is that the position will be moved to the HIM department.

Deliverables

Part 1

Create a plan for managing the critical conversation that needs to take place between Kate and Richard in regards to moving the position to the HIM department. Use Kate's perspective in developing the conversation plan. Refer to the steps for planning a critical conversation detailed in chapter 4 to make sure all aspects of the conversation plan are covered.

Part 2

1. Choose three different job analysis methods discussed in chapter 6 to collect data for the proposed new HIM application specialist position. For each method, explain the chosen method, and describe the method process for analyzing the application specialist position.

2. Create a new job title and job summary the human resources (HR) department will use to recruit for candidates for this new HIM position.

3. Result: The HR department posted the job internally but received no qualified applicants. The job was posted externally and there are three qualified applicants who meet the basic requirements of the position. The following resumes were screened by HR and meet the minimum requirements of the position:

    a. Rhonda, a 28-year-old Hispanic female who has worked with a health information systems vendor since graduating from a Registered Health Information Administration (RHIA) program five years ago. She has not specifically worked within an HIM department but she has worked with health information system installs at a variety of organizations. She is RHIA-eligible although she has not yet taken the RHIA examination. She does have several Health Information Technology Professional (HITPRO) certifications. Rhonda shared in her cover letter that she is a single parent and the caregiver for her elderly mother.

    b. Tom, a 55-year-old white male, recently graduated from the local community college with an associate's degree in health information technology. He passed the Registered Health Information Technician (RHIT) examination two months ago. Tom completed his practicum within the HIM department at University Hospital. He called in sick several times during his practicum because of chronic pulmonary issues. He also was often late to work. Prior to obtaining his associate's degree, he had worked within the IT department of a large manufacturer for approximately ten years.

    c. Laurie is a 39-year-old white female with a bachelor's degree in HIM and the RHIA credential. She has approximately ten years of experience as the coding manager at a large multi-specialty physician clinic. She recently relocated to town because of her husband's job transfer. She does not have much experience with IT other than coding products. Of note, her husband's best friend is the chief operating officer of University Hospital. He shared with Kate that Laurie has five children, ages 3, 6, 9, 10, and 12, who participate in many activities and her husband travels for his job so he is not home very often during the week.

Part 3

1. Develop three interview questions to ask of each candidate during a structured interview; each candidate will be asked the same three questions. Consider when developing these questions how to assess the candidates' actual computer technical skills in regards to maintaining HIM applications.

2. Identify, for each candidate, the topics that cannot be addressed during the interview process or considered when selecting an applicant for the position. Be sure to name the appropriate law which prohibits discussion of the topic.

3. Given only the information above, which candidate should be hired and why? Choose among the three candidates; continuing to recruit for the position is not an option. Remember that all three candidates meet the minimum qualifications for the position.

Chapter 1

1. C
2. D
3. A
4. B
5. A
6. B
7. A
8. C
9. B
10. C

Chapter 2

1. A
2. C
3. D
4. B
5. B
6. D
7. C
8. B
9. C
10. B

Chapter 3

1. B
2. C
3. C
4. C
5. C
6. B
7. A
8. C
9. A
10. C

Chapter 4

1. A
2. C
3. C
4. D
5. C
6. B
7. A
8. B
9. A
10. D

Chapter 5

1. C
2. C
3. B
4. A
5. D
6. C
7. A
8. B
9. A
10. C

Chapter 6

1. C
2. B
3. D
4. C
5. B
6. D
7. A
8. A
9. D
10. B

Chapter 7

1. C
2. C
3. D
4. A
5. D
6. A
7. C
8. A
9. B
10. B

Chapter 8

1. B
2. A
3. D
4. D
5. A
6. A
7. B
8. C
9. C
10. C

Chapter 9

1. A
2. B
3. B
4. C
5. B
6. C
7. A
8. B
9. C
10. D

Chapter 10

1. D
2. C
3. B
4. B
5. A
6. D
7. C
8. D
9. B
10. A

Glossary

Ability: The capacity to effectively engage in activities outlined by the job description

Acceptance view of authority: Management concept that is evident in organizations when an employee considers a request by the manager to be in the best interest of the group, is understandable, and meets the employee's personal interests

Active listening: Occurs when an individual makes a conscious effort to hear and understand the message being conveyed

ADDIE: An effective, step-by-step method of training program design; the acronym for the steps stands for analysis, design, development, implementation, and evaluation

ADKAR model: A change management model that is utilized to assess individual change management issues; five building blocks—awareness, desire, knowledge, ability and reinforcement in regards to the change initiative—are necessary components for individuals to understand in order to participate in change

Administrative management: A management theory that attempts to identify the design of an organization and is associated with the following principles: (1) requires a formalized administrative structure where there are clear lines of authority marked as a hierarchical structure; (2) defines a clear division of labor among workers; (3) reflects delegation of power and authority to upper management

Adoption of innovation: Relates to how individuals adapt to the situations presented to them

Affinity groups: Formed by employees with common interests, these groups come together for a specific purpose such as mentoring, continuing education, or participation in a service project

Age Discrimination in Employment Act (ADEA): Legislation that prohibits discrimination on the basis of age against individuals age 40 and older

Americans with Disabilities Act (ADA): Passed in 1990 and amended in 2008 with passage of the Americans with Disabilities Act Amendment Act (ADAAA), this legislation prohibits job discrimination against people with disabilities

Anchoring: Making the first offer in a negotiation and this is the foundation the rest of the negotiation builds upon

Arbitration: A proceeding in which disputes are submitted to a third party or a panel of experts and the arbitrator makes the final decision

Asynchronous: Web-based training that occurs at different times, meaning the instructor and students are not present at the same time

Audio conferencing: A learning technique in which participants in different locations can learn together via telephone lines while listening to a presenter and looking at handouts or books

Auditory learners: Learners who use the sense of hearing to best learn new material

Authoritarian leader: Leader who dictates activities to the workgroup but he or she does not participate in the completion of the activities; the authoritarian is very critical of the team's results

Authoritarian management: A management style in which the leader dictates policies and procedures, decides what goals are to be achieved, and directs and controls all activities without any meaningful participation by the subordinates

Authority: The right to make decisions and take actions necessary to carry out assigned tasks

Autocratic leadership style: Leadership style characterized by leader control over all decisions with no or very little input from the workgroup; this style is beneficial when decisions need to be made quickly by the leader

Backcasting: The process of deciding on a goal and then working backwards to determine from the current state what steps need to be taken to achieve the goal

Behavioral theories of leadership: Leadership theories that focus on the study of specific behaviors of leaders

Benchmarking: A measurement that takes into account the quality aspect of completing a job task from start to finish

Blended learning: A training strategy that uses a combination of techniques—such as lecture, web-based training, or programmed text—to appeal to a variety of learning styles and maximize the advantages of each training method

Bona fide occupational qualification (BFOQ): A job requirement that in most jobs would be illegal to discuss, but in specific jobs is a necessity

Bonus: A reward given related to the performance of an entire organization or individual

Bridge employment: A job that an individual takes between leaving their full-time position and beginning full-time retirement; the job could be part-time in the same organization or in the same field, part-time in a new field, self-employment, or even temporary work

Bridges' transition model: Developed by William Bridges and published in his 1991 book "Managing Transitions," this model provides a guide for how individuals' experience change by transitioning through different phases: Stage 1—Ending, losing, and letting go, Stage 2—The neutral zone, and Stage 3—The new beginning

Budget: A plan that converts the organization's goals and objectives into targets for revenue and spending; a budget describes, in dollars and cents, what fiscal resources will be necessary to meet the goals and objectives

C-suite: Position titles at this level are chief executive officer (CEO), chief operating officer (COO), chief financial officer (CFO), chief information officer (CIO), chief medical officer (CMO) and chief nursing officer (CNO); this level of management is responsible for decisions that affect the entire organization, focusing on the big picture and the long-term success of the organization

Chain of command: A hierarchical reporting structure within an organization

Change: To make or become different

Change agent: The individual or group that undertakes the task of initiating and managing change in an organization

Change initiatives: External or internal changes to the healthcare organization

Change management: The formal process of introducing change (becoming different), getting it adopted, and diffusing it throughout the organization

Charismatic authority: Embodies a leader who has the capacity to influence subordinates

Civil Rights Act of 1964: An antidiscrimination law that prohibits employment discrimination because of race, color, religion, sex, or national origin

Civil Rights Act of 1991: Upholds and strengthens the Civil Rights Act of 1964 under which an employee has the right to make a claim for discrimination against their employer; the EEOC then investigates the claim, and makes a decision and if discrimination is found to have occurred, depending on the charge, the employee could receive back pay, be reinstated, or awarded a promotion; the Civil Rights Act of 1991 takes possible actions by the employee farther, by allowing for jury trials and increased monetary awards for employees

Coaching: A method in which an experienced person gives advice to a less-experienced worker on a formal or informal basis

Coercive power: This type of formal power is granted to an individual who has the ability to punish employees for not doing what was requested of them; punishment my come in the form of a demotion, poor performance appraisal, or an undesirable work assignment

Collaboration: The relationships and interactions that occur between co-workers within an organization

Collaborative performance appraisals: Appraisals that engage employees within the process of evaluating work performed by requiring managers to solicit input from employees about actual work performance

Committee: A body of persons delegated to consider, investigate, take action on, or report on some matter

Communication: Process of using words, sounds, signs, or behaviors to exchange or share information

Compensable factors: Characteristics used to compare the worth of a job (skill, effort, responsibility, or working conditions)

Compensatory damages: Financial reward that cover the actual financial loss of the employee; compensatory damages could cover repayment for lost time off work, or payment for medical bills

Competency model: A method of evaluating competencies for particular job tasks and applying them within the job framework

Compressed workweek: A work schedule that permits a full-time job to be completed in less than the standard five days of eight-hour shifts

Computer-assisted coding (CAC): The process of extracting and translating diagnostic and procedural information from electronic health records into ICD and CPT evaluation and management codes for billing and coding purposes

Conflict: A clash between hostile or opposing elements, ideas, or forces; any difference in opinion, value, need, or want that causes frustration in one or more interdependent people and blocks them from achieving their tasks or goals

Conflict management: A problem-solving technique that focuses on working with individuals to find a mutually acceptable solution

Consolidated Omnibus Budget Reconciliation Act (COBRA): Legislation that offers continuing health insurance coverage for qualifying employees that have lost healthcare coverage

Consultative leadership: Task-oriented leadership that focuses on getting input from those who perform the tasks; the ultimate decisions for the group are still made by the leader but this leadership style takes into account the feedback provided by individual workers

Contemporary management: Management style that uses current or present period practices to plan, organize, and control individuals within an organization

Contingency approach: Approach to effective leadership that is dependent on matching the leader's style to the workplace situation

Contingent reward leadership style: An active and positive exchange between employees and managers whereby employees are rewarded or recognized for accomplishing agreed-upon performance objectives

Continuing education (CE): Training that enables employees to remain current with advancing knowledge in their profession

Controlling: The monitoring and correcting of organizational, departmental, and individual performance so goals and objectives are met; controlling is dependent on goals, objectives, and key indicators being set during the planning phase

Corrective action plan: A written plan of action to be taken in response to identified issues

Cost-of-living adjustments (COLA): Generally pay increases tied to a change in the consumer price index (CPI) published by the US Department of Labor, which measures purchasing power between time periods (usually one year)

Credential: A formal agreement granting an individual permission to practice in a profession that is usually conferred by a national professional organization dedicated to a specific area of healthcare practice

Critical incident method: Method that involves maintaining a log or documentation of critical incidences, both positive and negative, throughout each employee's performance cycle

Cross-functional teams: Teams that are made up of members from different departments; also known as interdisciplinary teams

Cross-training: A method in which employees learn a job other than their primary responsibility

Dashboard: A report of process measures to help leaders follow progress to assist with strategic planning; a quick snapshot of the status of key performance indicators

Delegation: The process by which managers distribute work to others along with the authority to make decisions and take action

Demand-control model of job strain: Originating from the use of the job content questionnaire, this scale is calculated from score results of the questions related to decision latitude and psychological demands of the job

Democratic leader: Leader who assists and encourages the workgroup, allows the workgroup to select activities to be completed as a group, and praises the group at completion of the work

Department-level orientation: Level of new hire orientation that follows the organization-level orientation to educate the new employee to the ways of the department in which he or she will be spending their work day

Development: The career-focused process of progressing within one's profession or occupation

Diary or log method: A job analysis tool that requires employees to complete a daily diary or log of all job tasks completed within a set period of time

Diffusion of innovation theory: Theory that explains how a typical population embraces the adoption of innovation or adoption of change

Distance learning: A learning delivery mode in which the instructor, the classroom, and the students are not all present in the same location at the same time

DMAIC approach: A Six Sigma problem-solving framework; it is an acronym that stands for: define the opportunity for improvement, measure current performance, analyze the opportunity, improve the opportunity, and control performance after improvements are made

Downward communication: Communication that occurs when information moves from the upper levels of an organization to the lower levels

Due process: The employee has the right to make sure their disciplinary action was carried out in accordance with the organization's policies and procedures

Dysfunctional turnover: Occurs when valued or highly skilled employees leave the organization or a number of employees leave a critical work area

Early adopters: Individuals who are the change leaders within the organization; they are a little more cautious than the innovators

Early majority: Those individuals within the organization who tend to adopt change quicker than the average person but are not considered innovators or early adopters

Electronic PHI (ePHI): Protected health information transmitted by electronic records or media, and maintained in electronic records or media

Emergent change: A continuous, open-end process of adaptation to changing circumstances and conditions

Employment-at-will: employees can be fired at any time and for almost any reason based on the idea that, in turn, employees can quit at any time and for almost any reason

Environmental scan: A systematic and continuous effort to search for important cues about how the world is changing outside and inside the organization

Equal Employment Opportunity Commission (EEOC): A federal agency with the authority to investigate discrimination claims, render decisions, and file lawsuits if necessary; the EEOC works to prevent discrimination through training and education on employment laws

Equity theory: Motivation theory that suggests that employees are motivated by the balance of their inputs in relation to their outputs as compared to both their employer and other workers

Essay evaluation method: Method that requires that the manager develop an employee appraisal by qualitatively identifying the strong and weak points of each employee's behavior and documenting each of these items in a written essay

Ethics: A field of study that deals with moral principles, theories, and values

Expert power: A type of personal power in which power is perceived in an individual, regardless of their position, who is a subject matter expert

External candidates: Job candidates who are individuals from outside of the organization

External change agent: individual such as an external consultant who is employed by the organization temporarily to escort the organization through the change

External forces: The influences, resources, and activities that exist outside of the healthcare organization but significantly impact and affect HIM

Extrinsic: External motivating factors are tangible and obvious to others

Factor comparison: Job evaluation method that breaks down each job into compensable factors and assigns a dollar value

Fair Labor Standards Act (FLSA): More commonly known as the wage and hour law, this federal law is the basis for many state wage and hour laws; the intent of the FLSA is to determine minimum wage and overtime pay rules as well as definition of a work week

Family and Medical Leave Act (FMLA): Legislation that allows employees to take unpaid time off work for specific family and medical reasons

Flextime: A work schedule that gives employees some choice in the pattern of their work hours, usually around a core of midday hours

Forced ranking: Methodology that ranks employees in terms of forced allocations meaning that only 10 to 20 percent of the employees' performance will fall into the higher levels of job performance, 70 to 80 percent will fall into the middle ranges of job performance, and the rest will fall into the lowest levels of job performance

Formal teams: Teams that structured, assigned a charter, and usually proceed with meetings, minutes, and agendas

Functional turnover: Occurs when poor performing or disruptive employees leave the organization or when an organization downsizes out of financial necessity

Gantt chart: A bar chart that allows project managers to plan and control projects at a glance

Goal-setting theory: Theory based on the premise that employees respond best when goals are clearly defined and feedback is provided about goal progress

Grade level assignment: Information that sets forth the criteria between or among the various levels of jobs within an organization that represent the pay level of the position

Graphic rating scales: The most common methodology employed in HIM departments, checks or monitoring are conducted on an employee's performance throughout the performance cycle; content of the performance monitoring includes quantity of work, quality of work, dependability, judgment and critical thinking, cooperation, and initiative or motivation

Great man theory: The most documented trait theory; it notes that certain traits within individuals can be identified as predictors for effective leadership and that by studying great historical leaders, individual traits can clearly be identified as keys for success in leadership

Headhunters: Professionals who seek out job openings and match specific individuals to specific jobs

Health Insurance Portability and Accountability Act (HIPAA): The federal legislation enacted to provide continuity of health coverage, control fraud and abuse in healthcare, reduce healthcare costs, and guarantee the security and privacy of health information; limits exclusion for pre-existing medical conditions, prohibits discrimination against employees and dependents based on health status, guarantees availability of health insurance to small employers, and guarantees renewability of insurance to all employees regardless of size; requires covered entities (most healthcare providers and organizations) to transmit healthcare claims in a specific format and to develop, implement, and comply with the standards of the Privacy Rule and the Security Rule

Herzberg's two-factor theory: Also known as the *motivation-hygiene theory*, Herzberg identified two motivational elements—motivators (satisfiers) and hygiene factors (dissatisfiers)

Hostile work environment: Environment that occurs when one employee's behavior is interpreted as being offensive by another employee

Humanistic management: Management theory in which individual human needs and human values are considered within the management of an organization and where three key dimensions must be considered: (1) human dignity is the key element of consideration; (2) ethical complexities are evaluated; and (3) all stakeholders must be involved in the decision-making process

Hygiene factors: Elements that can provide job dissatisfaction to employees and consist of company policies, supervision, working conditions, and financial rewards

Incentive effect: How pay influences the level or intensity of individual motivation toward job performance

Incentive program: Program intended to motivate employees where increased productivity results in an increase in pay

Inclusion: The differences between individuals are truly respected and valued in the workplace; inclusion is the result of successful diversity management

Individual orientation: One-on-one training that may be done by the employee's direct supervisor, or by the assigned veteran employee (buddy) and overseen by the supervisor

Informal teams: Employees who develop groups around shared interests that may or may not pertain to organizational business

Informational power: This type of power, which is short term and does not allow for continuing influence, is based on the leader possessing information (about a project, future plan, or new development in the organization); informational power is based on the content of the message as once the information has been shared, the power is gone

Innovation: The act or process of introducing new ideas, devices, or methods

Innovators: Individuals willing to step up to try the innovation or process first

Input-output process model: Developed by Joseph E. McGrath in 1964, this seven-component model evaluates the effectiveness of collaboration within teams; input refers to group composition and structure as well as the tasks required within a particular work environment; outputs are the group's tasks and performance, group development, and the overall effect of the group dynamics on individual team member's performance within a collaborative work situation

In-service education: Training that teaches employees specific skills required to maintain or improve performance, usually internal to an organization

Internal candidates: Candidates for an open position who are individuals already employed by the organization

Internal change agent: Individual who is employed within the organization and is familiar with the inner workings of the organization

Internal forces: The areas of focus the manager needs to address on a daily basis so the HIM department performs at its peak level

Intranet: A private information network that is similar to the Internet and whose servers are located inside a firewall or security barrier so that the general public cannot gain access to information housed within the network

Intrinsic: Internal motivating factors come from within the individual

Involuntary turnover: Employees leave the organization not of their own choosing, but because they are fired, laid off, or otherwise terminated

Job: A group of activities and duties that entail units of work that are similar and related

Job analysis: A structured approach utilized to identify the unique job tasks performed within each job

Job autonomy: Sense of individual control in a job

Job complexity: The quality or condition of being difficult to understand or lacking simplicity; the greater the level of job complexity, the harder is it is for an employee to acquire the skills necessary to perform the job and the more time it takes to adequately perform these tasks

Job content questionnaire (JCQ): A self-administered questionnaire, composed of questions that measure four main dimensions of the workplace environment: decision latitude, psychological demands of the job, physical workload, and job insecurity

Job context: The situations or conditions where the employee performs the job

Job crafting: The unsupervised or spontaneous changes to jobs that may or may not be congruent to the goals of the organization; redefinition of a job by an individual to incorporate his or her own motives, strengths, and passions

Job description: A detailed list of a job's duties, reporting relationships, working conditions, and responsibilities

Job design changes: Changes used to motivate employees by making their jobs more interesting and increasing an individual's usefulness throughout the organization

Job diagnostic survey (JDS): Developed to evaluate existing jobs to determine if jobs could be redesigned to improve employee motivation and productivity and to study the effects of job changes on employees, this questionnaire composed of core job dimensions, critical psychological states, and personal work outcomes assesses items within the core job dimensions like skill variety, task identity, task significance, job autonomy, and feedback from the job, management, and peers

Job enlargement: The concept that adding a variety of job tasks to an individual's job will decrease job monotony and thereby allow more job flexibility; a horizontal expansion of an employee's duties; tasks are added to the current job, but employees have the same degree of autonomy and responsibility

Job enrichment: A vertical expansion of a person's duties; generally, a new skill set is required and responsibility and autonomy are increased

Job evaluation: The process of applying predefined compensable factors to jobs to determine their relative worth to the organization

Job experience: The accumulation of job knowledge from action and practice and is linked to the tasks and duties associated with a particular job

Job grading: Assigning jobs to a pay grade; requires the establishment of predetermined categories and the various jobs sorted into these categories

Job performance: Work-related activities expected of an employee and how well the activities were executed during a set time frame

Job performance standards: Criteria that measure work performance and the stated expectations for acceptable quality and productivity associated within a job or job function

Job ranking: Process conducted by human resources with input from other departments as necessary, each job is ranked according to how valuable it is to the organization

Job redesign: The process of realigning the needs of the organization with the skills and interests of the employee and then designing the jobs to meet those needs

Job responsibility: A function that falls under the main job-holder's work-related tasks

Job retention: Keeping employees from seeking employment elsewhere

Job role: Different tasks or jobs that are completed by one employee; also known as a *position*

Job rotation: A method in which workers are shifted periodically among different tasks; employees learn new job tasks and job rotation offers a break from the monotony of a repetitive job

Job shadowing: A method in which one employee follows another employee to observe certain functions of their job

Job sharing: A work schedule in which two or more individuals share the tasks of one full-time or one full-time-equivalent position

Job specifications: Requirements section of the job description that outlines the knowledge and specific skills required for a position

Job summary: Describes the key tasks and responsibilities of a job; also known as job purpose or job scope

Job title: Title that comprehensively and clearly describes the level of skills and knowledge required for the role such as supervisor, coordinator, manager, director, analyst, or technician

John Kotter's change management model: An eight-step process, that management needs to perform in order to transform an organization through change; leadership needs to (1) establish a sense of urgency for change, (2) form a coalition, (3) develop a vision and strategy, (4) communicate the change vision, (5) eliminate the resistance to change, (6) generate short-term wins, (7) consolidate wins to create more change, and (8) adopt the change.

Key indicators: Quantifiable measures used over time to determine whether some structure, process, or outcome supports high-quality performance measured against best practice criteria

Kinesthetic learners: Learners who use the sense of touch to best learn new material

Knowledge: The formal organized body of factual information that must be present in order to be considered for the position

Kurt Lewin's three-stage change management model: Model that provides practical guidance for change initiatives; the three stages of this model are unfreezing, changing or transitioning, and freezing

Laissez-faire leader: Leader who does not participate in the selection of the group activities and does not provide praise or criticism to the workgroup; the laissez-faire leader provides the resources for the group's activities but does not interfere with how the group performs

Laggards: Individuals who resist change; they are bound by tradition and are very skeptical of change

Late majority: Individuals who are skeptical of change and will only participate in the change or innovation after it has been tried by the majority of the people involved in the change initiative or innovation

Leadership: The activity of guiding a group of people to a definite result

Leading: Influencing others to meet the goals and objectives of the organization by motivating subordinates, communicating effectively, and effectively using power; it is sometimes referred to as actuating, directing, or influencing

Leadership continuum: Theory that assumed that leadership behavior can be explained in seven steps of behavioral styles ranging from authority (boss-centered leadership) to delegation (team-centered leadership)

Lean: A management strategy that utilizes less to do more and is a process improvement strategy that can be utilized in any type of organization

Learning organization: An organization that quickly adapts to environmental changes and thus attains knowledge and skills that can be utilized in the future when experiencing change

Legitimate authority: Identifies individuals who have the right to demonstrate power over other individuals within a bureaucratic organization

Legitimate power: A type of formal power that is granted to an individual based on the position they hold in an organization

License: A legal authorization granted by a state to an individual that allows the individual to provide healthcare services within a specific scope of services and geographical location

Line management/hierarchical organizational structure: The traditional and least complex management structure in which top management has total and direct authority and employees report to only one supervisor

Management: The process of planning, organizing and leading organizational activities

Management by objectives (MBO): A management style in which the objectives of an organization are agreed upon by management and employees so that everyone is working toward common goals

Management theory: A collection of ideas which set forth general rules on how to manage a business or organization

Managerial grid: A behavioral theory that offers a two-dimensional behavioral approach that assists individuals with identification of an appropriate leadership style through the concern for people (people-oriented) or tasks (production-oriented); the objective of the managerial grid is to analyze and identify the type of leadership skills exhibited by the leader

Maslow's hierarchy of human needs: A theory developed by Abraham Maslow suggesting that a hierarchy of needs might help explain behavior and guide managers on how to motivate employees; as each need is met (physiological, safety and security, love and belonging, self-esteem, and self-actualization), the individual moves to the next level in an attempt to satisfy the next need

Market pricing: Determining the going pay rate for similar jobs in a particular labor market

Mediation: Both sides of the claim sit down with a neutral third party and reach an agreement; the mediator does not decide the issue, but rather helps both sides come to a solution together

Mentoring: A type of coaching and training in which an individual (protégé) is matched with a more experienced individual (mentor) who serves as an advisor or counselor

Merit pay: An increase to base salary (often annually) that is based on performance appraisal ratings by an employee's manager

Meritocracy: Employees are evaluated by positions and rewarded based on individual merits and contributions

Mission statement: A written statement that sets forth the core purpose and philosophies of an organization or group; it defines the organization or group's general purpose for existing

Morale: The feelings of enthusiasm and loyalty that a person or group has about a task or job

Motivation: The forces acting on or within a person that cause the person to behave in a specific, goal-directed manner

Motivators: elements that can provide job satisfaction to employees and consist of achievement, recognition, the work itself, advancement, and responsibility

Negligent hiring: Charge made against an organization if a current employee in some way harms a patient or another employee or commits a serious offense and the organization should have known about the employee's tendencies had a thorough background check been done prior to hiring

Negotiation: A formal discussion between people who are trying to reach an agreement

Needs assessment: A procedure performed by collecting and analyzing data to determine what is required, lacking, or desired by an employee, a group, or an organization

Networking: Cultivating a mutually-beneficial, active circle of acquaintances and associates

Noise: Any sound that undesired or interferes with one's hearing of something or concentration

Nonhierarchical organizational model: In this organizational model, there is no true line or hierarchy to reporting within the organization; these organizations reflect a combination of interconnected horizontal networks and this type of organizational structure combines aspects of functional and divisional hierarchies to create a rather complex structure where an employee may report to one or more managers

Normative decision model: Model that focuses on situational factors rather than leadership behaviors and it guides managers through the decision-making processes depending on the type of problem encountered

Observation: Method in which the HIM manager or HR consultant observes the employee or employees who are completing the job tasks

Occupational Information Network (O*NET): Developed and introduced by the US Department of Labor in 1995, this network is a standardized, comprehensive online system for performing worker and job oriented job analysis in the development of job descriptions

Offer of employment: A formal job offer usually in a letter or a telephone call followed by a letter; the offer of employment should include, at a minimum, the position title, salary, and start date

Office for Civil Rights (OCR): An agency of the Department of Health and Human Services that is responsible for enforcing civil rights laws that prohibit discrimination on the basis of race, color, national origin, disability, age, sex, and religion by healthcare and human services entities over which OCR has jurisdiction, such as state and local social and health services agencies, and hospitals, clinics, nursing homes, or other entities receiving federal financial assistance from HHS

On-the-job training (OTJ): A method of training in which an employee learns necessary skills and processes by performing, under supervision, the functions of his or her position

Operant conditioning: Behavior is associated with a positive or negative reward, and is modified or learned over time

Operational plans: Plans that are carried out within the departments, cover daily operations, and are in place for one year or less

Operations management: Management that deals with the design and management of products, processes, services and supply chains and considers the acquisition, development, and utilization of resources that firms need to deliver the goods and services clients want; it also evaluates tools that are needed to manage processes of interrelated activities

Organization-level orientation: A large-scale introduction to the facility

Organizational chart: A graphic representation of an organization's formal reporting structure that aids in understanding the reporting relationships and functional responsibilities throughout the healthcare organization

Organizational culture: Shared values and beliefs that guide behavior within organizations

Organizational development (OD): The application of behavioral science research and practices to planned organizational change

Organizational tenure: An accumulation of work-related information from job experience and the

information gathered is only relevant to the current organization climate or culture

Organizing: The coordinating of the activities of multiple people to achieve a common purpose or goal

Orientation: A set of activities designed to familiarize new employees with their jobs, the organization, and its work culture

Outsource: To designate certain positions or certain functions to be filled on a permanent basis by contracted employees

Participative leadership: A leadership style in which the leader allows the workers to provide input and make decisions about their work

Participatory management: A management style in which management allows employees to take an active role in decision-making processes that relate directly to their jobs

Path-goal theory: Originally developed by Martin Evans in 1970 and further expanded upon by Robert House in 1971, this theory suggests that a leader should develop a path for followers to achieve group goals

Pay for performance: Remuneration for job tasks completed throughout a certain time frame

Pay grade: Leveled system where each grade has a minimum, midpoint, and maximum range that allows an employee to progress, receiving pay increases for longevity or improving skills

Performance appraisals: An evaluation of an employee's performance during a designated period of time; also referred to as performance evaluations or performance reviews

Performance improvement plan (PIP): Initiated whenever an individual's job performance is substandard or the employee violates a departmental or healthcare organizational policy, the PIP is a strategic roadmap for the employee to utilize to achieve more positive results within his or her job

Performance management: A set of tools and practices for setting performance goals and designing sustainable job improvement strategies with employees, monitoring employee progress toward job performance goals with feedback, and coaching by managers and measuring individual or group performance

Performance standards: Criteria that measure work performance and the stated expectations for acceptable quality and productivity associated with a job or job function

Personal Interviews: Carried out by the HIM manager or HR consultant with employees who complete the job tasks being analyzed, these interviews should contain a list of structured questions that are asked of all the selected individuals

Personalization: In the workplace, allowing individuals to decorate or mark their workstation with items of interest (within reason) such as favorite quotes, family pictures, and sports team memorabilia

Phases of grief: In 1969, Elisabeth Kubler-Ross describes an emotional framework for grief in her book *Death and Dying* and that same construct has been noted in relation to how employees experience change within organizations; the five grief stages are denial, anger, bargaining, depression, and acceptance

Planned change: A formal process that is introduced methodically and is actively managed by managers or change agents

Planning: An examination of the future and preparation of action plans to attain goals; of the four traditional management functions, planning must be done first because it is the foundation on which the other functions operate

Point method: Method that places weight (points) on each of the compensable factors in a job and the total points associated with a job to establish its relative worth

Policy: A governing principle that describes how a department or an organization is supposed to handle a specific situation or execute a specific process

Population health: The capture and reporting of healthcare data that is used for public health purposes

Position: Different tasks or jobs that are completed by one employee; also known as a *job role*

Position analysis questionnaire (PAQ): A structured job analysis instrument used to measure job characteristics and relate them to human characteristics within the following five categories: information input, mental processing, work output, relationships with others, and job context

Power in negotiation: Refers to any unique attributes or position a particular negotiation party possess

Primary data sources for job analysis: Employees or managers who currently perform or oversee the job being evaluated

Privacy: The quality or state of being hidden from, or undisturbed by, the observation or activities of other persons; or freedom from unauthorized intrusion

Privacy Rule: The federal regulations created to implement the privacy requirements of the simplification subtitle of the Health Insurance Portability and Accountability Act of 1996; effective in 2002; afforded patients certain rights to and about their protected health information

Probationary performance review cycle: A set period of time that allows an organization to ascertain whether the new employee will be able to handle the job tasks and challenges associated with the new job

Procedure: A series of related steps given in chronological order that details the prescribed manner of performing work or implementing a policy

Progressive discipline: Method of discipline where the first few infractions are treated with less severity than later infractions

Protected health information (PHI): Individually identifiable health information

Punitive damages: Awarded to the employee as a way to further punish the employer and prevent the employer's discriminatory behavior from continuing

Quid pro quo: One person using their authority over another to demand some kind of sexual favor in return for job actions such as promotion, hiring, or continued employment

Rational-legal authority: Authority that is displayed as boundaries outlined within organizations, which rely on the rules and laws imposed by those in authoritative management positions

Reasonable accommodation: A change or adjustment to a work environment that allows a disabled employee to perform basic job duties

Recorder: Team member who creates a meeting agenda, takes and distributes meeting minutes, helps to create charts, and sends out necessary correspondence

Recruitment: The process of finding, soliciting, and attracting employees

Referent power: A type of personal power where leaders possess personal characteristics that make others want to be like them, to follow them, to want to be associated with them; leaders who have referent power do not necessarily do anything to earn their power, it is more about personality traits

Refreezing: Lewin's last stage of change in which the new behaviors are reinforced to become as stable and institutionalized as the previous status quo behaviors

Reinforcement theory: Motivation theory built on the incentive and reward concept; employees are motivated to perform in relation to incentives or positive reinforcement as well as disincentives or negative reinforcement

Reliability: A measure of consistency of data items based on their reproducibility and an estimation of their error of measurement

Reporting relationships: Component of job descriptions that defines the working hierarchy—who manages whom

Resistance to change: A force that slows or stops the motion of change efforts, which then increases the amount of work and energy needed to propel the efforts forward

Retaliation: If a person complains to their employer, files a claim of discrimination, or participates in an investigation of their employer charged with discrimination, the person cannot be fired, demoted or otherwise penalized for their actions

Reward power: A type of formal power granted to an individual who has the ability to reward employees for doing what is requested of them; reward may come in the form of a raise, promotion, time off, or other positive measure

Role-playing: A training method in which participants are required to respond to specific problems they may actually encounter in their jobs

Scientific management: Studying work processes and how they impact workers' productivity

Scorecard: A report of outcome measures to help leaders know what they have accomplished

Secondary data sources for job analysis: Information obtained from subject matter experts, human resource consultants, job data banks, or competency models

Sector changes: events triggered by new technologies, new or revised regulations, and new or revised accreditation or certification standards

Security Rule: The federal regulations created to implement the security requirements of HIPAA

Selection: The process of choosing the right person for the job

Self-directed learning: An instructional method that allows participants to control their learning and progress at their own pace

Semi-structured interview: A combination of the structured and unstructured interviews, the interviewer will have a few predetermined questions to start the interview, but then will respond to the interviewee's answers with more probing follow-up questions

Senge's theory of change: Theory that outlines disciplines that contribute toward a learning organization: personal mastery, mental models, building shared visions, and team learning

Servant leadership: A philosophy and set of practices that enriches the lives of individuals, builds better organizations, and ultimately creates a more just and caring world; servant leaders, unlike traditional leaders, share the power of leadership with those they serve

Sexual harassment: Unwelcome sexual advances, requests for sexual favors, and other verbal or physical conduct of a sexual nature

Similarity-attraction: Overall, people prefer to interact with others who are similar to themselves; when given a choice, people prefer to spend time with others whose attitudes and values are like their own

Simulation: A training technique for experimenting with real-world situations by means of a computerized model that represents the actual situation

Situational leadership theory: Developed by Paul Hershey and Ken Blanchard in 1969, this leadership theory proposed that leadership effectiveness depends on the leader's ability to change his or her behavior to meet the demands of the situation; it also takes into account the maturity of the followers in terms of their job ability and psychological willingness to work

Situational strength: The cues employees experience in their workplace that allow particular job performance behaviors to occur

Six Sigma: Disciplined and data-driven methodology for getting rid of defects in any process

Skills: The abilities related to the verbal, manual, and mental processing of data and information within a particular job

Social identity: A person's sense of belonging to a social group

Social power: The potential or ability of an agent [in this case, a manager] to bring change in attitudes, behavior, or belief by using resources available to him or her

Socialization: The process of influencing the behavior and attitudes of a new employee to adapt positively to the work environment

Sorting effect: The effect of pay for performance on the composition of the actual workforce

Span of control: The area of activity and number of duties and employees for which an individual or organization is responsible; also, the number of employees that a manager can efficiently handle while improving effectiveness

Spatial density: The number of items within a specific area or space

Staffing: A managerial function concerned with determining the most appropriate and cost-effective mix of individuals necessary to complete the job functions in a department; it includes recruiting, selection, compensation, evaluation of employees, and training and development

Strategic change: Change that involves improving the alignment of an organization's strategy, culture, and design

Strategic planning: The process in which the leadership of a healthcare organization develops the organization's overall mission, vision and goals to help guide the direction of the organization as a business entity

Strategic plans: Plan created by the organization's board of trustees, with the help of senior administration, which starts with the organization's mission and vision statements and communication of these to all employees; strategic plans are generally in place for three to five years, with annual evaluations

Stereotyping: Exhibiting cultural bias with generalizations about individuals based on their identity, group membership, or affiliations

Structured interview: Interview that focuses on the job to be filled, using the job description as the starting point; also called a directive interview

Structured questionnaires: Distributed to all employees completing the job tasks being evaluated, these questionnaires or checklists allow for a standardized method of collecting data on job tasks and questions related to job tasks can only be answered in one specific manner

Succession planning: A specific type of promotional plan in which senior-level position openings are anticipated and candidates are identified from within the organization; the candidates are given training through formal education, job rotation, and mentoring so they can eventually assume these positions

SWOT analysis: Analysis that looks at the internal strengths and weaknesses of an organization (or department), and the external opportunities and threats; it is a description of the factors that will impact a plan or project and should be done with input from all those affected by the plan

Synchronous: Audio and video conferencing that occurs at the same time, meaning that instructor and participants are present together for one- or two-way communication

Tactical plans: Short-term plans based on strategic plans that have a focus of one to three years and are created at the level of divisions and departments

Task analysis: A procedure for determining the specific duties and skills required of a job

Team: A group of people working together to achieve a common purpose for which they hold themselves mutually accountable

Team charter: Clearly defines the expectations of the team, details the mission and vision of the team, provides the scope, sets the boundaries, names the leader and members, and identifies the key outcomes

Team facilitator: Individual who understands the team process, and is available to assist with the mechanics of the team process, but who is not as concerned with the outcome of the project as much as he or she is concerned that the team functions productively; the facilitator is present at meetings, but is neither the leader nor a member; he or she provides coaching on how to run a meeting, assign tasks, and make decisions

Team leader: Usually selected by the sponsor, the team leader is responsible for the administrative aspects of team management like setting and running meetings, assigning tasks, keeping the team focused, resolving conflicts among members, communicating with the team sponsor, and making sure that the resources are being used efficiently

Team members: Individuals who do the work of the team such as participating in discussions, putting forth ideas, sharing solutions, carrying out assigned tasks, and supporting team actions in their individual work areas

Team sponsor: The individual who initially brings the team together and assigns their charter

Technical conference method: Method utilized for soliciting information about job tasks from a group of supervisors or managers who have knowledge about the job but do not actually perform the job

The Iowa Studies: Conducted in 1939 at the Child Welfare Research Station within Iowa State University by Kurt Lewin, Ronald Lippitt, and Ralph K. White, The

Iowa Studies were one of the first behavioral research studies focusing on leadership roles rather than the traits exhibited by leaders; these experimental research studies identified three leadership styles that are representative of the relations between leaders and the individuals being led: authoritarian, democratic, and laissez-faire.

The Michigan Studies: Undertaken in the early 1950s by researchers from the University of Michigan interested in understanding leadership behaviors in actual workplaces, these studies are more of a one-dimensional theory in that employee-centered leadership and job-centered leadership are opposing leadership styles and leaders are not able to focus on production and employees at the same time; they do not take into effect situational variances that may impact leadership styles and also noted that effective leaders utilized a participatory style of leadership where the leader involved a team of workers in decision making and problem solving in regards to work decisions

The Ohio State Leadership Studies: Conducted in the 1950s and 1960s by the researchers who were a part of the personnel research board at The Ohio State University, The Ohio State Leadership Studies delineated a two-dimensional theory of leadership behavior and assessed the dimensions of leadership concern over the task objectives (job tasks to be completed by followers) and the concern for relationship objectives (the relationship between leader and follower).

Theory X: A management theory developed by McGregor that describes pessimistic assumptions about people and their work potential

Theory Y: A management theory developed by McGregor that describes optimistic assumptions about people and their work potential

Thomas Kilmann conflict mode instrument: A questionnaire tool utilized to assess the manner in which individuals manage conflict; this tool assesses conflict management styles by using two parameters—assertiveness and cooperation—which manifest in five distinct styles: to avoid, compete, collaborate, accommodate, and compromise

360-degree interview: Process that involves three different interviews with the supervisor of the position, the peers of the position, and the subordinates of the position

360 performance appraisal: A methodology most often used in conjunction with other more traditional methods such as graphic rating scales and critical incident methods, it measures the manner and capacity of work performance and concentrates on the more subjective areas of work such as teamwork, character, and leadership; it requires that employees obtain confidential and anonymous assessments from their colleagues

Timekeeper: Team member who is responsible for keeping meetings on track by managing time

Traditional authority: When authority is inherently understood within an organization or group

Training: The set of activities and materials that provide the opportunity to acquire job-related skills, knowledge, and abilities

Trait theory of leadership: Theory that attempts to define the general qualities or traits that need to be present within an individual to be a leader

Transactional leadership: In this type of leadership, there is a hierarchy within the organization where leaders clarify goals and objectives for followers and followers receive some kind of reward in exchange for performing work satisfactorily; the types of rewards elicited within this leadership model are items such as a promotion, pay raise, or personal recognition

Transformational leadership: The act of changing or transforming from one current state to another state; it focuses on leaders' attempts to motivate followers to achieve at a higher level or to perform at a level beyond expectations

Transitioning: The second stage of Lewin's change process in which change is a process rather than one single event; this is the inner movement employees make in reaction to change

Turnover: Employees leaving the organization

Undue hardship: In the context of reasonable accommodation, the accommodation cannot be too disruptive or expensive for the employer to implement

Unfreezing: The first stage of Lewin's change process in which people are presented with disconcerting information to motivate them to change

Unstructured interview: Interview where no questions are planned in advance, although certain topics may be targeted; also called a nondirective interview

Upward communication: Occurs when information moves from the lower levels in an organization to the upper levels

Validity: The extent to which an instrument measures what it purports to measure

Value: A principle or ideal intrinsically valuable or desirable (human rather than material)

Values-based leadership: A style of leadership built on a foundation of personal values, principles, or ethics

Video conferencing: Learning technique in which participants in different together adds the ability to see and hear the instructor and uses satellite, television, or computer capabilities

Virtual teams: Teams whose members are geographically distributed, requiring them to work together through electronic means with minimal face-to-face contact

Vision statement: A short description of an organization's ideal future state

Visual learners: Learners who use the sense of sight to best learn new material

Voluntary turnover: Employees choose to leave the organization

Web-based training: Instruction via the Internet that enables individuals to learn in a structure that is self-paced while interacting and collaborating with other students and the instructor via a conferencing system

Webcast: Video conference using the Internet in which a broadcast is done similar to a television show

Weber's theory of bureaucratic management: Management theory that notes there are two essential components to a bureaucratic organization, (1) organizations are structured into hierarchies arranged at an organizational level of authority as demonstrated in an organizational chart, and (2) the organization and its work group are governed by clearly defined decision-making rules that are outlined in policies and procedures that are managed by levels of authority within an organization

Webinar: Video conferencing that uses the Internet for transmission

Work design questionnaire (WDQ): Questionnaire that surveyed a variety of workers in different settings in order to assess specific characteristics related to job tasks; the outcome of the study was that the WDQ results showed good promise to assist practitioners in the design and redesign of jobs in the organization

Workflow: Any work process that must be handled by one or more employee

Work environment scale (WES): Developed by Rudolph Moos based on his research of development of a conceptual framework that assesses the interplay of individuals and their work environment, the WES was designed to measure the social environments of different types of work settings through completion of a questionnaire; it assists organizations to evaluate employee productivity, assess employee satisfaction, and clarify employee expectations to ensure a healthy work environment

Work-life balance: A balance between an individual's work and personal life

Work sampling: A statistical method that reviews a select portion of tasks performed and provides baseline data for further job performance assessment

Workplace diversity: The set of individual, group, and cultural differences employees bring to an organization

Zone of indifference: The range in which a manager's orders will be perceived as legitimate and the employee will act on or perform the request without a great deal of thought

Index